A Question of Ethics

Case Conferences in Everyday Ethical and Legal Issues

Professor
Errol Walrond

Dedication

To all of those colleagues, fellow health workers, students, and patients who may have been in the path of any lapses in the author's conduct over the years, be assured that those experiences were part of the author's development. To my late wife Beverley, who had to put up with the long hours of research and writing when she thought I had retired.

A Question of Ethics: Case Conferences in Everyday Ethical and Legal Issues
Copyright © 2020 E.R. Walrond
ISBN 978-976-8265-83-8 (paperback)
Design and layout: GENESIS Graphics
Pre-press/printing: COT Holdings Ltd.
Publisher: Margaret Hope

Table of Contents

Preface

Since the publication of Ethics in Everyday Health Care, UWI press 2005, the author has been collecting the case conferences on the issues encountered and discussed by the staff in a general hospital in the Caribbean. Attempts to involve those outside of hospital have been unsuccessful as has been the involvement of some departments in the hospital. The lack of involvement of some disciplines is not for the lack of encouragement, or the lack of issues, for some issues have surfaced even in the public domain, and it is evident at interactions with the departments that do acknowledge and present problems for discussion. There has also been a notable absence of administrative personnel from the conferences even when they have played crucial roles in the cases discussed and have been advised of the discussions.

It could be said that these issues may be because the conferences are seen as student instructional exercises. Another answer may be that the conferences have been held outside of the Monday to Friday work hours and some staff may not be willing to sacrifice that time to these issues. Nevertheless, there have been many staff members who have attended regularly and contributed to the discussions on all types of cases.

One would like to thank all those staff that have become adept at raising relevant issues that have enhanced the discussion of the cases presented.

Professor Sir Errol R. Walrond, KA; BSc Hons; LRCP, MRCS; MBBS; FRCS; FACS; FCCS;
Emeritus Professor of Surgery

Disclaimer: Any names used in case reports are entirely fictional and are only used to enhance the narrative.

Biographical Note

Professor Errol Walrond's career in medicine would not have been possible had he not won a Barbados Scholarship in 1953 at age 17. Mickey as he was known from childhood, came from a poor family, and his situation did not allow him to consider anything else but a career as a teacher, while dreams of others for him included the priesthood.

He applied to go to England despite the strange advice from the headmaster that he would not be able to gain entry there, but firm of the view that he would return to serve the people of Barbados on qualifying. He was drawn to the concept of service by the distant presence of his father he had known little of, who when he was four years old had volunteered and joined the RAF in Britain in 1940 at the beginning of World War II; and was killed in action three years later and was celebrated as a hero in his village.

He was admitted to Guy's Hospital Medical School in London, where after gaining the prize in Anatomy, he was invited to do an intercalated BSc degree which would extend his course by one year. Pointing out that his scholarship would not accommodate an extra year, and that his family had no resources to fall back on, the university authorities persuaded him to go ahead and apply to government who they said usually granted such requests. The extended year had almost finished by the time the Barbados Government responded that the request was not granted. Professor Walrond thus faced the first major challenge of his life which was to go through the last year of his medical studies without any financial support. The challenge was met by doing odd work at night, such as waiting at table, and some luck at the card tables.

After qualifying as a doctor he chose to ignore the letters reminding him that the government bond had to be fulfilled and determined that given the previous history, the bond should be deferred until his early career goals had been met. He therefore completed his internship and went on to qualify as a surgeon in 1964, in the minimum four years required to qualify.

Armed with his qualifications he then decided to return home to fulfil his bond and was appointed to work as the junior to the Visiting surgeons, who were general practitioners practising surgery once a week in the hospital. During this year Professor Walrond would have the opportunity to do a wide range of surgery, and make his first academic contributions to the international medical literature. However, he was not considered for a newly established consultant's post, on the grounds that his specialist qualification was too recent.When he was made aware that the post was being reserved for someone who was still studying for his specialist qualification, he decided to look for other opportunities, and responded to an advertisement for a position at the University Hospital in Jamaica, and for a Commonwealth fellowship to study thoracic and cardiac surgery, which were not available in Barbados at that time. Both opportunities were offered, and he decided to take up the offer in Jamaica in the first instance. After leaving Jamaica to do the Commonwealth fellowship, he was invited to join the University staff in 1968.

The rest of his career was spent in the Faculty of Medicine in the University of the West Indies, first in Jamaica until the end of 1973, and in Barbados from 1974 until retirement in 2001 as Dean of the Faculty. These posts involved a full service load of surgery in both Jamaica and Barbados, and in addition he treated many patients from other parts of the Caribbean.

During his career Professor Walrond has had over 150 academic publications and done, as well as supervised innumerable operations; has contributed to the development of medical practice in the region, by the expansion of medical training, the establishment of postgraduate specialist training in many fields, and by being a scientific secretary to the regional medical research council.

In Barbados, Professor Walrond's university career was also marked by extensive community service which included a full-time service load as a general surgeon, which at that time encompassed all of the specialty areas that would later emerge. He was also the President of the Barbados Association of Medical Practitioners when it became a trade union, and lead the national response to the AIDS pandemic; first leading BAMP's task force, then the National Advisory Committee on HIV/AIDS and represented the region on the Global Programme on HIV/AIDS. It was in this battle to educate the public and the profession and to protect those affected from blatant discrimination that ethics had to be brought into the mainstream of medical and community education. In this regard the ethics case conference was introduced as part of the teaching of ethics in medical teaching in Barbados and Professor Walrond has been called upon to be the lead discussant at such conferences many years after his retirement. For his contribution to medicine, the Barbados Government in 2011 conferred on him the Knight of St. Andrew.

Professor Walrond has also been Chairman of the Medical Council of Barbados from time to time, and was Chairman at the time of the introduction of the new Medical Registration Act in 2011 and relinquished that position when he retired from clinical practice in 2015. During his tenure as Chairman of the Medical Council, the

Council published for the first time a Code of Conduct for members of the profession. In retirement from the University, Professor Walrond was asked to lead the formation of the Caribbean College of Surgeons, and was its Foundation President. The College has incorporated an ethics case presentation as an integral part of its annual conference. Professor Walrond was also invited to be a Trustee of the Arnott Cato Foundation and later to be its Chairman on the death of its founder Sir Carlisle Burton.

Professor Walrond's professional journey was supported in the last 45 years by his marriage to Beverley, an attorney whom he met in the last of his seven years living in Jamaica. They raised their two children while both for the most part had their full-time professional careers, which involved frequent absences. Both children became Barbados Scholars, the first, Maurice, studied medicine and also decided on a career in surgery; Maya pursued an undergraduate degree in business and engineering, and later an MBA at Harvard.

The concept of ethical conduct has forged Professor Walrond's philosophy of life and his career and was deeply rooted in the fundamental belief that fairness to all is the platform on which the practice of medicine should be based. He has been called a man of ethics by colleagues. Work in this publication indicates how this has been applied in everyday medical care situations.

Acknowledgements

This collection of cases would not have been possible without the courage of the practitioners working in public hospitals in the Caribbean, to bring cases that they felt had some ethical or legal issues that needed to be discussed and be given wider exposure. Sometimes the practitioners found themselves at the uncomfortable end of the discussion but more often than not felt that they learned from the experience. Finding such practitioners on a monthly basis was the unenviable task of a member of the Faculty of Medical Sciences at the Cave Hill Campus of the University of the West Indies. Over the 20 years of these conferences the coordinators have been Prof. Harley Moseley and Dr. Ramesh Jonnalagadda, both now retired and most of all Dr. Maisha Emmanuel, who have encouraged the author to continue as the discussant over this period. This collection would not have been possible without their hard persuasive work.

Thanks also has to go to those persons who edited this work, Ms Sonia Mills, Mr Carl Moore and Ms Margaret Hope who had to put up with medical jargon and faulty language and the uncomfortable realities of what can go on in medical practice.

CONSENT

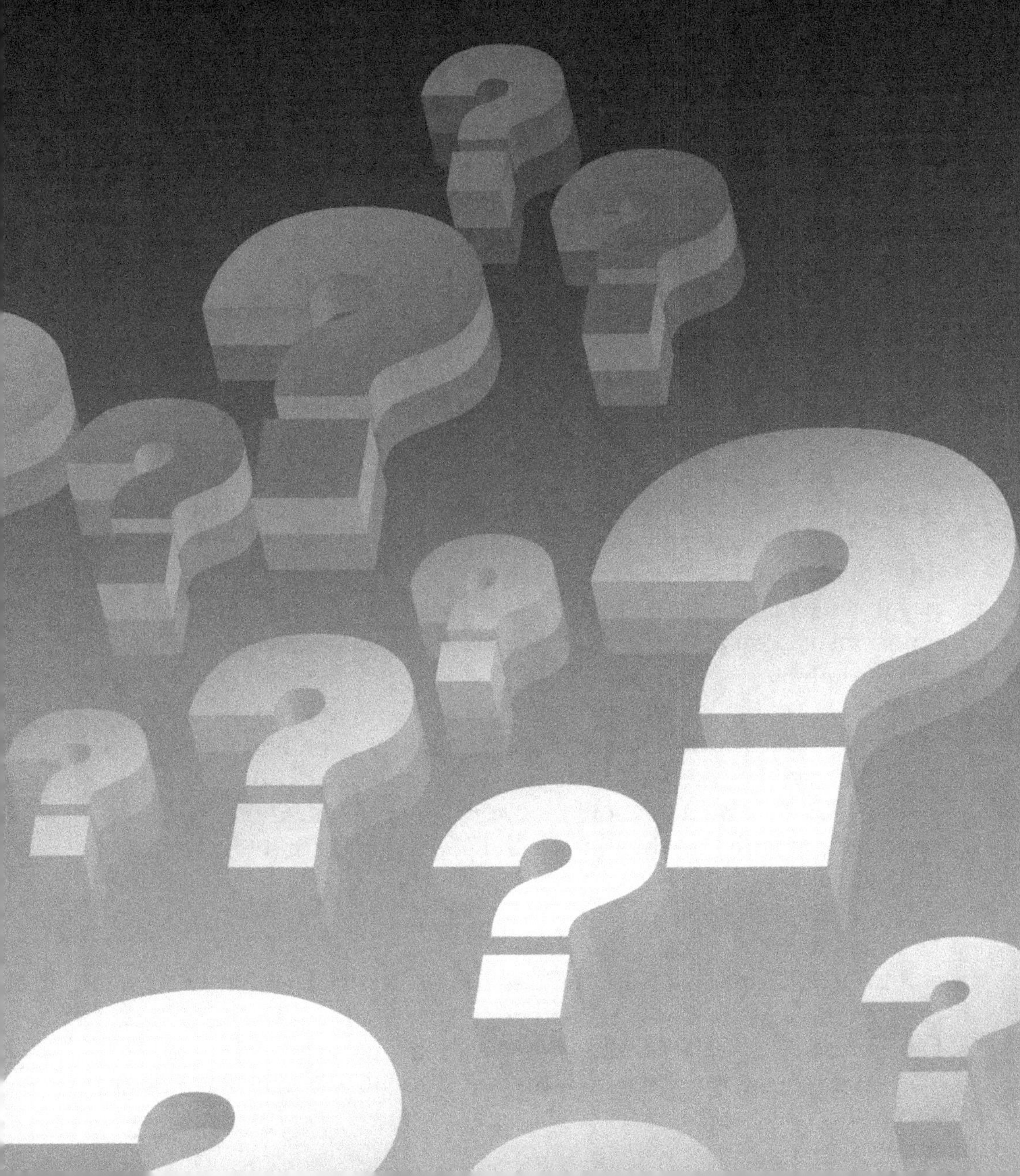

Parental Refusal to Treat a Child

Case report 1:

A male infant born during the 23rd week of pregnancy is placed on a ventilator because his lungs are immature. The infant develops intra-cerebral bleeding and his parents are told that it is unlikely that he will survive the next few weeks. They are also told that if he does survive, he will probably be handicapped, both mentally and physically.

After a week, the infant's condition worsens and is diagnosed as having a serious infection of the bowel. A surgeon is consulted and gives the opinion that removing the inflamed bowel would give a small chance of survival, but without an operation there is no chance of recovery. The infant's parents are informed of the situation and asked to give consent for the operation. After consulting, the parents refuse consent to the operation stating that they do not want the child to suffer further pain, particularly when the quality of his life will be so poor. The paediatrician thinks that the operation should be done, and discusses with the surgeon how to deal with the parents' refusal.

Case report 2:

An infant was delivered by caesarean section at 33 weeks gestation because of pre-eclampsia, to a gravida 7 para 5+2 mother. The infant was admitted to NICU for observation re prematurity, and the baby was started on antibiotics with the mother's consent. Antenatal care was unremarkable apart from the mother's refusal of antenatal HIV testing. There had been three previous antenatal HIV tests recorded, but only one negative result was found in the notes. There was no record of previous antenatal or postnatal HIV treatment. Both parents refused permission for HIV testing of the baby.

The CEO of the hospital was informed and asked to speak to the parents, who reaffirmed their refusal of consent. The Child Care Board was contacted but declined to intervene. The hospital's attorney was asked to take the matter before the court, and responded that after a conversation with the Chief Justice the parents' right of refusal had been upheld.

Case report 3:

A four-year-old patient was admitted for an elective adeno-tonsillectomy. Pre-operative assessment revealed no history of blood dyscrasia or family history of such, and the pre-operative Hb was 11.7 Gm./dl. The operation was performed with informed consent, adequate haemostasis was achieved and the patient was sent to the recovery room and later transferred to the ward. One hour after return to the ward, the patient developed a nosebleed; the doctors were called and considered the bleeding significant enough to warrant a return to the operating theatre. The vital signs were pulse 114 b/pm, BP 96/52 mm Hg.

The anaesthetist saw the child and discussed with the parents the possibility of a blood transfusion being needed. The mother responded immediately that the child was not to have a blood transfusion under any circumstance. The anaesthetist asked her why since it was stated that their religion was Anglican. The mother simply repeated her statement at which point the father started crying and left the room. The anaesthetist then got the mother to sign a note stating her wishes and instructions, and the patient was taken to surgery. The surgery was done to arrest the bleeding and there was an uneventful recovery. In the postoperative period the Hb was 7.3 Gm./dl.

Case report 4:
A five-year-old child was noted by her mother to have a painless swelling in the abdomen. She was diagnosed as a possible Wilm's tumour. A CT scan showed a large mass arising from the lower pole of the right kidney with intravascular extension. Funding was raised and she was referred to a surgeon in a nearby island. The child was seen, a biopsy consented for and done, and she was evaluated with a view to preoperative chemotherapy. The child's mother refused to accept chemotherapy for the child. She was counselled by the surgeon, as well as the paediatric and haematology staff about the importance of chemotherapy to reduce the size of the mass prior to surgery. There was a child on the ward who had a similar tumour who had had preoperative chemotherapy, successful surgery and was now in to have further chemotherapy. The mother was invited to talk to that child's family but declined to do so.

At a subsequent family meeting, the child's aunt was the main spokesperson, and cited research she had done on the Internet that showed good results by doctors in the USA who used herbs to treat this condition. She described chemotherapy as poison and stated that she was living proof that herbs and diet could cause tumours to shrink.

After a long conversation in which the results of treatment and its prognosis were discussed, the mother was connected to speak to the referring paediatrician in her country. She was asked to give her decision independently of the aunt, and responded that she was still of the same mind. She said they had brought the child for surgery and since she was now being told that the tumour needed to shrink before surgery, they would go back home and use herbs to shrink the tumour. She then asked what size should the tumour be before the child was brought back for the surgery. The child was discharged back to the referring doctor who was informed of the mother's decision.

Case report 5:
A 16-year-old delivered her first child in hospital; two days later she developed psychotic behaviour and was seen by a psychiatrist. Before instituting treatment, her parents were contacted to obtain their consent for treatment. When the parents came, the father was inebriated and the mother was hostile and attempted to remove her daughter from the hospital. The staff recognized the mother as a previous psychiatric patient, and had her restrained by the security staff. She was persuaded by the psychiatrist, whom she knew, to have her daughter stay and be treated.

The patient's mental condition improved on therapy but she had a persistently raised blood pressure, which was investigated. After three days, the patient's mother again insisted on her going home and she was taken home, against medical advice. The matter was referred to the social services department and an application made to the court to make the patient and her infant wards of state. This was granted by the court. The patient returned to the hospital accompanied by a paternal aunt and was readmitted.

Issues raised

- ***Prognostic factors in infants***
A baby born prematurely has a smaller chance of survival than a full-term infant. Prematurity is defined by both gestational age and weight, which, depending on the country, varies from 20-28 weeks and a weight of 400-500gms. In contrast, a stillbirth is defined by country as being dead at birth providing that the gestation age was greater than 20-28 weeks; below that it is classified as a miscarriage.[1]

Neonatal mortality defines death within the first month of life and is used in many countries as a measure of the efficacy of the antenatal, obstetric and neonatal services.

In the jurisdiction in which the first case reported was encountered, the cut-off point for statistical purposes is 28 weeks. However, the obstetric and paediatric

---

[1] Stillbirth rates: delivering estimates in 190 countries; C. Stanton, J. Lawn, H. Rahman, K. Wilczynska-Ketende, K. Hill The Lancet, Volume 367, Issue 9521, Pages 1487-1494

*services considered a gestational age of 24 weeks and a birth weight of 500 gms as
sufficiently viable for delivery in high-risk pregnancies. With a gestational age of
23 weeks, the chances of survival for the infant in the first case reported are poor,
and appear to be good for the infant in the second case report.*

*It was not stated what resources other than ventilation were available to
treat the premature infant, for without highly developed neonatal intensive care
resources, the paediatrician's determination to treat at all costs may be overly
optimistic, or driven by the philosophy that life should be preserved regardless of
the likely outcome of severe disability.*

- ***Should parents be only given the chance for survival and not likely
outcomes?***

In obtaining consent, a balanced picture of the risks as well as the
advantages of the treatment or procedure must be given. It is also
appropriate to discuss with parents what facilities are available to treat or
ameliorate the problems discussed.[2]

*From the report given of the first case, it appears that as a result of the poor
prognosis given to them, the parents do not wish treatment to continue. They
may have come to their conclusion after taking into account more than whether
the infant lives or not, whilst the paediatrician seems to consider being alive the
most important factor. Any further discussion with the parents should be done
with the aim of listening to and responding to their concerns, and should not be
entered with a view of making them feel guilty about the decision they have made.*

*In the other case reports, the prognosis of the child does not take centre stage
at the time, and it is the beliefs of the parents that dominate how the child should
be treated.*

- ***About what risks should the patient be informed before an
operation?***

A physician must "advise the patient of those material facts, risks,
complications and alternatives to surgery that a reasonable person in the
patient's situation would consider significant in deciding whether to have
the operation."[3]

In the case of blood transfusion, it is prudent to inform any patient
or parent of the possibility of having to use a blood transfusion where
there is a reasonable possibility that it may be needed; this is particularly
important with the fear of HIV transmission. Anaesthetists should
consult with the surgeon as well as the patient / parent about the

---

[2] Informed consent -Mosby's Medical Dictionary, 8th ed. 2009; Elsevier
[3] Gouse v. Cassel, 532 Pa. 197, 615 A.2d 331, 334 (1992)

need for blood transfusion. There are other requirements that may be preparatory to operation such as biopsies, other consultations, or other treatments including downgrading of tumours through chemotherapy or radiotherapy. Patients have challenged decisions about treatment and its outcome on the grounds that they were not fully informed when they consented. Courts generally uphold that all reasonable risks should be explained to the patient and that very rare risks need not be disclosed unless specifically asked for by the patient, or that they are of such a serious nature that it could influence the decision of the patient to have the operation. It is prudent to record in the notes when specific risks have been discussed with the patient. In the case of Jehovah's Witnesses, who are well known to refuse transfusion of blood and blood products, rare risks of bleeding that may require transfusion therapy should be explained.

A doctor who agrees to do an elective operation on a child without giving a blood transfusion, and the child dies from bleeding when the child's life could have been saved by blood transfusion, remains at risk for a suit of negligence, or even manslaughter if evidence could be adduced that the doctor knew the risk to be unacceptably high.

Chemotherapy is generally well known to cause persons to feel ill and to lose their hair, and patients are often reluctant to have chemotherapy, on the grounds that it will harm them more than help them.

In the first case reported, the poor outcome for the infant had already been impressed upon the parents, and they made the decision that further invasive therapy would produce more suffering without any prospect of a better life.

In the second case report, the physicians were unable to convince the parents of any benefit that HIV testing would bring to the infant and they withheld their consent for this test alone.

In the third case described the parents were not initially informed about the risk that the child may require blood transfusion. The doctors were surprised about the mother's refusal because their religion was stated as Anglican; however, there are other reasons and beliefs for refusing blood transfusion or other treatments.

In the fourth case, consent was given for an operation, but the prospect of preoperative chemotherapy was met with a blunt refusal, and a strongly expressed belief in the efficacy of herbal therapy. All prerequisites to treatment should be discussed in obtaining consent.

In the fifth case, the rationale for the refusal of treatment of the minor appeared to be rooted in the parent's own illness or previous experience with treatment for her own illness.

• *What should be done when parents refuse treatment of their infant?*
A parent's right to refuse treatment for their child can only be overridden
by the court. It is therefore incumbent, particularly in urgent situations, to
try and persuade the parents to change their minds. As much information
as possible should be given, including all the risks particularly as
they relate to a child of a given age. Information should also be given
when necessary about the possibilities available to overrule the
parents' opinion.

There are times when there is a failure of, or inadequate
communication with the physicians dealing with the parents and the most
senior physician or surgeon involved may have to intervene. In some
situations, a patient advocate or counsellor may be used to liaise with the
parents. Physicians are obligated in some jurisdictions to perform life-
sustaining treatments on premature infants with serious developmental
or physical impairments, even if it goes against the parents' wishes.[4] If the
doctor does not feel it is safe to conduct treatment, they should decline to
treat the child and advise the parents to seek other opinions.

When a doctor decides to petition the court to override a parent's
decision they should do so preferably through the institution. Institutions
should have an ethics review mechanism that can be called upon in
urgent situations. The physician should be prepared to justify to the
institution why court action is being invoked. The reasons most likely to
be persuasive to a court are that the parents are projecting their religious
values, or that their idea of the child's suffering is in reckless disregard
for the child's life. Where time permits the institution should give the
parents or their representatives the opportunity to present their case with
the clear understanding of the purpose for the enquiry. Where the child
is of an age and in a condition to understand, their independent view
should also be heard and taken into account in decision-making.[5]

A patient, a parent or a legal guardian has a right to refuse treatment
of any sort without giving any reason. Jehovah's Witnesses are well
known for their refusal of blood transfusion but health personnel should
not assume such refusal. The refusal of blood transfusion or any other
treatment in any critical situation should be clarified and a record made
of the discussion and decision. Caution should be taken to ensure that
such critical decisions are made without undue pressure from others.[6]

---

[4] Overriding Parental Decision to Withhold Treatment, M Woods; Amer. Med. Ass. Virtual Mentor.
2003, Vol 5, No 8
[5] Children and Consent to Medical Care; Canadian Bar Association Script 422; updated 2010
[6] Jehovah's Witnesses' refusal of blood: obedience to scripture and religious conscience. Ridley DT. J
Med Ethics. 1999 (6): 469-72

All strongly held beliefs are not related to accepted religions, there may be other less well-known religions, or beliefs in alternate medical practices, which may not have gained wide acceptance in the community.

In the first, third and fourth cases reported there is no consideration of taking the parents' refusal to the court and the physicians use their persuasive powers to prevail.

In the second case, the hospital's lawyer takes the matter before a high court judge and the application to overrule the parents' decision is not allowed. It is likely that the parents' rights were upheld since the child was not in any immediate danger.

* ### *The rights of mothers vs fathers*

In most jurisdictions parents who have legal custody of their children have equal rights in decision-making about their children. These legal rights exist whether the parents are married or not. There are some Muslim majority countries where the right of women in relation to decision-making remains subservient to that of their husbands.[7] If there is disagreement among parents and consensus cannot be reached, only a court can decide. The court can give sole or qualified custody to one parent, or make the child a ward of the court or other agency such as a child protection service. Normally the court will give most weight to the parent who normally provides care for the child, and taking into account the nature of the dispute, decide what is in the best interest of the child.

In the third case the father of the child was distressed at the decision by the mother to refuse blood transfusion, but decided not to challenge her decision.

In the fifth case report, the father did not appear to be in a state to participate in the decision-making process.

* ### *If parents are unavailable and an emergency arose what should be done?*

The parents' expressed wishes must be respected, including that implied by stating they are Jehovah's Witnesses. Any move to give blood transfusion to a child of a Jehovah's Witness parent should be sanctioned by the court. If there is no express or implied direction the doctor should do whatever is necessary to save the life of the child.

---

[7] Gender equality and social institutions in United Arab Emirates ; http://genderindex.org/country/united-arab-emirates

In the case described where blood transfusion was objected to by the child's mother, there was nothing in the notes to suggest that a blood transfusion should not be given.

- ***HIV testing -Voluntary vs. Mandatory vs. 'Routine'.***
AIDS was first diagnosed as a pattern of fatalities due to immunodeficiency illnesses among male homosexuals.[8] The societal and professionals' reaction was one of discrimination, exclusion and avoidance of affected individuals, and was described as the third epidemic by the director of the WHO's Global Program on AIDS.[9] As the disease was studied further, particular groups were singled out as at higher risk: these included Haitians, Africans, prostitutes, IV drug abusers and persons receiving multiple blood transfusions.[10] When the causative virus was discovered and a test for it developed, the epidemiology and natural history was elucidated to show that the virus could be transmitted from mother to infant, during pregnancy, at birth and during breast-feeding.[11]

However, the antibody test used would prove to have the problems of false positives and negatives and a window period of a few weeks to months in which the infection could not be discovered by production of antibody.[12] The tests for antigens and the virus itself were subsequently developed, but would prove to be more difficult and costly as screening tests. These testing difficulties would complicate how HIV infection would be diagnosed, including infection in infants born to HIV positive mothers.[13]

The overwhelmingly negative reaction to HIV/AIDS patients drove those affected underground into the shadows of society, and opened the debate as to how affected persons should be best diagnosed, and treated. Voluntary vs. mandatory testing was widely discussed and the overwhelming public health consensus was that voluntary testing with pre- and post-test counselling was the most effective means to reach the most at-risk persons for HIV infection, as well as reduce their risk

---

[8] A Timeline of HIV/AIDS - AIDS.gov; https://www.aids.gov/hiv-aids-basics/hiv-aids.../aids-timeline

[9] Mann, J. (1987). Statement at an informal briefing on AIDS to the 42nd session of the United Nations General Assembly

[10] Current Trends Prevention of Acquired Immune Deficiency Syndrome (AIDS): Report of Inter-Agency Recommendations; MMWR; March 04, 1983 / 32(8); 101-3

[11] European Collaborative Study. Children born to women with HIV-1 infection: natural history and risk of transmission. The Lancet, (1991) 337(8736), 253-260

[12] What is the window period for an HIV test? i-base.info/guides/testing/what-is-the-window-period

[13] Laboratory testing for the diagnosis of HIV infection: updated recommendations; 2014, http://dx.doi.org/10.15620/cdc.23447

of transmitting HIV to others, including mother to child. As effective treatment for HIV emerged in the form of HAART therapy,[14] there was a call to try and diagnose more asymptomatic HIV positive patients, by encouraging more voluntary testing without the necessity for pre-test counselling. This call was not widely heeded and efforts to test more persons would extend to advocacy for routine 'opt out' testing of all persons attending health facilities.[15] The methodology proposed was that all patients would be told that they would have an HIV test unless they explicitly forbade such testing to be done. HIV positive patients would then be referred to specialized HIV treatment centres. The manner in which patients would be informed of the results of the tests was left to the doctors required to do such 'routine' tests, and the consequences would only be explained if positive patients reached the specialized treatment service.[16] The consequences of an individual opting out of testing are not addressed in the proposal put forward but become apparent, where an individual because of a state of mental incompetence, is not capable of exercising an option. The question then arises as to whether the patient's confidentiality should be broken and the 'opt in' option exercised by their next of kin? The consequences of opting out also arise in the case of pregnant mothers, for the possible consequence of undetected HIV infection may fall upon the infant.

In the second case report the parent was adamant that she was opting out of HIV testing, and both parents refused to have their newborn infant tested for HIV, although they accepted other tests. The reaction of the paediatrician was that HIV testing of the infant should be mandatory and requested that the matter be put before the court.

- ***What is the responsibility of a doctor to act against a parent's wishes?***

Any physician has a responsibility to assess a situation and try to clarify the patient's/parents' position and point out the risks to the patient/child. If the parents persist in their opinion, it should be written in the notes and they should be asked to record their decision in writing.

---

[14] HIV Treatment: The Basics | HIV/AIDS Fact Sheets ...https://aidsinfo.nih.gov/.../hiv-treatment--the-ba

[15] WHO | HIV testing services; www.who.int/hiv/topics/vct/en/

[16] Revised Recommendations for HIV Testing of Adults, Adolescents, and Pregnant Women in Health-Care Settings; MMWR, Sept 22, 2006 / 55(RR14); 1-17IVM/AIDS Basics / Prevention :IV Opt-Out Testing

Except in emergencies, testing without consent should be carried out when a patient is in mortal danger, and the legally competent person to give consent is not available or mentally competent to do so. Otherwise, testing without consent can be carried out under a mandatory testing statutory requirement, or by an order of court. An order of court may be required when a parent or legal guardian of a child or a mentally incompetent adult, refuses testing where HIV infection is suspected clinically.

In the case of a possible HIV infected infant, the infant is not in any immediate danger of an HIV related illness. Furthermore, with the availability of current HIV treatment or any other treatment that may arise, the later emergence of an HIV related illness is likely to be effectively treated if detected early. On the other hand, immediate treatment of an HIV infected infant may bring about the elimination of HIV from the infant's blood, but the virus is likely to re-emerge after cessation of treatment.[17]

This situation may arise where the patient has been sexually abused or assaulted or the patient is the infant of an HIV positive mother. In the latter case, the HIV antibody test will be positive with or without the infant having HIV infection, and the crucial decisions to be made are related to advice about breast-feeding and the use of antiretroviral therapy in the infant. A court decision making the infant a ward of the court would be required to prevent the mother from breast-feeding and to institute antiretroviral therapy in the infant against the parents' wishes. There has been no work to show that the benefit of mandatory screening in identifying more HIV positive persons, outweighs the disadvantages, such as not attending antenatal or other clinics, and a possible lack of cooperation / compliance with offered HAART treatment.[18]

In the case of sexual transmission of HIV, it is important to elucidate the history of the sexual partners; and in cases of pregnancy it cannot be assumed that the spouse is the father. Such realities may impact on the decision of persons to be tested for HIV, and the danger of transmission of HIV to other persons may impact on a court's decision as to whether to remove the autonomy and confidentiality of a person. The danger to another person of maintaining such confidentiality lies in whether the danger is a mortal one.[19] Confidentiality of HIV status in a pregnancy

---

[17] HIV Detected in "Cured" Mississippi Baby, 2014www.scientificamerican.com/.../hiv-detected-in-cured...

[18] Prenatal HIV screening in pregnant women: a medical-legal review. Oldenettel D1, Dye TD, Artal R. Birth. 1997 Sep; 24(3): 165-72

[19] Tarasoff v. Regents of the University of California, 17 Cal. 3d 425, 551 P.2d 334, 131

applies not only to the pregnant mother and the infant but also to the father, who may or may not be the spouse. Therefore, some enquiry should be made of the father of an HIV positive pregnant mother and infant, and to do so requires maintaining the confidence and trust of the mother. Expert counselling and protection from the consequences of any 'betrayal' of confidential information about their sexual partner/s gains such trust.[20]

If the doctor feels that a child's life is in grave danger, they have a responsibility to place the issue before the court, whilst at the same time trying all other measures available to save the child's life. Appearance before the Court should be made through an institution and the motion made to make the child a ward of the court. The court then makes the decision as to what treatment the child should have.[21]

In the cases reported that were taken to the court the minors' lives were not in danger. In the first case the petition to overrule the parents' decision to not test for HIV was rejected by the court. There was no information offered to suggest any suspicion of new HIV infection in the mother, except to state that the pregnancy was with a new partner, a Rastafarian priest.

In the fifth case reported, neither the minor nor her infant is in mortal danger, but the behaviour of the parents suggests that they may be put in danger when under their care.

- *Counselling – what is required and by whom?*

Counselling at varying levels of intensity is required for all medical actions. However, intense counselling is required when risks are high. At the advent of the HIV/AIDS pandemic, the risks were high for death and social ostracism, so high that pre- and post-test counselling were advocated for HIV testing. As HAART treatment became available, pre-test counselling was deemphasised and was often reserved for those who refused testing, such as at antenatal clinics; post-test counselling became largely confined to specialised HIV units. Advocacy for 'routine' HIV testing with an opt-out provision makes no specific provision for counselling and the follow-up of persons who opt out.[22]

In the circumstances described in the second case report, counselling was done by the senior doctor on the obstetric service. No information was recorded re

---

[20] Routine antenatal HIV testing: the responses and perceptions of pregnant women and the viability of informed consent. A qualitative study; P de Zulueta and M Boulton; J Med Ethics; 2007; 33(6): 329–336. doi: 10.1136/jme.2006.015750

[21] Parents know best: or do they? Treatment refusals in paediatric oncology. Alessandri AJ. J Paediatr Child Health. 2011; 47(9): 628-31

[22] Guidance on provider-initiated HIV testing and counselling; www.unicef.org/aids/files/PITCGuidance 2007

reasons for refusal of testing, and no other socio-cultural information other than the parents are Rastafarian. Rastafarians may feel discriminated against and may feel compelled to stick to their beliefs despite professional advice. Other than HIV testing, no other testing or treatment advice had been refused. There appeared to be no ethical committee that both sides could have consulted to try and resolve their differences. The doctors resorted first to the CEO of the hospital and then to the hospital's lawyer and the court to find support for their preferred course of management.

In the fifth case report a psychiatrist who had previously treated the mother was able to alter her objection to treating her daughter, albeit temporarily. When her objections were renewed, the matter was placed before the court and the minor and her child were made wards of the court.

- ***Institutional mechanisms before recourse to the court.***

Major health care institutions should have an experienced ethicist or an ethical committee that staff can discuss issues with, and that can offer insight into approaches that can be taken in seeking to resolve issues between professionals and between professionals and patients.[23] Such persons should also be knowledgeable in the legal statutes, processes and services that are available in relation to particular problems. Such mechanisms are not a replacement for the courts, and should be explicit in this regard when consulted. Ethics committees should also be constituted in such a manner that they can be seen as, and trusted to be, an impartial sounding board for disputes, seeking to resolve issues or forge compromise, rather than appear to be an adjudication body giving direction to either party.[24]

Social services departments are the interface between the hospital and the community, and the professionals within them may be asked to investigate the circumstances of patients, so that their care can be better understood and coordinated.[25]

When such mechanisms fail to resolve disputes between the professional and the patient or parent, the institution should then be in a better position to put forward the case of the professionals before a court, and the patient would also be better prepared to set forth their reasons for refusal of care before the court.

---

[23] Medical Ethics » AMA Code of Medical Ethics » Opinion 9.11-Ethics Committees in Health Care Institutions; http://www.ama-assn.org/ama/pub/physician-resources/medical-ethics/code-medical-ethics/opinion911
[24] Ethics Committee Handbook - Center for Practical Bioethics https://www.practicalbioethics.org/.../ethics-committee/Ethics-Committee-H
[25] Medical social work; http://en.wikipedia.org/wiki/Medical_social_work

In the reports given, there is no mention of an ethical committee in the institution.

In the second case report the clinician has turned to the CEO and then to the institution's lawyer. The CEO is not described as having either clinical or ethical expertise, and the intervention proves ineffective. The lawyer is described as not making a written submission to the court, and reports that the approach was unsuccessful.

In the fifth case report it appears as if the social services referral was a prelude to bringing an action before the court and to remove parental responsibility for the patient.

- ### *Considerations in court*

A judge is expected to take into account the immediate risk to life of the child, as well as the most likely outcome in the quality of life projected. In emergency situations a judge is most likely to opt for the life-saving option presented by the physicians, and thus give the opportunity and time to sort out other issues later. The judge should go beyond the emotional or religious convictions of the parents or the professionals, and enquire into the family's and the society's ability to cope with the expected outcomes in the patient.

A judge's decision should be made within the law in the jurisdiction for the protection of children.[26] Where specific law does not exist the judge should try to determine what is the best interest of the child, rather than the sole interests or beliefs of the parents, the physicians or of the institution.[27] The unifying standard a court should adopt to compel medical action on a patient is that the action must be in the best interest of the patient.[28] Determining the best interest of a patient does not rest on the opinion of the professionals alone; for no matter how compelling the data presented, a medical professional cannot guarantee a favourable outcome of any treatment in a particular individual. The determination of best interests is made by parents, next of kin or legal guardians, as well as professionals.[29]

When the decision of a parent or other surrogate differs from that of the health professional, the professional may turn to the court to impose their point of view. This is most likely when there is a threat to the life

---

[26] The Child Care Board Act, Barbados 1981 Ch 381
[27] Withholding and withdrawing life-prolonging medical treatment: guidance for - British Medical Association 3rd Ed 2007 Pt. 8
[28] Determining the Best Interests of the Child - Child Welfare ...https://www.childwelfare.gov/.../best
[29] Best Interests Guidance on determining the best interests of .T Joyce www.scie.org.uk/.../BPS-best interests...

of a minor and the parent / guardian refuses to have the child treated.[30]
When the court undertakes guardianship it assumes all of the legal
rights of that individual. In exercising those responsibilities, the court
will appoint guardians who may be individuals or organizations such as
a child care board or a psychiatric hospital.[31] In a few instances this has
been done in adults.[32]

An infant is best left with its mother, particularly if it is being breast-
fed. However, the mother may be on medication that may affect the
infant. The father is the next person who is legally responsible, but
may be denied custody if he is unable to care for the child. A close
female relative is usually preferred if the child's parents are thought
to be unsuitable, and failing that the infant is taken into care by a
responsible agency.

In deciding on medical treatment, the court may make a direct order
or may rely on the judgment of the appointed guardian. Being a ward of
state may end when a particular objective is achieved, or it may extend
until the end of childhood, but may be challenged by an application to,
and the determination by the court.

The court may also be petitioned by a patient's legal guardian /
surrogate to order that treatment be stopped, e.g. treatment that is
prolonging the life of a patient who is in a persistent vegetative state and
there is no demonstrable chance of recovery.[33]

*In the first case described, should the parents hold fast to their opinion it
would seem injudicious to place the matter before the court given the poor
outcomes expected. However, if the situation is urgent, and depending on the
arguments put before the judge, the judge may opt for the life-saving option.*

*In the second case reported, this was placed before a judge; the child was
not in danger and it is not surprising to have had the parents' strongly held
views upheld.*

*In the third case reported, the contentious situation arose during an
emergency, and the treating physicians decided to have the child's mother write
down her refusal of blood transfusion before proceeding with the emergency
surgical procedure.*

---

[30] Overriding Parental Decision to Withhold Treatment; M. Woods, Am. Med. Ass, J. Med. Ethics;
2003; Vol 5; 8
[31] Ward of court http://www.judiciary.gov.uk/glossary.htm#MainControl_Glossary_ZoneMain_
GlossaryPlaceholderControl1_ctl00_PresentationModeControlsContainer_SECTION_W
[32] Overriding a Patient's Refusal of Treatment; D. Casarett, and L. F. Ross, N Eng. J Med 1997;
336:1908
[33] Ethical Issues In The Persistent Vegetative State Patient; J L. Bernat http://www.aan.com/globals/
axon/assets/6114.pdf

In the fourth case report, no consideration appeared to have been given to compelling treatment through making the child a ward of the court. Such a consideration was probably complicated by the fact that the child was domiciled in a different jurisdiction. Nevertheless, a petition to compel treatment was likely to succeed in the face of the parents wishing to rely on herbal medicine as an alternative to effective chemotherapy.

In the fifth case a successful application was made before the court to remove parental responsibility and to make the minor and her child wards of the court. The social services department's assessment of the parents' capacity to look after their ill daughter and her infant would have played a pivotal role in the judge's determination. There was no mention of a father in the report given.

- ***What are the rights of a child in relation to a parent's decision?***
A child has a right to life and health and is entitled to protection from anyone who endangers it, including its parents. Authorities including medical and other health personnel have a duty to bring to the attention of appropriate authorities, the courts or the police, either directly or through an agency such as a child protection agency, any suspicion of endangerment of a child.

The concept of the liberated minor can also play a role in such decisions where the minor is of an age that their views on their treatment should be taken into account.[34] The 'Gillick' case set a precedent making it clear that doctors could make decisions against the parents' wishes, and in agreement with the wishes of children old enough to understand the decision being taken. Although such decisions are defensible in court in accordance with the 'Gillick' precedent, such decisions should probably be made by the court to avoid subsequent litigation.[35]

In the instance of an older child, the doctor should comply if the child and parents agree. However, whenever there is doubt about such agreement further opinions should be sought.

The child in case report five is the only child in the reported cases that could fall under the Gillick precedent. The others are too young to understand the issues and participate in the decisions made for them. She could also be considered a liberated minor by virtue of being a mother. However, her psychotic illness may preclude her from being able to make decisions for herself.

₃₄ Minors' Rights in Medical Decision Making; K Hickey, JONA'S Healthcare Law, Ethics, and Regulation; 2007/ Vol 9, No.3
₃₅ Gillick v West Norfolk and Wisbech Area Health Authority [1985] 3 All ER 402 (HL). ...

- ***If a court decides against the parents, what is the future of the child?***
Parents can appeal the decision of the court and can petition for the
return of the child to their care. If the parents decide that they no
longer wish to care for the child on religious grounds, then the court
has to provide for the care and protection of the child, which includes
finding foster parents, who are suitable and willing to undertake the
responsibility of parenting the child.

Although a doctor may be sued under such circumstances, the defence
would be that they are carrying out the will of the court. However, the
court cannot protect the doctor from a suit of negligence, should they
deviate from the standard of care and the patient is harmed as a result.

*In the fifth case report where the court has removed parental responsibility,
the minor patient and her infant have been placed as wards with the hospital.
When the patient has recovered a further determination will have to be made by
the court.*

Brain Death

Case report:

A three-year-old child was involved in an accident in which it was said that he had been struck and dragged along the road by a motorcycle. He was taken to the Accident and Emergency Department where it was observed that he was deeply unconscious. X-rays confirmed that he had a haemothorax and a fractured femur. His thorax was drained, his leg splinted and he was intubated, hyperventilated and admitted to the Paediatric Intensive Care Unit.

A CT scan of the brain demonstrated cerebral oedema and he was placed on mannitol and dexamethasone. On review the following morning, no pupil response, deep tendon reflexes or spontaneous respiratory efforts were observed. In the following days a repeat CT scan demonstrated cerebral oedema; he became anaemic and diabetes insipidus developed resulting in hypernatremia. The patient was transfused, the hypernatremia corrected, the diabetes insipidus treated with desmopressin and he was started on dopamine because of an unstable blood pressure.

One week after admission caloric tests to determine cerebral reflexes were performed and were negative, apnoea tests were aborted because of the patient's circulatory instability and serial electroencephalograms showed no baseline brain activity. The intensive care consultant and a neurologist reviewed the studies and both concurred that the child was brain dead. Over the next two weeks the child remained hemodynamically stable whilst on dopamine but developed progressive hypernatremia.

The child's parents said that for religious reasons [Muslim] they did not want an autopsy performed in the event of the child's death and were prepared to sign a DNR order and to have ventilator support withdrawn as long as they could have the child's body to be buried within 24 hours. The advice of the Attorney General's office was sought and the response was that there was no precedent in the country's law to withdraw ventilator support and attempts would be made to review relevant law in similar legal systems.

Three weeks after admission, the patient desaturated, became hypotensive and bradycardic while still on medication and after a few hours the heart stopped and death was certified.

Issues raised:

• *Was the child brain dead on admission to the Accident and Emergency Department?*
Brain death is the absence of neurological activity and spontaneous respiration is therefore not possible. Without respiration life is not possible and cardio-respiratory death occurs within minutes of its cessation. Therefore, brain death is diagnosed in patients on ventilator support and can be supported with 'objective' confirmatory tests over a period of time. It is an anomalous state in which a professional determination of death is made but the body cannot be delivered for burial because the heart is beating.

In the case described there is no observation recorded to suggest brain death when the patient was admitted. Although deeply unconscious the patient was breathing spontaneously and X-rays were done before the patient was intubated. Therefore, the diagnosis of brain death would have had to be confirmed later over a 24-48 hour period.

• *What is the law related to brain death?*
The formulation of criteria for brain death was first done in a report of an ad hoc committee of the Harvard Medical School in 1968 and the criteria were adopted that year at the 22nd World Medical Assembly .The criteria used were independently observed clinical evidence of no neurological activity, which could be confirmed by a flat EEG on repeated readings or no demonstrable cerebral circulation on angiography or radio-nucleotide scan.[36]

The purpose of making such a determination was to have a definition of death that would allow the transplantation of the heart and to procure other organs for transplantation in better condition than waiting for the natural cessation of the heartbeat. Anencephalic babies were reportedly used as donors as early as 1963 for renal transplantation,[37] and in 1966, a heart transplant was attempted from such an infant.[38] The first successful heart transplant in 1967, and those that followed, raised questions as to whether murder had been committed since a beating heart had to be taken from the donor. With the provision of a definition of 'brain death' doctors were empowered to be able to turn off the respirator in the circumstance of brain death with the backing of agreed professional

---

[36] A definition of irreversible coma. Report of the Ad Hoc Committee of the Harvard Medical School to Examine the Definition of Brain Death. JAMA 1968; 205; 337-40
[37] Human renal transplantation; Goodwin et al J. Urol. 1963; 89:13
[38] Transplantation of the heart; Kantowitz A.J et al. Cardiol 1968; 22; 782-90

opinion. However, it must be emphasised that such action was done with the concurrence of the responsible relatives or legal guardians who gave permission for the transplantation of organs.

The diagnosis of brain death had been made prior to the beginning of heart transplantation and in fact could only have been used prior to donation of the heart. It had been widely used as a prognostic tool and as a guide to when treatment was futile. The establishment of criteria for brain death provided the professional backing for turning off the ventilator in such cases, for it could be deemed a waste of resources. It is difficult for the relatives of a patient to accept that a person with a beating heart is dead; particularly when a patient who is brain dead can look remarkably normal. Therefore, both staff and relatives must be made aware of the patient's condition and how the diagnosis was made and confirmed, if they are not to feel that some wrong is being suggested or perpetrated when withdrawal of treatment is raised. Ventilator support is seen as the ultimate in preserving life, and turning off the ventilator without the full concurrence of relatives could lead to questions and /or legal actions; these could be defended but at the cost of time, anxiety and money. Most patients diagnosed as 'brain dead' die within 72 hours of the diagnosis being confirmed, and the 'withdrawal' of supportive measures other than ventilation usually speeds this up further. Therefore, except in an acute shortage of resources, it is unwise to turn off a ventilator without the concurrence of relatives and should probably only be initiated if it has been agreed that the patient will be an organ donor.

In the United States the need to seek the concurrence of relatives in withdrawing ventilator support was regularised in 1981 with the passage in some states of 'The Uniform Determination of Death Act'.[39] This act defined death, including criteria for brain death, and stated that the physician may stop all treatment on the diagnosis of death. Laws are not only derived by statute but also in a body of common law supported by judicial precedent. In the common law a registered medical practitioner certifies death and thus physicians could and did declare a person brain dead before statutes were passed. A number of countries now have statutes defining brain death, however, in countries where there is no statute, brain death would have to be considered within the practice of the common law and precedents set by the judicial bodies.

The practice in common law for determining medical practice is the usual accepted standard among a body of practising medical

---

[39] 2009 California Health and Safety Code - Section 7180: Article 1. Uniform Determination Of Death Act

professionals. The clinical criteria used for brain death were in practice in the UK, but were only given formal approval in 1976 when the Royal Colleges of the UK issued guidelines for the Diagnosis of Brain Death; these were reviewed in 1995.[40] [41] In the UK, the Privy Council accepts for judicial purposes the ordinary standard of care in the profession, and pronouncements by such a combined and authoritative body of opinion would be accepted by the Lord Justices. Thus, a practitioner in the UK could reasonably expect that stopping treatment in cases of brain death would be defensible in law.

Utilising brain death criteria can be abused. There are allegations that the criteria may not be faithfully followed in order to procure organs for transplantation. Persons who have drugs circulating are alleged to have had this happen, and in a number of instances 'donation' has gone on without the consent of relatives. There is no recourse for the 'brain dead' if it is determined that they were not really brain dead after they have given up their heart as well as other vital organs.[42]

When insurance payments are not guaranteed or likely to be obtained, it has been alleged that criteria have not been faithfully followed to allow ventilation to stop and death to occur. There are also reports that doctors have used the definition of brain death to reaffirm their power of decision-making without the consent of relatives, and to withdraw ventilation support without their knowledge or over their objections. Although this is what the law may empower physicians to do, challenges to how the criteria were followed and to the technology used in any confirmatory tests are possible. Therefore, it is wise to involve relatives and care-givers in the decision-making process.

In the case described were the criteria used appropriatly, and were they applied properly and independently? The criteria given in defining brain death specifically exclude their use in infants and although this child is over one year old – it is just three years old – and it is well acknowledged that the determination in small children can be more difficult than in adults.[43] The patient developed hypernatremia and the determination cannot be made with electrolyte disturbances, however, it is said that at the time of the determination that the hypernatremia had been corrected, although it is noted to be present after the determination. The methods used to correct hypernatremia and what effect these have on cerebral oedema or the cerebral circulation must be taken

---

[40] Diagnosis of Brain Death, Lancet 1976 ii 1069-70
[41] J Royal Coll. Phys. Lond. 1995; 29; 381-2
[42] State of Montana vs. Madill, (Billings, MT) DC-84-210 and State of South Carolina vs. Matthews (Charleston SC) 1985
[43] Guidelines for the determination of brain death in children. ...Clin Perinatol 1997; 24: 859-882 and Shemie SD, Pollack MM, Morioka M, Bonner S. Diagnosis

into consideration. In the case report there was no mention of a neurosurgical consultation on how the evidently very severe injury should be treated. However, the methodology and the time taken over separate observations in the case were appropriate.

- **Was the diagnosis of brain death correct and for what purpose was it made?**

There are three reasons for making the diagnosis of brain death:
   i. To provide a prognosis for the guidance of relatives and care-givers.
   ii. To consider organ donation, and
   iii. To make equipment available for other patients.

The correctness of the diagnosis of brain death can be raised because the patient survived for two weeks after it was recorded that the EEG was flat, for brain dead patients usually die within three days in spite of supportive measures. However, it is known that children do survive on average longer than adults. It also raises the point of why was the diagnosis being made?

The prognosis was evident in this case on clinical criteria and the use of confirmatory tests should only have been employed as confirmation of the intent to carry out one or both of the two other considerations. There was no consideration of organ transplantation in this case and nothing was said about the urgent need for the ventilator. However, when urgent needs will arise is unpredictable and one should be as prepared as possible.

Withdrawal of life support could provide emotional closure for the relatives but in this case closure appeared to be conditional on religious needs in not having a post-mortem to allow a quick burial. These are situations where an ethical committee should be consulted and where any necessary clarification of the law sought. What question was asked of the legal authority is not clear from the case report, and the answer given that there is no specific statute should have been known to those involved in making such determinations.

- **What is the legal issue?**

There is no legal issue related to the withdrawal of ventilator support in a brain dead patient where the relatives have been informed of the determination and raise no objections. However, in the case of an injury where a felony such as manslaughter or murder may have been committed, then the questions related to defining brain death and withdrawal of ventilator support could jeopardize the defendant as well as hampering the prosecution. These are matters that are properly enquired into by the coroner. Only the coroner or a judge in the High Court should make a decision to withdraw ventilation in such a case. In a case reported in the medical law literature in 1992, a 19-month-old child was declared

brain dead after a suspected non-accidental injury; the doctors wanted
to turn off the ventilator and an emergency order was granted to require
consent from the guardians before doing so. Subsequently a High Court
judge declared that the child was 'undoubtedly dead' and the doctors
could if they deemed it appropriate withdraw ventilation. The point is
that under circumstances where a felony may have been committed it is
best to get the authority from the judicial authority, which is either the
coroner or a judge in the High Court.[44]

*In the case as described the relatives were prepared to consider withdrawal
of ventilation but on conditions which could probably only be adjudicated on by
the coroner.*

• ***Should ventilation not be stopped when the diagnosis of brain
death is made?***
As already discussed, the law by explicit statement or implication allows
for the physician to stop ventilation on the diagnosis of brain death.
However, to do so without the consideration of other factors could
lead to unwanted publicity as occurred where a doctor was accused of
withdrawing a ventilator from a patient in order to put the relative of
a colleague on it. Thus the criteria for brain death should not only be
carefully followed and documented independently of the care-givers
and other interested parties, but the purpose for withdrawing ventilator
support must be clear to all involved, relatives and care-givers alike, as
outlined in the human tissue transplant regulations of the country.[45]

In the absence of specific law relatives and guardians should be
persuaded to consent to the withdrawal of ventilation. This is difficult
given the emotions of the moment and in particular when the event was
unexpected, or hope for recovery had been given. Broad institutional
information/guidelines available to staff and the public before such
tragedies occur, provides a platform on which to start this difficult
conversation. Such guidelines should address all of the issues of end-
of-life care and should encompass Advance Directives /Living Wills,
Do Not Resuscitate Orders, Persistent Vegetative States / On Being a
'Vegetable', as well as Brain Death.

*In the institution in which the case described occurred there is no specific law,
neither are there any guidelines or information available to either the staff or
the public.*

---

[44] 3 Med Law Review 1992 303-5
[45] Laws of Trinidad and Tobago. 2. Chap. 28:07

- *Can religious requirements override the law in the diagnosis of brain death?*

Most religions have come to accept the concept of brain death in relation to the availability of organs for transplantation. Orthodox Jews have difficulty in accepting the concept of brain death and therefore do not allow the withdrawal of ventilator support; nevertheless, accommodations have been reached to allow the transplantation of organs from persons who have had ventilator support withdrawn. On the contrary, a Jehovah's Witness accepts the concept of brain death and withdrawal of ventilator support, but has had to come to accommodations about the transfer of tissues and accept transplantation of organs.[46]

In this case it has been suggested that the Muslim parents, having accepted brain death, wished to abide by other religious observances such as no post mortem and burial within 24 hours. There are other religions that also practise a quick burial and these include Jews and Hindus, and clearly any wait for a post mortem is a problem for them. Under the circumstances where a felony may have been committed, there is no discretion on the part of the doctors or the family or the Attorney General, it is the coroner who has the responsibility to have a post mortem carried out and only the coroner could determine otherwise. Nevertheless, the emotional needs of the family must be considered and it would seem that an approach to the coroner to waive or arrange a post mortem as soon as the heart stops would give the family an opportunity to be able to deal with the burial in the required time.

- *Was futile treatment carried out or were the doctors and family frustrated?*

Ventilation is not the only futile treatment even though it holds the public's attention. The variety of drugs given to maintain circulation in a brain dead patient must also be considered.

It is difficult to escape the conclusion of a futile course of management in this case. Given that the diagnosis of brain death is correct, treatment could have been withdrawn up to two weeks before death was accepted. This would have provided earlier closure.[47] [48]

---

[46] Ethical issues in neurology; James L. Bernat; 3rd ed Lippincott. 2008
[47] Prognostic significance of a dead brain stem, Pallis C, BMJ 1983; 286; 123-4
[48] Brain Death with prolonged somatic survival, Parrish G.E. et al NEJM 1982; 306; 14-6

Case report 1:

An 80-year-old man was admitted complaining of a painful leg for two weeks. He had been seen by his general practitioner and prescribed medications for his circulation. His family found him in extreme pain and he agreed to come to hospital.

He was well looking but had a cold left leg, with gangrenous toes and necrotic patches from ankle to shin. His pain was controlled without sedation and he refused amputation. His eldest son was contacted but was reluctant to encourage his father to have the amputation, stating that the hospital had a reputation for doing unnecessary amputations. He added that he would call his siblings in England, and arrange for his father's transfer there.

On the third day the leg was worse and he again refused amputation. The nursing staff stated that he was disoriented when the doctors were not on the ward. His son was contacted again and although agreeing that an amputation was needed, he would only sign the consent if his father became disoriented. A psychiatric consultation was obtained and it was stated that the patient was not competent to consent to or refuse treatment. The patient's son was contacted with this information but stated that his father was heard shouting that no one was to "cut off" his leg and he would not go against his wishes. On day five of admission the patient appeared lucid; he said he understood the need for amputation and agreed to sign the consent form. He was unable to write his full name but made a mark. The psychiatrist reviewed the patient again and reasserted that he was not competent to accept or refuse treatment. However, the surgical team deemed that the patient was coherent when he agreed to have surgery and that his consent remained valid. The patient underwent surgery that day, and died the following day.

Case report 2:

A 65-year-old man was referred for surgical repair of a ventral hernia. In surgical outpatients he was not responding to several calls of his name and when identified it appeared that he was deaf mute. He was alone and a history was attempted with gesticulations and by writing to no avail. In trying to communicate with the doctors the patient pointed to various parts of his abdomen and chest, including the hernia.

On examination, an uncomplicated ventral hernia was found. The notes showed that the patient had had a previous admission for blunt abdominal trauma, and an attendance in the eye outpatients department.

No mention was made in the notes of his being deaf mute. Several attempts to call the telephone numbers listed for a next of kin and for someone in the hospital who could perform sign language, proved futile.

The surgeon wrote a note to be delivered to the next of kin listed in the notes, asking whether they could accompany the patient on the next visit. The concern of the surgeon was how to obtain informed consent for an elective operation for a non-life threatening condition.

Case report 3:

A 60- year-old man was admitted with an infected wound on his leg. He had sustained a fall one week before and struck his left ankle on a stone. He was diabetic and hypertensive, non-compliant on medication. Despite initial management with debridement and antibiotics his condition deteriorated within the next 24 hours and he became obtunded. A decision was made to do an emergency below-knee amputation.

Multiple attempts to contact his wife via the telephone were unsuccessful. The CEO of the hospital was informed and the patient was taken to the OR for the amputation. The nurse in the OR questioned the validity of the consent given by the consultant in charge of the patient.

Case report 4:

A 90-year-old man was admitted to the Surgical Intensive Care Unit after being struck by a car. He had sustained a head injury, a fractured right femur and multiple fractured ribs. He was intubated and sedated and it was decided that he needed an operation for fixation of his fractured femur, and a tracheostomy for ventilation. He had no known next of kin. The consultant orthopaedic surgeon gave consent for fixation of the femur, however, the ENT surgeon refused to give consent for the tracheostomy procedure.

Case report 5:

A 50-year old man, a chronic alcohol user, presented with sudden onset of epigastric pain and vomiting. He was a known epileptic and had had a number of admissions for alcohol-related complications. After examining his abdomen a diagnosis of acute appendicitis was made, but at operation no abnormality was found.

His post-operative course was complicated by seizures, aspiration pneumonia, diarrhoea, an upper GI bleed and delirium tremens. On day 20 post-op the abdomen remained distended and a decision was made to re-operate; at operation only dilated small bowel was found. Four days later he developed pneumonia; a CXR was interpreted as consistent with pneumocystis carinii pneumonia and an HIV test was requested.

At this time his mental state was altered, he was being treated for delirium tremens with sedation, and his consent was not obtained to do the HIV test. He had two regular visitors, a brother and a sister, neither of whom was consulted. The HIV test came back positive. His pneumonia resolved on treatment with septrin. When his mental status improved he was counselled re HIV testing; after some hesitation he gave permission to have the HIV test done, and asked for the results to be told to his relatives. He recovered and was discharged from hospital and referred to the HIV treatment clinic.

Case report 6:

A 55-year-old man on holiday in an English-speaking Caribbean island is admitted to hospital with an acute abdominal emergency. He does not speak English and a man who accompanies him states that he is his spouse and will act as his interpreter. The consultation takes place with the 'spouse' as interpreter and it was decided that an operation was necessary. It appears from the interaction that the patient agrees to the operation and his spouse/interpreter was asked to sign the consent form on the patient's behalf.

Issues raised

- ### Consenting to treatment

Consent is an agreement or permission for someone to do something to another. Treatment in the context of patient care means anything done in the course of addressing an illness. The persons entitled to treat patients are registered health professionals including doctors, dentists, some nurses and others, such as chiropodists, depending on the jurisdiction.

A patient or their legal guardian has an absolute right to consent to, or refuse, anything that is done to them; this includes matters that may appear non-threatening or trivial to the health care staff, as well as those matters that may threaten the patient's life. Competence to consent is assessed in both legal and mental terms.[49]

Legal competence resides in any adult, i.e.18 years and older in most jurisdictions, who is capable of understanding the matter to which they are asked to consent.

---

[49] Competency to Make Medical Decisions; http://www.stanford.edu/group/psylawseminar/Competency.htm

A parent or legal guardian consents on behalf of a minor. In some jurisdictions, like the UK, a minor aged 16 years may consent to medical treatment.[50] If an adult patient is unable to consent, the next of kin, the person in charge of the institution responsible for the patient, or a legally appointed guardian consents for the patient. The next of kin varies in different jurisdictions, but generally it would be a spouse, followed by adult children, parents, siblings and other relatives.[51]

Legal guardian. A person may make an advance directive or 'living will' where they give the power of attorney/ legal guardianship to a surrogate to make medical decisions for them when they become incompetent to do so.[52] A legal guardian may be appointed by the court to deal with the affairs, medical and otherwise, of a mentally incompetent person. Where there is no next of kin or legally appointed surrogate and a mentally incompetent patient is in an institution, the head of the institution may assume the role of the guardian of the patient for the purpose of consenting, in urgent situations, or as otherwise stated in the law.

Mental competence is a prerequisite for a patient to be able to consent to treatment. Mental incompetence is usually determined by the doctor treating the patient, e.g. the patient is in a coma, is unconscious or delirious without a clear understanding of their surroundings. When mental competence is related to a mental disorder, the opinion of a psychiatrist should be sought to determine whether the illness is of such severity that the patient cannot consent for their treatment. If a patient's mental illness is of such severity that they are a danger to themselves or others, there are usually provisions in mental health statutes to have the patient involuntarily admitted to a psychiatric facility and treatment ordered for the patient without their consent or that of their relatives.[53]

Anything done to a patient who, because of their mental incompetence, cannot consent for themselves must be done in that patient's best interest and not for the convenience of the parent / guardian, the health care staff, or the institution in which they are being treated.[54]

Minors: All persons below the age of 18 years, except by specific statute, require consent to be given for them by one of their parents or their legal guardian. Some minors have the capacity to consent to

---

[50] Family Law Reform Act 1969; UK C 46; section 8

[51] Next of kin; http://en.wikipedia.org/wiki/Next_of_kin

[52] Advance health care directive; http://en.wikipedia.org/wiki/Advance_health_care_directive

[53] The Mental Health Act 1980 - Laws of Barbados; Chapter 45

[54] Guidance on determining the best interests of adults who lack the capacity to make a decision (or decisions) for themselves; T. Joyce; The British Psychological Society; http://www.briscomhealth.org.uk/files/Best_Interests_Guidance.pdf

treatment in certain instances that are established in law or judicial precedent. The Gillick precedent established certain general ground rules whereby a minor can consent to treatment and override the wishes of the parents.[55]

- The minor must understand the advice being given.
- The minor does not wish the parent to know and cannot be persuaded otherwise.
- The minor was likely to continue with the risk behaviour and this behaviour was likely to produce harm to the minor.
- The best interest of the minor would be served in spite of parental disapproval.

Although the legal age of consent for sexual intercourse in many jurisdictions is 16 years old, a person that age would not, except by special statute, have the legal capacity to consent to the treatment of a sexually transmitted disease or its consequences. On the other hand, in one jurisdiction a 16-year-old can consent independently of her parents to a termination of pregnancy of 12 weeks or less duration under the Termination of Pregnancy Act 1983.[56] However, that same young person would be unable to consent to a caesarean section being performed. After giving birth the 16-year-old mother can consent for the treatment of her child but is not entitled to consent for her own treatment.

Court orders. When in doubt, legal advice should be obtained or a court asked to adjudicate. Orders of court are sometimes used when relatives or doctors cannot agree on the best course of treatment for the patient; these are rarely used for mentally competent patients. In such cases the court will seek to determine what is in the best interest of the patient, rather than the interest expressed by their relatives or the professionals involved.[57]

- *Refusal to consent*

Any competent patient, parent of a minor or legal guardian can refuse investigation or treatment. Such refusal can only be overridden by a court of law and would only occur in unusual circumstances. A patient or their surrogate can refuse treatment at any time, even after the treatment

---

[55] Gillick v West Norfolk & Wisbech Area Health Authority [1985] UKHL 7 URL
[56] Laws of Barbados; Medical Termination of Pregnancy Act No. 4; 1983
[57] Guidance on determining the best interests of adults who lack the capacity to make a decision (or decisions) for themselves; T. Joyce; The British Psychological Society; http://www.briscomhealth. org.uk/files/Best_Interests_Guidance.pdf

or procedure has started. It is wise to have such refusal recorded and witnessed.[58]

- ***Treatment without consent***

Any doctor may act in the best interest of a patient in a life-saving emergency situation.[59] Anything done to a competent patient without their consent, whether it is an emergency or not, is an assault in law. The remedies available to the patient are a criminal charge of battery or a civil action for negligence.

- ***Forms of consent***

Consent can be implied, given orally or in writing.

Implied consent is given when a person offers themself to have a blood sample taken. However, if the person discovers that the test that was done was not something that they wanted done, then such 'implied consent' is invalidated.

Oral consent is commonly applied for most medical treatment and should be obtained for tests or 'minor' procedures depending on the seriousness of the expected result. Harm to a patient can be psycho-social, e.g. diagnosing diseases like HIV that carry a significant stigma in the community, or malignancies that strike fear in some patients. In such instances there is no place for implied consent, but oral consent could suffice.

Written consent is usually obtained for surgical or other invasive procedures where the risk of physical harm is obvious. However, it must be remembered that such documents are only indicative of the patient's awareness of the event and should not be seen as sanction to do something that may harm the patient.

Informed consent. The term informed consent has come to be associated with interventional research on human subjects as well as surgical procedures, and implies a written record of the explanation given about the intervention to be employed and its risks. All consent must be informed in the sense that the patient should know and understand what is to happen to them. This means that the diagnosis, general nature of the procedure proposed, the anticipated benefits and risks, as well as the alternatives should be explained. Explanations should be in terms that the patient can understand, rather than terms that are only clear to other

---

[58] Rationality and the refusal of medical treatment: a critique of the recent approach of the English courts. M Stauch; J Med Ethics. 1995; 21(3): 162–165

[59] Exceptions to Informed Consent in Emergency Medicine; K M. Hartman, B A. Liang, Hospital Physician, 1999 http://www.turner-white.com/pdf/hp_mar99_emergmed.pdf

professionals. A judge in explaining consent related to surgery said that
one should:

> "Advise patients of those material facts, risks, complications and
> alternatives to surgery that a reasonable person in the patient's
> situation would consider significant in deciding whether to have
> an operation."[60] Treatment or investigation could be substituted in
> this advice.

Informed consent with a written record is necessary in clinical
situations where events, no matter how rarely they occur, may have a
serious and permanent effect on the patient. On the other hand, there
is a fine line to be drawn between outlining all the risks of a procedure
and calling to the attention of the patient the possibility of unusual but
specific events that may occur. For example, it is prudent to warn every
patient undergoing amputation about the possibility of phantom limb
pain whilst it is not necessary to stress, unless asked, that they may suffer
a cardiac arrest during the surgical procedure or the recovery period and
die, for the latter risks are rare and not specific to this procedure.

Situations of uncertainty. There are some situations that may not be
clear, either because the legal parameters are not well defined, or where
practice varies in different countries or institutions. In such situations
advice should be sought from whatever legal or ethical resources are
available to the practitioner. In hospital practice two such well-recognised
situations relate to organ donation and to the cessation of life support.

Organ donation. In countries where there is no specific law governing
organ donation, consent should be obtained from the next of kin, or
from the coroner in those cases of death that come under the coroner's
jurisdiction. A donor card carried by a patient is indicative of their
willingness to donate their organs and should be viewed as persuasive by
both the next of kin and the coroner of the person's wishes.[61]

Cessation of life support becomes a consideration for persons diagnosed
as 'brain dead' or those who are severely and irreversibly brain damaged.
It is wise to obtain the agreement of the next of kin with any decision to
cease life support in such cases.[62] There are jurisdictions where the law
defines brain death and the practitioner is thereby entitled to cease life-
support having made the diagnosis.

There are situations where the question is raised as to whether life
support measures should be started in the event of the patient becoming

---

[60] Gouse v. Cassel, 532 Pa. 197, 615 A.2d 331, 334 (1992)
[61] Consent for Organ Donation - Balancing Conflicting Ethical Obligations; R D. Truog,
N Eng. J Med 2008; 358:1209-1211
[62] Discontinuation of ventilation after brain stem death J M A Swinburn, BMJ 1999; 318:1753

severely ill or incapacitated. While the issues of consent remain the same, prior determinations may be indicated through the use of 'living wills' and DNR (do not resuscitate) orders.

Living Wills are legally made documents in which the patient gives prior directions as to what measures may or may not be taken in the event of their becoming incapacitated. Such documents should be placed in the patient's record, but like any other will it has to be executed by the next of kin or the health personnel who are aware of its existence.[63] In emergency situations the existence of the document may not be known. Therefore, a living will can only be considered indicative of a patient's wishes and cannot override clinical judgment.

Do not resuscitate orders are similar to Living Wills in that prior directions are determined. Although such notations are placed in patient's notes they may be ignored when the emergency arises because the staff present were either not aware of the determination or were unconvinced as to its correctness.[64]

- ### Consent and emergencies.

An attending doctor has a duty to treat a patient in an emergency situation to preserve their life. In such situations the patient is seldom able to consent. However, if a patient was clearly able to discuss and understand the life-threatening nature of their illness and made a clear decision against a course of action, then that decision should be honoured even when the patient eventually becomes incapacitated by the illness. The use of parents, guardians or surrogates in emergency situations is fraught with difficulty, particularly if they do decide against the emergency treatment required. Any contested decision can be defended on the basis that it was made in the best interests of the patient. If it is thought by an attending doctor that a decision made by a parent or guardian is not in the best interest of the patient, the doctor has to decide whether a court convened in emergency session should override the wishes of the parent or the surrogate of an adult.

In all the cases presented except for the second one the doctors are faced with consent issues in emergency situations. In the first case the judgment that the patient was mentally competent to consent can be faulted on the basis of the available psychiatric assessments.

In the third case, the surgeon has decided to proceed without the consent of the next-of-kin on the basis that the procedure was life-saving. It is not appropriate

[63] Advance health care directive; http://en.wikipedia.org/wiki/Advance_health_care_directive
[64] Do not resuscitate; http://en.wikipedia.org/wiki/Do_not_resuscitate

to delay treatment if that judgment is correct. The head of the institution was appropriately informed and was available to respond to the urgent situation. Nevertheless, an objection was raised by a member of the nursing staff about the lack of consent by the next of kin. This suggests either a lack of knowledge or a breakdown in communication within the caring team.

The differences in knowledge/perception of how to proceed in emergency situations is illustrated in the 4th case where emergency treatment is required in an elderly man without known next-of kin. One surgeon responded without consent to the emergency, whilst another did not.

In the fifth case the situation was complicated by issues related to confidentiality and the stigma and discrimination that can be associated with a diagnosis of HIV. However, in this condition the diagnosis of HIV could be regarded as only supportive of the clinical diagnoses being suspected and which needs to be acted on. If it was thought that specific treatment of HIV infection was necessary then testing had to be done and it should have been discussed with the relatives, unless there was specific institutional advice to the contrary. Given the state of stigma and discrimination that may exist it was reasonable not to approach the relatives without a more thorough examination of the social and sexual history of the patient. Once the decision has been made, how it should be handled is the next problem. Although the patient is temporarily deceived, the decision to counsel and persuade the patient to have an HIV test appears to be the right decision. The difficulty would have arisen if the patient had insisted that he did not want to be tested. The doctor would be theoretically open to a charge of battery, and the defence would be that the test was a medical necessity. However, if the defence of medical necessity were used it would be difficult to justify why the patient was not told as soon as possible without going through the subterfuge of seeking consent.

In the sixth case the patient has a language barrier and the doctor accepts the imprimatur of a same-sex spousal relationship to act as both interpreter and guardian of the patient. Such acceptance requires trust, which might only be broken if treatment goes badly wrong.

- **Is a psychiatric assessment the final determinant is assessing mental competence?**

Illness with delirium or hypoxia, use of drugs, sedative medicines and alcohol, and psychiatric illness such as dementia or psychosis may temporarily render a patient mentally incompetent. Attending doctors must make these decisions in ill patients taking into account any previous history of mental disorder, drug or substance use.

Psychiatrists are usually called upon for advice on the diagnosis and treatment of a patient thought to have a psychiatric illness. Like other specialist opinions they are considered more persuasive than those of other physicians when dealing with a patient's mental competence, and, in the case of a severely mentally ill patient, designated psychiatrists may treat such patients for their psychiatric illness without their consent within the limits of the law, such as a Mental Health Act.[65] Nevertheless, the court may be called upon to make a judgment on the determination made by attending doctors or psychiatrists, when persons who represent the patient's interests make a challenge.[66]

In the first case described, it appears that the surgeons are unclear about the mental competence of the patient to refuse the proffered operation and seek a psychiatric opinion on the matter. The specialist psychiatric opinion that the patient is mentally incompetent does not solve the problem, for the next of kin will not sign the consent form over what is seen as the clear refusal of his parent. The surgeon seizes on a moment of 'lucidity' of the patient, and in spite of a further psychiatric opinion to the contrary, gets the patient to 'consent' to the operation.[67]

- ***Coercion and obtaining consent***

Coercion of patients in the course of their care may come in many forms. A patient may fear that if they do not agree to the proposed treatment incorrect or unkind treatment may occur; and they may also fear opposing well-known or dominant professional figures. Giving sham treatments for pain, or giving an unrealistic prognosis for the proffered treatment are indirect forms of coercion. On the other hand, coercion of a patient to accept life-saving therapy could be defended ethically but not necessarily legally.[68]

Offers of benefits or rewards, for example to incarcerated and other disadvantaged persons for research purposes, and the illegal purchase of donor organs can also be considered as examples of coercion in medical care.

In the narrative of the first case given, the patient was probably coerced into signing consent on the basis of a moment of lucidity, yet was too ill to sign his name. If it can be shown that the patient could normally sign his name, making a mark would be the most telling evidence of the incapacity of the patient and therefore an assault on the patient when surgery was done.

---

[65] Mental health law; http://en.wikipedia.org/wiki/Mental_health_law
[66] Competency to Make Medical Decisions; http://www.stanford.edu/group/psylawseminar/Competency.htm
[67] Assessing patient's capacities to consent to treatment; P.S. Applebaum and T. Grisso; N.E.J.M. 1988; 318; 1635
[68] The morality of coercion; S M Glick J Med Ethics 2000;26:393-395

- *Do 'extraneous' factors influence obtaining informed consent?*

Presenting credible information about the necessity, risks and alternatives to a proposed operation is the essence of informed consent.[69] Credibility depends on both the manner in which information is presented and the ability to present facts in a convincing way and to counter any disinformation that may have been presented to the patient. It also depends on the ability of the patient to be able to understand and reason when alternatives are given. The ability to understand and reason is affected by many factors including age, physical and mental status, beliefs, as well as the relationship with the persons giving advice, as well as the involvement of relatives and friends.[70] Distrust of the professional's advice can be an important factor in patients refusing treatment.[71]

Another factor that reinforces the perception of the patient and the public is the way in which the professionals react to the patient and their relatives when advice is refused. Dismissive or withdrawal reactions on the part of the professionals are not usually persuasive to the patient, whilst coercive or deceptive actions are fraught with legal pitfalls should anything go wrong.

In the narrative given in the first case report there is little doubt that the patient and his relatives distrust the professionals when they state that an amputation is the only alternative available. The son believes that the leg may be saved elsewhere and speaks of making arrangements for the patient to be treated in another country. When the surgeon obtains consent, this goes against the psychiatrist's assessment of the patient's mental capacity to consent.

In the third case report, a nurse challenges the validity of the institutional consent obtained for the patient who is incapacitated and the relatives cannot be found in an emergency situation.

- *On being mute*

Being unable to speak cuts off a major avenue of human communication, and has a major impact on all aspects of a person's life, their development, and their ability to access medical care, particularly as an adult.[72] In making a medical evaluation of a mute adult, it is important to understand the genesis of the person being mute, for it will determine whether the person's intellectual status is such that they will be able

---

[69] Bolam v Friern Hospital Management Committee [1957] 1 WLR 582

[70] Mental Capacity, Consent, and Undue Influence; http://www.preventelderabuse.org/issues/capacity.html

[71] Patients Who Refuse Treatment in Medical Offices; J. E. Connelly, C. Campbell, Arch Intern Med. 1987; 147(10): 1829-1833

[72] Implications of Prelingual Deafness. Margolis Lancet 2001; 358:.p 76 http://www.thelancet.com/journals/lancet/article/PIIS0140-6736(00)05294-6/fulltext

to understand and be able to consent to the treatment being sought; or whether, like an infant or a young child, this responsibility has to be undertaken by a legal guardian.

Being mute may mean that no sound is uttered at all or that the sounds uttered are unintelligible. It is possible that with no physical abnormality an infant brought up without any verbal or sound communication would not have learnt how to speak, but would make noises to itself. The common problem is that of congenital deafness, so that the child hears no sounds and without special training will not learn how to speak.

Apart from congenital deafness there may be other abnormalities in the organ chain that learning to speak requires, such as in the vocal organs and the frontal lobe of the brain.[73] Damage to the brain may occur early or late in life and becoming mute may be part of a psychiatric illness, or may be drug induced.

In the second case described a history could not be taken by any of the means available at the time. Although a hernia was observed, the responses of the patient were not consistent with the observation made, making it difficult for the surgeon to know if it was indeed the patient's problem, and to obtain consent for surgery.

- *Obtaining consent*

Consent should be explicitly informed particularly in dealing with a condition that does not threaten life. Informed consent cannot be obtained without good communication, which may be obtained with the assistance of an interpreter or care-giver. When a proxy is used in communicating with a patient it has to be made clear to them that they should not substitute their own responses, but those of the patient, however illogical they may seem at the time.

When a proxy is used consent should always be in a written form, in the language that the patient understands, and in translation for the doctor concerned. An interpreter may act as a witness, but should not also act as a proxy for the patient. Where there is no translatable language the patient's legal guardian should be the one to consent in elective non-life-threatening situations. When there has been a refusal of treatment, it is equally important to have this in a written witnessed form.

In the cases reported there is some problem in obtaining consent. In the first case the patient is assessed to be mentally incapable of consenting, but is rejecting an amputation thought necessary by staff. Unfortunately, the next of kin would not accept responsibility.

---

[73] Cerebral organization for language in deaf and hearing subjects: Biological constraints and effects of experience. Neville, H. J; Proceedings of the National Academy of Sciences 95 (3): 922–929. doi:10.1073/pnas.95.3.922

In the second case report there was no prospect of obtaining informed consent, given the fact that no means of intelligibly communicating with the patient had been found and a search was being made for a next of kin.

In the third, fourth and fifth cases the treating physicians having determined that there is an emergency situation undertook the responsibility of carrying out treatment or investigation without seeking or awaiting consent from next of kin.

In the sixth case the language barrier has led the surgeon to deal with an adult patient as if they were a child and have the patient's spouse act as both interpreter and 'parent' in signing the consent form.

- ***Challenges to consent***

Any member of the health care team, a relative or guardian of a patient, may challenge the consent given on the grounds that the person giving the consent was not competent to do so, or that the consent was not informed. Written consent forms are usually witnessed to attest to the action of the person signing the consent. A witness to a signature may be any legally competent person willing to do so. Challenges can usually be resolved after a discussion and clarification of the concerns expressed. However, time for discussion may be severely limited in an emergency situation and should only be entertained for the objections by the next of kin if the patient is not or was not competent to give the consent.

A patient's mental state is, like their symptoms, social history and previous illnesses, important in making a full assessment of the patient. The assessment should include their ability to be able to make important decisions, including consenting to treatment. Mental competence or incompetence, and the perception of it, can be fleeting, and may depend on both physical and mental illness. It is therefore important, whenever there is a doubt, to have the mental status of the patient formally assessed.[74]

It is not possible to obtain informed consent from an uncommunicative patient and physicians must marshal the skills and resources to deal with the problems the patient presents. The reason for a patient being uncommunicative should be diagnosed and be taken into account during the entire course of care of the patient. Information should be passed between the health care professionals as to how to communicate with the patient.[75]

A history is not only important in making a diagnosis it is vital in deciding on the best course of treatment. Taking a history requires

---

[74] Assessment of Patients' Competence to Consent to Treatment; P S. Appelbaum, N Eng. J Med 2007; 357:1834-1840

[75] Deaf & Mute Communication; M. Andrews; http://www.ehow.com/facts_6739722_deaf-mute-communication.html

a language whether by signs, writing or graphic representation.[76]
The history may be obtained from a caregiver or observer, or with
the assistance of an interpreter or translator. The elicitation of signs
is dependent on accurate observations and is less dependent on
communication with the patient.

*In the cases presented, the capacity to consent is compromised by the mental
state of the patient produced by an acute illness or the patient's inability
to communicate.*

*In the first case the surgeon ignores a psychiatric assessment and the objection
of the next of kin to operation, and chooses a moment of 'lucidity' to declare that
the patient has consented to the operation.*

*In the second and sixth case reports the consent process is compromised by the
inability of the patient and the surgeon to communicate. The solution in the 6th
case of using a spouse as if he were a parent is predicated on the trust involved in
dealing with the doctor-patient relationship.*

*In the third case the surgeon has judged the patient's condition an emergency
and with the inability to reach the next of kin determined that the head of the
institution be apprised of the situation and proceeded. However, the surgeon was
challenged by the nurse in the operating room on the validity of the surgeon's
authority to consent for the patient.*

*In the fourth case treatment was urgently required and there were no known
relatives. One consultant surgeon decided that he had the authority to proceed,
whilst another did not. Since this was an urgency rather than an emergency,
the head of the institution could have been asked to act as guardian or have one
appointed by the court.*

*In the fifth case doing an HIV test without seeking the consent of the
available next of kin was done to protect the confidentiality of the patient with
a sensitive diagnosis. The subsequent action of pretending that the test had not
been done had the potential if discovered to undermine the trust in the doctor-
patient relationship.*

- **Can a mentally competent adult be asked to give up their right to
consent?**

A mentally competent adult can only be compelled to give up the right
of consent by a Court. This is rare, but has occurred in circumstances
where the adult has refused to be treated for a curable condition and the
court has been petitioned that the patient should not be allowed to die by
refusing standard treatment such as blood transfusion for the condition. It
is not so rare when a parent is refusing treatment for their child, and the

---

[76] Language Acquisition by Deaf Children; R. Meier, American Scientist 1991; 79 (1)

court is petitioned to take the child into its care and remove the parental right to consent to treatment for the child.[77] Competent patients must be given the opportunity to give their consent in a manner and language that they understand, or be asked to assign a power of attorney to the person that they would wish to exercise that right for them.

In the sixth case reported it does not appear as if the patient was given the opportunity to consent for himself, presumably on the grounds that he did not understand the consent form. An alternative would be a bilingual consent form, and the spouse could act as the interpreter and be witness to the patient's consent.

- **What is the role of an interpreter in a patient being properly informed?**

An interpreter should ideally be totally detached from the patient and the doctor, so that they do not inject their own personal interpretation or preference into the consultation. Interpreters should also be asked to sign a confidentiality form.

Spouses or other relatives who act as interpreters should be treated with caution in critical or emotive situations.

On the other hand, medical consultations may involve very confidential information and the patient may or may not be more comfortable with a relative, particularly if a health professional interpreter is not available.[78] In situations where there are no alternative interpreters available, the doctor should be cautious and assess whether the information being given is tainted with personal interpretation.

In the second case report an interpreter is not available and the consultation is compromised.

In the sixth case, it appears that there was no independent/health professional interpreter available and the patient's spouse is used as both interpreter and guardian. The illness did not appear to have any emotive component that could lead to misinterpretation.

- **Does one legally recognize a same gender spouse?**

Same sex marriages or civil unions are not recognized in all jurisdictions and where recognized, spouses should have all of the rights of spouses

---

[77] Overriding Parental Decision to Withhold Treatment; M. Woods, Am. Med. Ass. J. Med. Ethics; 2003; Vol 5, No8

[78] Using Medical Interpreters; D Hart, J Bowen, R DeJesus, A Maldonado, and F Jiwa, http://www.minnesotamedicine.com/CurrentIssue/ClinicalHartApril2010/tabid/3373/Default.aspx

of heterosexual marriages.[79] In jurisdictions where such marriages are not recognised, health professionals should accept such declarations for visitors as for any other person, i.e. a declaration of close personal relationship akin to common law marriage. In elective care situations such spouses could consider giving their partners the power of attorney to make decision for them.

In the sixth case report the doctors have accepted the word of the English-speaking partner that he is the spouse of the patient, to the point that they ask him to sign the consent form for the partner. The situation is an emergency and no legal pitfalls have been anticipated.

- ***Does a spouse have the legal right to take over a patient's right of consent?***

A spouse where they are the legal next of kin only has the right to take over the legal right to consent of their partner when that partner is mentally incompetent and unable to give informed consent. In some jurisdictions, a partner, although not formally married, can be recognized as a spouse in relation to rights to property under common law provisions.[80]

A spouse is not necessarily the next of kin depending on the jurisdiction. In many 'western' countries, the spouse is the next of kin, followed in legal hierarchy by the eldest adult child, the parents, siblings and other relatives. Under Sharia law a female spouse is not the next of kin; this may be the eldest adult son or brother.[81] Persons of Muslim faith may have to be reminded of the law in the jurisdiction in which they are, if a dispute arises about who bears responsibility for the patient.

The legal/declared next of kin automatically becomes the legal surrogate of a mentally incompetent adult. A surrogate who is not the next of kin may be appointed by executing a living will, which becomes valid only when the patient becomes mentally incompetent.

In the cases described there was no difficulty in deciding who the next of kin was. However, in the sixth case the marriage would not have been considered valid in the jurisdiction and the decision to treat the partner as if he were a legal spouse was compassionate, but could be challenged when allowed to sign the consent for his mentally competent partner. The alternative course would have been to record that the partner acted as the interpreter, and he should have been asked to act as the witness to the patient signing the consent form.

---

[79] Civil Unions & Domestic Partnership Statutes; National Conference of State Legislatures. 2012 http://www.ncsl.org/issues-research/human-services/civil-unions-and-domestic-partnership-statutes.aspx
[80] Succession Act, Cap. 249 Laws of Barbados 1975
[81] Islam and Healing. www.bu.edu/bhlp/Resources/Islam/health/guidelines.html

- ***The best interests of the patient***

The best interests of the patient are the sole standard for determining and giving consent to treatment for another person. Mental Health Acts proscribe the way in which patients who are mentally incompetent from a psychiatric illness may be treated; this is usually by admission as an involuntary patient.

Where there is no next of kin, the institution in which the patient has been residing or is being treated takes on the responsibility for the patient. Some institutions seek the appointment of an independent legal guardian to carry out these functions and thereby seek to avoid any taint of conflict of interest. Courts may be asked to determine what is in the best interest of a child or when there are unresolved disputes related to mentally incompetent patients.[82] However, there are other situations where it is best to keep the following statement in mind -

> "The medical judgment that treatment is indicated does not entail the ethical judgment that it ought to be administered to a particular person. Judgment of medical indication does not command the patient [or doctor] categorically, but gives medical advice." D.L. Miller[83]

In the cases reported there is every indication that the attending doctors considered their decisions in the best interests of the patients in spite of any difficulty they may have encountered in the process of obtaining informed consent. In cases 3 and 4 the situation is judged as a life-saving emergency and the surgeon assumes appropriate authority.

The surgeon in the first case report was clearly determined that an amputation should be done and could be challenged over the consent obtained. On the other hand, in spite of the outcome, no other alternatives were offered to treat the patient's condition.

---

[82] *In Re Quinlan*, IN THE MATTER OF KAREN QUINLAN, AN ALLEGED INCOMPETENT 70 N.J. 10, 355 A.2d 647 (1976), N.J. LEXIS 181; 79 A.L.R.3d
[83] Factors Influencing Physicians in Recommending In-Hospital Cardiopulmonary Resuscitation D. L. Miller, et al Arch Intern Med. 1993; 153(17): 1999-2003

Case report:

A 15-year-old schoolgirl attends a clinic and says she wants a prescription for 'the pill' to prevent her from becoming pregnant in case she is the victim of sexual assault. She states that becoming pregnant would stop her going to school and end her ambition to become a doctor. Asked why she thinks she will be sexually assaulted, she replies that her sister, who is one year older, is having a baby for her mother's boyfriend. Her sister told her that he refused to wear a condom when he was having sex with her. Asked if her mother knows what's going on, she replies that a year ago she heard her mother and her sister quarrelling and the mother said, "What wrong with you; you better off giving it to him than those snotty-nose boys you like talking to down by the corner". She thinks her mother is going to have the same attitude to her, and the man has been "pulling" at her ever since her sister started to show. When asked if she ever thought of reporting the man to the police, she says she is afraid what her mother and the man would do and she has no one to go to.

Told that contraceptives cannot be prescribed at her age without her parents' consent, she blurts out 'that she does not want her mother to know and she does not see her father too regular'. Pressed as to why she thinks her mother would object, she states that her mother is very religious when it comes to that and is always saying that a man does not stay if he thinks a woman is a mule. Although suspicious of the girl's statements, the doctor admires her determination to avoid pregnancy, and asks her to come to the clinic with her mother so that they could have a discussion about her health in general and her plans for going to university. Three days later she returns alone and says that her mother says "she don't have time to waste at the clinic unless someone is really sick".

Issues raised

- *What was the girl's full history?*

A thorough medical, family, social, and sexual history, as well as a thorough examination, is vital to being able to reach a good decision when faced with a problematical case from a clinical, ethical and legal point of view. Health care workers working in crowded clinics become accustomed to making rapid assessments used in emergency situations but these are not appropriate in detecting subtle illness or problems.

In the narrative given there was no sexual or other history taken from the patient, nor was she examined. The girl's demeanour, the clarity of her story and her lack of physical complaint may have led the physician to accept her story without further examination. The physician then proceeds to reach for a solution for the minor's legal incompetency and asks her to attend with her mother.

- ***Was the girl's sister being abused and should this be reported?***
Reports of abuse whether sexual or otherwise should be treated seriously and investigated by appropriate means. The profile of the alleged victim and the history of the allegations must be obtained to ensure that an offence has been committed. In accusations of sexual abuse, it is important to determine at what age the alleged abuse started and whether there is any element of coercion in the relationship.

There are jurisdictions where childhood abuse must be reported to the authorities, but there are others without this provision and it may be more appropriate to have the matter investigated through a social service agency, before determining what is the best course of action for the protection and welfare of the victim of the alleged abuse.[84]

In the instance reported there was no attempt made to get details or clarify an accusation of childhood sexual abuse, and there is clearly no intention to initiate action against the alleged abuser.

- ***Was the approach to getting the girl's mother to the clinic the correct one?***
Health care staff act within the letter of the law when they ask that parents should attend to discuss and to consent to medical treatment for their minor children. However, the laws do vary in jurisdictions and there are laws and precedents that allow health care professionals to treat minors without the consent of their parents. Staff have to make judgments based on their assessment of the minor's capacity to understand their illness, a thorough assessment of the minor's problem, and an informed assessment of the parent's behaviour and attitude towards the minor.

When a minor has sought a service without the consent of their parents, the health professional has an obligation to investigate the medical and social issues involved, using the resources available. When this has been done, the best interests of the minor should be determined including the need for respecting the confidentiality of the minor in sensitive situations.

From the account given it is clear that the minor did not trust her mother to

[84] World report on violence and health; Sexual violence
http://whqlibdoc.who.int/publications/2002/9241545615_chap6_eng.pdf

*agree to the request she was making. Testing the veracity of the statements made
by the minor would require a much more extensive history than was taken and
on independent enquiries.*

*It appeared unlikely that the girl would bring her mother to the clinic, and a
more direct approach to the mother could have been made. The minor returned
with a story that fits in with her original statements, and there is no further
information to verify the minor's account. Further enquiries can still be made of
the minor and through the social services.*

• *Can a minor be treated without the consent of their parents?*

A minor should not normally be treated without the consent of their
parents. However, the prescription of contraceptives for the protection
of minors was the basis for the judicial precedent where the judge
determined that if the minor was capable of understanding the situation,
had been counselled and objected to the parent's involvement, and if it
was in the minor's best interests, contraceptives could be prescribed for
that minor without the parent's consent.[85]

In some jurisdictions a minor aged 16 years can consent to and obtain
medical treatment as if they were an adult;[86] and in another jurisdiction
a minor aged 16 years who is 12 weeks or less pregnant may seek a
termination of her pregnancy without the knowledge or consent of her
parents.[87]

*In the report given there is not sufficient information obtained from either
the history or the physical examination to verify that the minor can be safely
given oral contraceptives. It is certainly not in the girl's best interest to become
pregnant, and she needed to have had her sexual history explored and be
counselled in relation to sexual intercourse at her age with anyone. One also
needs to consider whether it is in the girl's best interests to accede to her request
that she 'gives in' to sexual assault and the alternatives explored. In exploring
alternatives one should be sensitive to the family situation and explore this
further before any decision is taken. It may be that the sister may have to be
sought for an interview before that of the parents. Social service professionals are
best able to handle these kinds of enquiries.*

• *Should the confidentiality of a minor be respected?*

The issues of consent and confidentiality of a minor are inextricably
linked, particularly when sexual issues are involved. Whilst it is clear that

---

[85] Gillick v West Norfolk and Wisbech Area Health Authority and another. HOUSE OF LORDS [1986]
1 AC 112, [1985] 3 All ER 402, [1985] 3 WLR 830, [1986]
[86] Family Law Reform Act 1969 - Legislation.gov.uk. www.legislation.gov.uk/ukpga/1969/46
[87] Medical Termination of Pregnancy Act, No 4 1983, Barbados

a parent cannot influence a situation with their child without knowledge of the situation, it is also clear that an insensitive parent could make a sensitive situation worse. Therefore, an assessment of the parent's attitude needs to be made before a minor's plea for confidentiality is ignored. Laws vary and may make exceptions for such situations as contraceptive use by minors.[88]

When a minor appears before a court as a defendant, a complainant, or as a witness, provisions are made to protect the identity of the minor from the public in accordance with the United Nations Convention on the Rights of the Child.[89] However, the minor's identity cannot be shielded from an accused person, who has every right to be able to defend themself.

In the situation described there is nothing from the girl's story to suggest that the parents are sensitive or caring. Nevertheless, it would be unwise to take the child's word alone and other enquiries could be made through social services or other family sources before asking that the mother be brought to discuss the situation.

• *What is the health worker's role in pursuing a suspicion of child abuse?* In situations of childhood abuse a wide array of health professional skills is required before conclusions and actions are taken. The professionals involved should be the clinicians to whom the situation is presented, their forensic skills in diagnosis and marshalling evidence that is required for treatment and evidential purposes; it must also include the psychology professionals and social services professionals skilled in garnering knowledge and the assessment of family and social situations outside of the clinical setting. Law enforcement and other skills also have to be used when appropriate.[90]

In the case described none of the required skills in dealing with childhood abuse appeared to have been deployed.

• *What responsibility does a health worker have to report a possible felony?* In general, a health worker has a responsibility, like any other citizen, to report a felony to the police. However, the health professional could be said to have a higher degree of responsibility than the average citizen because of being in a position of trust with both the patient and the

---

[88] Minor's Rights Versus Parental Rights: Review of Legal Issues: Privacy and Confidentiality for Minors; A Maradiegue, http://www.medscape.com/viewarticle/456472_6
[89] Convention on the Rights of the Child; UN General Assembly resolution 44/25; 1989
[90] Child Protective Services: A Guide for Caseworkers D DePanfilis www.childwelfare.gov/pubs/usermanuals/cps/cps.pdf

police. They must therefore act on more than just superficial duty, based on suspicion. In reporting a felony they should be in a position to back their reporting with evidence. When the report is likely to have adverse consequences for the patient, the health professional has to balance their duty as a citizen with that of their duty to preserve the confidentiality of the patient. It is therefore prudent to inform or discuss with the patient any report to the police that is being initiated by a health professional.

When a minor is in danger from the abuse or neglect of their parents or guardian, the health professional may refer the case to the appropriate Child Care Agency, who after enquiry may take the minor away from the parents and guardians for their protection. Having done so the appropriate agency has to justify their action before the court in a prescribed time, giving the parents the opportunity to challenge the determination. Abuse by parents may be physical, emotional, sexual, or exploitative for financial gain such as child prostitution, or forcing the child's co-habitation or marriage with an adult. There are criminal statutes where parents can be brought before the courts when they have contributed to the delinquency of a minor.[91]

Health care professionals should be wary of suggesting to patients that they make accusations of criminal or civil misconduct before acquiring the evidence that could make such accusations successful; to do otherwise can place the patient in jeopardy.

In the case described there is an accusation of possible statutory rape of a sister, but no evidence is adduced that could form the basis for an enquiry by the police. Nevertheless, the health professional made a suggestion to the patient of going to the police without exploring with the patient the kind of evidence and support the patient would need in making such an accusation.

In this instance the child has described an exploitative situation by her mother with her sister, in which there is a possibility that there has been childhood sexual abuse. The child states that she wishes to protect herself from similar sexual abuse, which she sees as inevitable, but has not asked for help in avoiding the situation. If the child is to be believed and action taken, including the prescription of contraceptives, further enquiries should be made including her current sexual activity. Her story may be to deflect blame from herself and to evoke a sympathetic response. There is little one can do to compel the parent to attend to the child's problem unless an emergency, medical or otherwise, arises.

---

[91] World report on violence and health; Eds. E G. Krug, L L. Dahlberg, J A. Mercy, A B. Zwi and R Lozano Ch 3. CHILD ABUSE AND NEGLECT BY PARENTS AND OTHER CAREGIVERS; http:// whqlibdoc.who.int/publications/2002/9241545615_chap3_eng.pdf

Refusal to Consent

Case report 1:

A 70-year-old man who lived in a shed in his sister's yard, was brought by ambulance to the Accident and Emergency Ddepartment. On a visit his daughter had noticed an offensive smell coming from his foot. On examination he was unkempt, not ill-looking but was febrile; there was wet gangrene of his left forefoot up to the mid-calf. Pulses were felt in both limbs except for the affected foot.

He was advised to have a below knee amputation which he refused. It was noted that he was uncooperative but quiet, refusing to talk at times. He was placed on antibiotics and a dry dressing applied. The day after admission his relatives advised the doctors that the patient had a history of psychosis, and had been institutionalized in the UK fifteen years ago. He had had no psychiatric follow-up since repatriation from the UK. He was referred for a psychiatric consultation and was assessed as having paranoid ideation, with some insight into his current medical illness, but said, "I don't trust anyone."

A week later the offensive smell persisted, and in spite of urging from his relatives he continued to refuse amputation. The psychiatrist concluded that his psychosis prevented rational decision-making. Another surgical opinion agreed that amputation was necessary and suggested that the limb be exposed so that the patient could see how bad his foot was. After five weeks, a psychiatric second opinion suggested that anti-psychotic medication be started, hoping that the patient would gain insight into the potentially lethal nature of his problem. After a week he remained grossly thought disordered, was less objectionable but remained adamant that he did not want surgery. By the eigth week the forefoot was mummified and the psychiatrist advised that he be involuntarily committed.

Case report 2:

A 70-year-old woman with a longstanding history of diabetes, hypertension and chronic renal failure, was noted on follow-up to have worsened to a point where she required dialysis. She refused dialysis despite stating she understood the consequences of doing so. A formal psychiatric assessment was not done, as she appeared to be completely oriented.

She was later admitted for treatment of hypercalcaemia and again refused dialysis. She was discharged but readmitted four months later with severe uraemia, she was disoriented with clear features of uremic encephalopathy and was unable to consent for emergency dialysis. Her relatives stated that just prior to her becoming disoriented she had changed her mind about dialysis, but offered no confirmation that she had changed her mind. The question remained as to whether she was of sound mind at the time of the recantation. The decision was made to dialyse her as an emergency; she improved and has since accepted further dialysis.

She was later referred to surgery for an ischemic right leg with dry gangrene, as well as with a diagnosis of parathyroid adenoma. She refused surgical intervention and was referred for a psychiatric opinion. She was assessed as being mentally incompetent to accept or refuse treatment and for being at risk of developing organic brain syndrome from her multiple medical problems. It was advised that proxy consent of her next of kin be obtained for further medical interventions.

Her husband refused surgery and stated that although he thought it necessary, he did not want to risk upsetting her by going against her will. This was the overwhelming sentiment of the rest of the family as well. She was discharged to be followed up in the nephrology outpatient clinic.

Case report 3:
An 80-year-old man was forcibly brought by his daughters to the Emergency Department. He had a six-month history of weight loss and lethargy, six-weeks of difficulty in swallowing, nasal obstruction and two episodes of fainting, and had refused to seek medical attention. He had a long history of heavy cigarette and alcohol use. He was very upset with his daughters and said he preferred to stay at home and die. On examination he was cachexic, there was a large friable mass in his mouth that extended into the nasal cavities. He was diagnosed with advanced carcinoma of the hard palate and advised admission, which he refused. He was seen by the consultant surgeon and told firmly that he was to be admitted for resuscitation, investigations and biopsy and he complied. Investigation confirmed a locally advanced cancer, and he was referred for palliative radiotherapy, and nutritional supplementation via gastrostomy. He refused the gastrostomy and said he wished to go home. He was not allowed home and was seen by the gastroenterologist for insertion of the gastrostomy but he again refused. He was referred for a psychiatric opinion and was assessed as competent to make his decisions. After three weeks he agreed to have the gastrostomy, but developed a uremic encephalopathy secondary to dehydration and obstruction from an enlarged prostate. A family meeting was held and the decision was made by them to perform a tracheostomy and open gastrostomy. The

surgery consultant deemed him unfit to give consent, but was reassured that consent had been given previously. He was reassessed by psychiatry, deemed competent and his consent was obtained. By this time the family made it clear that they did not want any surgery done and that he should be allowed to die peacefully. The ENT surgeon insisted that he had consented and that the procedures would be performed. The surgery was done and he died in hospital three weeks later.

Issues raised.

• *What is the law regarding refusal of treatment by a patient?*
A legally and mentally competent patient has an absolute right to consent to anything that is done to them. Consent to treatment includes matters that may be considered non-threatening or trivial to health care staff, as well as matters that may threaten the patient's life. Treatment can be refused at any time even after a procedure has started. Refusal of treatment by a competent patient to investigation or treatment can only be overridden by an order in court. In agreeing to the treatment suggested by the doctors the court may order that it be carried out or state that the appointed guardian makes the decision.[92] The remedies available to the patient whose wishes are ignored are a charge of battery or a suit of negligence against the health practitioners involved.

In the cases presented the patients have refused specific treatments offered but have accepted other treatment measures. Psychiatric opinions have been sought when treatment has been refused, but except for when the patient has a reversible problem, the opinion in all three of the reported cases is that the patient was competent to make their own decisions.

In the first case report, after weeks of psychiatric medication and the patient's continued refusal of surgical treatment, the psychiatrist concluded that involuntary commitment should be the course of action.

In the second and third cases reported the patients are said to have reversed their refusal of treatment at some point, but this cannot be confirmed at the time treatment was to be carried out. When the relatives are asked to take responsibility for making the decisions, they decide to go with the previously expressed wishes of the patients even though they may have disagreed with them.

• *What is meant by informed consent?*
To have validity in law, consent must be informed in the sense that the

[92] Competency to Make Medical Decisions.www.stanford.edu/group/psylawseminar/Competency.htm; 2011

patient should know and understand what is to happen to them. This means that the diagnosis, general nature of the procedure proposed, the anticipated benefits and risks, as well as alternatives should be explained. Explanations have to be in terms that the patient can understand, rather than those that are only clear to other professionals.[93]

In the cases presented questions were raised as to the mental competency of the patients to make informed decisions about their care. In each case there was a psychiatric consultation, presumably to assess the patient's competence to give their consent to treatment. The psychiatrists who were consulted conceded that the patients had enough insight into their illness and therefore were able to consent or refuse treatment.

In the first and third cases the specific treatments refused are operations, but in the second case, renal dialysis is also an invasive procedure that is being refused. In the third case one consultant insists that the patient had consented to the procedures although he was not currently competent to do so, and had previously been adamant that he did not want surgery.

- ***The mentally incapacitated patient and the law related to consent.*** If an adult patient is unable to consent, for example, if they are in a coma, the next of kin or the person in charge of an institution responsible for the patient may consent. The mental capacity of a patient can change from time to time, and their ability to understand simple situations may be different from those that are more complex.

Under Mental Health Acts there is usually provision for a person to be involuntarily admitted, and can be deemed by the psychiatrist in charge as being incapable of giving informed consent; in such instances, psychiatric treatment can be administered without the patient's or their relatives' consent.[94] However, mentally incapacitated patients may have to be treated for conditions other than psychiatric illness, when such treatment is in their best interest. It is best to have a legally appointed guardian or power of attorney to handle the affairs of such persons, including health care decisions. If necessary, the best interests of the patient may have to be established in court if there is a difference of opinion between the family, guardians or other community interests and the health professionals.[95] It is preferable to come to an agreement without invoking the law.

Clinicians find it easier to determine mental incapacity to consent in a patient who is delirious from sepsis, rather than the patient who

---

[93] Bolam v Friern Hospital Management Committee [1957] 1 WLR 582
[94] Mental health atlas; World Health Organization; Geneva; 2005
[95] The moral character of clinicians or the best interests of patients? L Doyal, BMJ, 1999;318 : 1432

is mentally ill. Psychiatrists and others can make rapid assessments of mental capacity using standardised questionnaires.[96]

In the first case two psychiatrists differed on whether the patient's psychosis required treatment. After weeks of medication, involuntary admission documentation was initiated. This patient illustrates that the capacity to consent is not easy to assess in a mentally ill patient who clearly refuses a line of treatment but is not a threat to themselves or others.

In the second case there is no documentation indicating that the patient changed her mind about dialysis, but she accepts it after having it in an emergency situation. However, she remains adamant about other recommended surgery and her family respects her wishes even though they agree she would benefit from the procedures.

In the third case presented it appears that the patient may have been bullied or given in to having procedures that he clearly doesn't want, but the caring team thinks will make him more comfortable. Whether he is made more comfortable is not stated, but he is left unable to communicate in the last few weeks of his life.

- **How does the law apply in emergency situations?**

Any doctor may act in the best interests of a patient in an emergency situation when the patient's life is threatened. Best interest should not be seen as embarking on futile previously declared unwanted treatment, or not using a ventilator or other treatment because it is anticipated that someone 'more worthy' will require it.[97]

What course of action should have been taken if a patient with a gangrenous limb who had refused amputation had become septicaemic and their life was in immediate danger? In the UK, a court found in favour of a man in this situation, and issued an order preventing the hospital from amputating the gangrenous limb should his mental condition make him incapable of refusing treatment at the time; the principle being that mental illness does not automatically call a patient's capacity into question.[98]

In the cases presented the initial judgment of the doctors is that a specific treatment is needed urgently but the patient's condition was not an immediate threat to life.

---

[96] Mini-mental state". A practical method for grading the cognitive state of patients for the clinician. Folstein MF, Folstein SE, McHugh PR Journal of psychiatric research 1975; 12 (3): 189–98
[97] Code of Ethics for Emergency Physicians; ACEP, 2011
[98] Adult: Refusal of Treatment. All England Reports 819; 1994

In the first case report the patient was not incapacitated by delirium from his sepsis and although he expressed paranoid feelings, particularly about the doctors, he appeared sufficiently clear to all concerned that he understood what an amputation was and that he did not want it performed.

In the second case the patient appeared sufficiently clear in her decision that the doctors accepted her refusal of dialysis although it was clearly indicated. However, when her uraemia incapacitated her and threatened her life, her relatives accepted responsibility stating that she had changed her mind before she became so ill.

In the third case the patient has clearly stated that he did not wish to be treated. He was probably coerced into having procedures that may have prolonged his life for a few weeks, but compromised his quality of life for he was unable to communicate and was being kept alive by tube feeding.

- ***Should a patient's wishes be followed when they can no longer consent?***

Given the patient's right to autonomy over their body, their clearly expressed wishes should be respected. This situation usually arises when a decision has to be made as to whether a patient should be resuscitated or placed on ventilation should a life-threatening situation arise. This is the purpose for which advanced directives such as living wills have been used.[99] Living wills like 'Do Not Resuscitate' orders have not been respected in a number of situations, for health care workers faced with emergency situations often feel compelled to act to safeguard themselves legally, and then argue about the living will or the do-not-resuscitate order later.

In cases of refusal where there is an unresolved question, the only safe course would be to let a court decide. Courts are unlikely to be invoked unless the doctors feel that the stakes in relation to the patient's life are high. A high priority on life in cases before the courts usually involve the life and welfare of children, or a clash of religious beliefs. However, when the situation is an urgent one, there may not be enough time to argue before the court. If the patient's next of kin and relatives are clear that they would like the doctors to proceed in spite of the patient's wishes, the legal ground is firmer to stand on, but will not prevent a legal challenge by the patient on recovery. This raises the question as to whether the doctors, by consenting to the patient's wishes, can be considered to be a party to 'a suicidal act by the patient'.

---

[99] Time for a new law on health care advance directives. Alexander, G.J, Hastings Center Law Journal. 1991;42(3):755-778

In the first case presented the patient has clearly expressed his wish not to have an amputation. The gangrenous limb did not present a threat to his life at any stage in his hospitalisation, and because of his mental state there was no determination as to whether he would continue to refuse if his life was threatened.

In the second case reported there was no attempt made to determine whether she would continue to refuse dialysis when her life became threatened. Her relatives declared that she had changed her mind and would accept the treatment.

In the third case the patient appears to be aware of the seriousness of his illness and expresses the desire to go home and die. He is offered operations, which he does not want and which would render him uncommunicative and dependent on tube feeding, but there is no prospect of treating his disease. He appears to have given in after being 'persuaded' but neither he nor his family express any satisfaction with his condition after the operations that were performed.

- **Should a patient be allowed to "commit suicide" by refusing treatment?**

Suicide is an illegal act and doctors, apart from saving lives, should prevent and not be a party to illegal acts wherever possible. However, suicide is done by an act of commission, it is not normally considered to be done by an act of omission. Man is mortal and will die from an illness of some sort, and there are few who will argue that a person should not have some say in the manner in which they will die.

There is a community interest in preventing unnecessary deaths, and there is an equally strong individual interest in the quality of one's life. Therefore, each patient should be considered on the merits of their individual case. Normally a court will allow a competent adult to refuse treatment even if it means that it will result in their death. The courts try to decide what is in the best interest of the patient; this must take into account the patient's mental and physical status and the effect that any actual or anticipated disability will have on their quality of life. For example, a court in the US had ordered that a woman, a Jehovah's Witness with dependent children, should have a blood transfusion against her wishes, in order that she might live for the benefit of her children. In a similar case the ruling was different because it was pointed out that the children would be well looked after by relatives and that the patient had a right to refuse treatment even if it would save their life.[100]

---

[100] Norwood Hosp. v. Munoz, 409 Mass. 116 , 122 (1991)

In the cases presented the situation of suicide by refusing treatment does not arise. In each case the patient appears to want their illness to take its course without invasive surgical treatment in particular. It would be entirely speculative as to what arguments would be put before a court that these patients' wishes should not be respected.

It appeared from the description of the first patient's living conditions that an amputation could make his situation worse. However, living conditions can be improved and services provided to make an amputee have a good quality of life. It could be concluded that to override this particular patient's wishes, the relatives or the community should be obliged to improve the conditions in which he lives and to provide him with treatment for his mental condition.

In the second case, the treatment offered promises a better quality of life, but it clearly was not deemed better by the patient.

In the third case the treatment offered was to facilitate palliative treatment of the disease, but it made the quality of the patient's life unacceptable.

• **What measures can be used to get a patient to change their mind?**
In order to persuade a patient towards a physician's judgment a variety of measures are utilised: counselling by health care workers, relatives, priests, friends and second opinions are all clear and acceptable methods. However, counselling has its risks if done inexpertly and where the best interests of the patient are not the primary objective. Coercive measures such as withholding medication or other items of care, or discharging the patient are not acceptable ethically. Because medical treatment is not absolute some measures, which are 'coercive' in one circumstance, may be within the normal standard of practice in other situations; it is the intention of the advice that is the ethical issue.

The physician should also be wary of deliberately using sedation to alter the judgment of the patient, and under its effect obtain consent to a procedure.

In the first case reported the second psychiatric opinion advised medication with the intent of altering his mental state to see if he would become compliant with advice. Such an intention could be hazardous both ethically and legally, particularly if the patient is 'sedated 'and makes their decision under sedation, or the patient's wishes are overridden whilst incapacitated by sedation. In the event, the medication had the effect of making the patient more approachable but he did not change his mind. The second surgical opinion confirmed the surgical advice and advised that as a 'persuasive' measure the gangrenous limb should be exposed so that the patient could see how futile refusal was. Exposure of a gangrenous part is an acceptable and standard treatment in some instances whilst awaiting demarcation of the dead part, the issue that arises is that this was not the intention of the exposure. In the event, exposure did not alter the patient's mind but may have offended others in the ward. This raises the question as to whether treatment can be mandated for the 'protection' of others.

In the third case reported, it appears as if the patient is prevented from discharging himself and bullied into making the decision that the physician wanted.

• ***Can a patient's refusal of treatment be ignored as being a threat to others?***

There are provisions in both Public Health Regulations and in Mental Health Acts to protect the public from patients who are a risk to the public and who refuse treatment for their condition. The medical authorities have the power under public health regulations to confine or isolate patients for prescribed communicable disorders and to enter premises or destroy property that is deemed to be a public health hazard. Mental Health Acts and the courts provide for the restraint and treatment of a mentally ill person who is a deadly threat to a third party, the community or themselves.

"The physician knows the many clinical distinctions that tell him when death is imminent or hope abundant; when to treat and when to wait; when to sedate with drugs and when to sedate with words; when to stop treatment change or add; when to treat aggressively for cure, palliatively for relief and consolingly for comfort. ... But he cannot express these specifically or consistently." Feinstein[101]

In the first case reported the public nuisance of a smelly gangrenous limb in an open ward was probably made worse by the advice to expose the gangrenous smelly limb. However, medical treatment accepted by the patient did eventually reduce the infection and the consequential public nuisance.

In the third case the admitting surgeon is convinced that the procedures recommended are in the best interest of the patient but is unable to convey this to the patient in a convincing manner.

---

[101] Miller, F.G. 'The concept of Medically indicated Treatment' J. Med and Philosophy 1993; 18; 81

Case report:
An 80-year-old man with a history of atrial fibrillation, on anticoagulation, Digoxin and Lasix presented with a one-day history of bleeding per rectum. The bleeding had occurred after stool and there were no other symptoms. He had a previous history of myocardial infarction and a stroke from which he had recovered. He was alert, cooperative, but pale with an irregular pulse rate of 92 b/min, and a BP of 114/65. Examination found the cardiovascular system, chest, abdomen and rectum normal. Initial investigations showed a SpO2 97%, Hb 13.0 gm/dl, PT 23/12 and INR 3.8.

He was assessed as bleeding secondary to over anticoagulation or diverticular disease. He was placed on antibiotics, IV fluids and O2 and blood cross-matched. The following evening he had further bleeding, his vital signs remained unchanged, but his Hb dropped to 9.1 gm/dl. The next day he had a larger bleed and it was decided to transfuse him. A nurse brought to the doctor's attention that he was listed as JW -Jehovah's Witness. The pros and cons of blood transfusion were discussed with him in the presence of his daughter, and he agreed in her presence to have the blood transfusion.

While the transfusion was in progress, one of his sons visited and objected to the blood transfusion. The duty doctor was called and after outlining the poor outcome if transfusion was rejected, the patient said he had changed his mind but would not sign the offered waiver rejecting the transfusion and said that his son could sign it. The son signed the waiver and the transfusion was stopped. That evening the patient had a massive bleed, and became shocked. He was taken to theatre and had a sub-total colectomy done. He remained shocked in spite of vasopressors, had a cardiac arrest, could not be resuscitated and died.

Issues raised

• *Should blood be cross-matched for a patient without their consenting to it?*
The doctor in ordering blood to be cross-matched before ascertaining whether the patient would accept a blood transfusion is acting in a routine manner, but has done nothing wrong. However, blood transfusion carries a number of risks and its use needs to be considered carefully, taking into account the factors which could be safely employed without resort to blood transfusion. Thus, there are ways to stop bleeding

including medication and surgery which can be employed as early as possible, particularly in a patient who is anti-coagulated and will require to be anti-coagulated again.

In the case presented the patient was willing to accept a blood transfusion until the 'intervention' of his son. He clearly felt some element of coercion by his son for when asked to sign the waiver stating that he refused transfusion, he did not do so and stated that his son should do so.

- ***Should abbreviations be used for critical information in patient care?***

The use of abbreviations for critical information produces a hazard for both the patient and the doctor, particularly in emergency or busy situations. The use of handwritten abbreviations creates an even greater hazard since they may be mistaken for something else, and are well known to cause errors in prescription writing. Abbreviations even when clearly written can mean different things in different disciplines. Nevertheless, they are in common use and when someone recognises they have been misunderstood it is proper to bring it to the responsible person's attention.

In the case described, the omission should not be crucial for the patient was mentally competent at the time, and would have been able to ask for the blood to be not given if that was his wish. If the patient had not been alert, it would have been prudent to discuss the matter with the patient's next of kin.

- ***How does one decide on a patient's mental and legal competence?***

An adult patient, unless otherwise declared by law, is legally competent to make decisions for themselves. Depending on the jurisdiction, there are some minors who can make decisions for themself.[102] There is no upper age where patients cannot consent for themselves if they are mentally competent to do so.

A patient may be mentally incompetent because of a long-standing illness; for example, brain damage or a psychiatric disorder. In the case of a brain-damaged adult, the courts could be petitioned to appoint a legal guardian who would be entitled to make decisions for the patient. In addition, where there is a psychiatric illness the patient's competence to decide for themself is laid down in procedures in mental health laws. The provisions in such laws are not uniform and may vary from country to country. In most countries, for patients who are senile and have not been

---

[102] Competence and consent to treatment in children and adolescents, M Shaw, Advances in Psychiatric Treatment (2001) 7: 150-159

formally declared mentally incompetent, their next of kin are expected
to act on their behalf. Next of kin may be relatives or formally and
legally appointed by the patient when they were mentally competent.[103]
In the absence of an authoritative psychiatric evaluation within the
parameters of the law, the decisions of the next of kin could be subject to
legal challenge.

The attending doctor on the basis of the clarity and orientation of the
patient and their consistent rational responses makes a decision on the
mental competence of a patient. There are situations due to hypoxia,
stable mental illness or short-term memory loss, where it might be
unclear whether the patient is fully mentally competent.

When the situation is not urgent, a psychiatric consultation or a rapid
mental assessment test should be done.[104] Otherwise, the next of kin could
be invited to participate in the decision.

*In the case described, the attending doctor has assessed that the patient is
mentally competent. However, it must be borne in mind that there could be
short-term memory loss in an eighty-year-old. Fortunately, the discussion with
the patient was in the presence of one of his children who raised no alarms about
his decision-making ability.*

• *Who makes the decisions in regard to care for the incompetent
patient?*
The next of kin is the legally competent person to make decisions for an
incapacitated patient, unless the patient had previously made a legal
declaration stating otherwise. Where there is no next of kin or legal
guardian, the head of the institution where they are normally domiciled
or where they are being treated becomes the responsible entity. In life-
threatening emergencies the attending doctor has a responsibility to go
ahead and save the patient's life without any consent from others.

In most jurisdictions the next of kin has a legal family hierarchy,
usually the spouse is the next of kin and absent a spouse the oldest child.
In Islamic jurisdictions the next of kin could be the oldest male child
or the oldest male relative. From the point of view of medical decision-
making in the UK, a next of kin has to be legally declared prior to the
illness, otherwise the decision is that of the physician.

---

[103] Mental Capacity Act 2005; UK
[104] Assessment of Patients' Competence to Consent to Treatment P S. Appelbaum, N Eng. J Med 2007;
357:1834-1840

- *Should a Jehovah's Witness give written consent for a blood transfusion?*

It is prudent in discussing blood transfusion with a Jehovah's Witness to invite them, if they so desire, to have their family, friends or priests to help them in making a decision. All of the available alternatives should be discussed and this in itself may lead the doctor into changing their strategy on management. For example, it may be decided that urgent investigation and operation should be done rather than waiting to see whether there will be another bleed.

Consent can be given orally, by implication or in writing. The objection of Jehovah's Witnesses to blood transfusion is well known and it is therefore prudent to ask for consent in writing whatever the decision.

In the case described a discussion has occurred with a mentally competent patient in the presence of a close relative, therefore the consent can be considered clear and witnessed. In such circumstances written consent was not thought necessary. However, when the decision was changed it was essential to get written confirmation. A further question is the appropriateness of acting on the objection of a relative when a clear and competent patient has given consent.

- *Can a surrogate impose their personal view on the patient, and has the doctor any alternative but to agree to a surrogate's viewpoint?*

In any emergency life-threatening situation the doctor is entitled to make a decision for the incompetent patient, unless they are aware of the prior contrary wishes of the patient. In less urgent situations the next of kin or the legal guardian is the appropriate person to give consent. When there is a problem and there is contention among the relatives it is appropriate to determine who is legally the next of kin.

Surrogates should not seek to impose their personal, including religious, views on a patient competent or otherwise. It should be made clear to all parties that all decisions and actions should be in the best interest of the patient. If there is a situation where the patient had clearly made a decision whilst they were competent, and a surrogate wishes to make a contrary decision, the doctor need not accede to the surrogate's wishes, and may only be compelled to do so by an order of the court.

Family interactions in times of crisis are unpredictable and subject to a variety of factors. For example, an elderly person may oppose a relative's viewpoint in maintaining a sense of independence and control, or they may acquiesce for fear of loss of economic or other support. Imposing religious viewpoints by relatives is particularly troubling, for the patient may hold to religious tenets generally but not in every circumstance. Patients find it difficult to summon the courage to go against a religious belief in a time of crisis.

Doctors should try to influence the family interaction when they perceive that the patient's life is being put in immediate danger. However, in less immediate situations strongly held viewpoints should be discussed with the help of independent persons such as ethicists. If the doctor feels that decisions made by a surrogate are not in the patient's best interest then they can take the matter to the court and seek to overturn the surrogate's decision. Such court action has usually been brought on behalf of a minor, seeking to overturn a parent's decision, but has also been done in cases of incompetent adults and even more rarely against a competent patient.[105]

In the case described the patient's son has persuaded him to change his mind about the blood transfusion while it is in progress. The doctors involved did not appear to feel strongly enough about the change of heart to challenge it. The patient was stable at the time when the decision was changed and the situation may not have been considered life threatening at the time. The doctor could have insisted that the patient sign the withdrawal rather than the son. The refusal to sign does not invalidate the withdrawal of consent and a note should have been made of the circumstances. The absence of written consent to give the transfusion in the first place further complicates the matter when the consent is withdrawn.

- **Should a doctor 'on-call' change management without consultation?**

It is prudent if a new doctor sees a patient in a difficult situation that they do not alter the management, which they think incorrect, without seeking to consult with the attending doctor. This applies in particular to non-emergency situations and in those situations where one has agreed to give a second opinion.

In the situation described it would have been prudent to try to find the managing team to ascertain what were the circumstances that led to the Jehovah's Witness patient receiving blood before engaging in any action at the behest of a relative on the matter.

- **What are the rights and responsibilities of the various parties involved?**

The rights of the patient are paramount, and they may consent or withdraw their consent once they are legally and mentally competent to do so. Patients are not always aware of their rights to accept or refuse treatment and these should be explained free of the pressures of others unless it is their wish to have others involved.

---

[105] Norwood Hosp. v. Munoz; Mass., 1991

The right of the family and in particular the next of kin or legal guardian is to act as a surrogate for the mentally or legal incompetent patient. They have a grave responsibility to act in the best interests of their charges and not to impose their views, religious or otherwise, on the patient. Doctors have the right to act in the best interests of the patient, and are entitled to do so in life-threatening situations. The well-known religious view of Jehovah's Witnesses about blood transfusion must be taken into account in deciding what is in the patient's best interest. If the doctor feels very strongly that the patient's best interest is not being served, the doctor may petition the court to impose treatment on such a patient. It is rare for a court to overturn the wishes of a mentally competent adult in regards to their own treatment.

The society also has an interest to ensure that each individual enjoys the rights guaranteed in the constitution and the law; and through the organs of opinion or the law, to ensure that incapacitated patients are not harmed by their relatives or subjected to overzealous measures by their doctors.

It is unfortunate that the doctor who was asked to come and deal with the son's objections did not try to ascertain from the admitting team what were the circumstances and to try and ascertain the wishes of the patient free from the pressures of the objecting relative. The patient appears to have feared what he might have to face from his son and their religion on his recovery.

• ***Should a decision be overridden when a life is in immediate danger?*** Although in a life-threatening situation a doctor is entitled to administer what they consider life-saving treatment, such treatment should not be administered over the previously known wishes of the patient. If time permits a court could be asked to issue an emergency order to overturn the patient's wishes.

In the situation that emerged the doctor decided to forego blood transfusion and try to save the patient's life by stopping the bleeding by operative means. The treatment proved unsuccessful and would have had a better chance of success when the patient was stable.

Validity of Consent

Case report:

A 75-year-old man was admitted with profuse rectal bleeding. He had no previous illness and was on aspirin daily. He was alert, pale, BP100/75 mms Hg, pulse rate 90 b/min. Clinical examination was normal but for blood on rectal examination. A diagnosis of bleeding diverticular disease was made. The Hb was 5gm/dl and he was told that if the diagnosis was confirmed and bleeding recurred he would require surgery to remove his colon. Meanwhile he would require blood transfusion.

His wife intervened stating that he was a Jehovah's Witness and would not have blood. The doctor responded that further bleeding could endanger his life if there wasn't a blood transfusion. A barium enema confirmed the diagnosis, but a colonoscopy was abandoned for lack of cooperation. In the presence of his relatives, he stated that he would not accept a blood transfusion under any circumstances. The surgeon in charge advised that blood was to be cross-matched in case he changed his mind.

The anaesthetist saw the patient, noted that he was shocked and disorientated, that the Hb had dropped to 3Gms/dl, and stated that the patient could not undergo a major operation without blood being available. The surgeon decided to contact the patient's eldest son and asked him whether he would sign for the operation and the use of blood on his father's behalf. The son responded that he did not want to accept that responsibility but would try to get his father to change his mind. The surgeon decided to talk to the patient who agreed to have the operation and signed the consent form with a shaky X. The patient was taken to the operating theatre right away, and on emerging from the theatre with a blood transfusion going, the son expressed concern that he had not been informed. He was shown the consent form and declared 'That is not my father's signature.'

Issues raised

  • *Confidentiality and relatives*

The support of relatives is to be encouraged particularly in sudden illness, but one must not assume that their presence is always welcomed by patients for there may be matters that may arise that the patient may wish to keep confidential. It is therefore important to ask relatives to leave the room before or during a consultation and to ascertain from the mentally competent patient if and when they would wish a relative or friend to be present.[106] It is equally important to try to give 'mature' minors some degree of privacy particularly in dealing with the history of the illness. This does not mean that the parent should not be involved, they have the right to be, but this can be done separately.

In the case described the patient's wife intervenes whilst the doctor is outlining the management plan to the patient and purports to speak on his behalf. This intervention could have altered the decision that the patient would have made and he should have been given the opportunity to hear the medical advice, ask questions, and to consult with his family or others as he wished.

- ### *Exploration of alternatives*

In obtaining informed consent a judge stated that the doctor should "Advise patients [guardians/ surrogates] of those material facts, risks, complications and alternatives to surgery that a reasonable person in the patient's situation would consider significant in deciding whether to have an operation".[107]

In describing the alternatives, the risks and complications of the alternatives should be discussed, including their availability.

In the case presented blood transfusion was refused. While there was an explanation of why a transfusion was advised, there was no discussion of the alternatives to operation or blood transfusion and the availability or otherwise of those alternatives. In discussing alternatives, the patient should have been given the opportunity to make up their own mind without the presence of others, unless they had specifically requested otherwise.

- ### *Are there limits to a patient or surrogate accepting or refusing treatment?*

A competent patient [parent/ guardian/ next of kin/ surrogate] has the right to accept or refuse treatment and this right can only be challenged in the court. Such challenges rarely succeed when the patient is a mentally competent adult; they are usually made when parents or other surrogates have made a decision, which in the opinion of the doctors will result in the death of the patient rather than giving them a chance to live. In some instances, the challenge is made by others to the decision made by the patient [surrogate] and the doctor. This is usually related to the ending of the life of the patient by withdrawing life support treatment,[108] or to the practice of euthanasia, which is illegal in most jurisdictions.[109]

---

[106] Confidentiality guidance: Sharing information with a patient's partner, carers, relatives or friends; General Medical Council, U.K. http://www.gmc-uk.org/guidance/ethical_guidance/confidentiality_64_66_sharing_information.asp

[107] Gouse v. Cassell (615 A.2d 331) 1992

[108] Schiavo v. Schiavo, 2005 WL 665257 (11th Cir. (Fla.) Mar 23, 2005

[109] People v. Kevorkian; Hobbins v. Attorney General, 527 N.W.2d 714 (Mich. 1994).]

A doctor has a duty to institute life-saving treatment in the event of
a life-threatening emergency. However, if the patient whilst mentally
competent expressly forbade that in the event of such an emergency they
did not want to be treated, their wishes should be respected. The patient
can express such wishes in the form of a living will, or by expressly
stating their wishes to the attending doctors.[110] These declarations by the
patient are often not carried out because the life-threatening emergency
may occur when other care-givers are in attendance and may not know of
the patient's wishes.

*In the case report given, the patient while judged to be mentally competent
has refused the use of blood transfusion. His declaration has been tainted in the
sense that he was not allowed to make the initial declaration uninfluenced by his
wife's assertion of what he would not accept. There is no mention of a written
declaration that he will not accept blood transfusion if his life is threatened,
and the attending doctors proceed to try various means of trying to reverse
his decision.*

- *Challenging religious beliefs*

The religious beliefs and practices of a mentally competent person
should be respected, provided they are not illegal or impact on the
rights of others. Such beliefs impact on medical care, particularly but
not exclusively, in the termination of pregnancy and in the use of blood
transfusion.[111]

Religious beliefs impact during medical care, not only on patients but
also on care-givers and on the decisions made on behalf of patients by
parents, guardians, next of kin or other surrogates. Care-givers have a
right to their religious beliefs but have no right to impose those beliefs on
patients; this includes not proselytizing their beliefs to patients during the
vulnerable period of an acute illness – physical or mental.[112] On the other
hand a care-giver can express a conscientious objection to participating
in any procedure that is contrary to their beliefs, providing that such
objection does not endanger the life of the patient, and that they can
provide the patient with competent doctors and care-givers who can treat
their condition without a similar conscientious objection.[113]

Parents, guardians, next of kin and other surrogates also have a right
to their religious beliefs but must be cautioned that they should not

---

[110] Kutner, L. The Living Will: a proposal. Indiana Law Journal. 1969;44 (1):539-554
[111] Two Christian groups that oppose medical care; http://www.religioustolerance.org/medical2.htm
[112] Religion, Spirituality, and Medicine: Application to Clinical Practice; Harold G. Koenig; JAMA. 2000; 284(13):1708
[113] Conscientious objection in medicine; J Savulescu, BMJ. 2006; 332(7536): 294–297

seek to impose their own religious belief on the patient that they have responsibility for. It must be made clear that the decisions made must be in the best interests of the patient, and if known, in accordance with the wishes of the patient. If it is thought that a decision is being made that is not in the best interests of the patient and persuasion fails, then the parent or surrogate could be challenged in the court to have their decision reversed. Court challenges are seldom mounted in emergency situations.[114]

In the case described there is a religious objection to blood transfusion, and the doctors apparently feel that the patient should be persuaded to abandon his beliefs in order to save his life. However, questions can be raised as to whether the patient was coerced into changing his mind, or whether he was mentally competent when doing so.

- ***The interface between persuasion and coercion.***
There is an imbalance of knowledge and power between the doctor and the patient which is somewhat balanced by the legal right of the patient to consent to whatever treatment is to be carried out on them. Therefore, in situations where the patient or their surrogate is unwilling to accept the recommendations of the doctor, the doctor's ability to persuade is put to the test. There is no greater test of the ability to persuade than when the advice given presents major risks, or goes against strongly held beliefs.

In order to overcome the fear of risks, the doctor must not only be knowledgeable about the likelihood of the risk occurring, but be honest if challenged about their experience and results in similar situations. The doctor must find the time to answer all questions, provide information on alternatives and offer the patient second opinions where possible.

Dealing with religious beliefs should start with the reassurance to the patient that their beliefs will be respected. However, if a challenge is being made to those beliefs the patient must be given the opportunity to make their decision without being pressured by their relatives or fellow believers, but be able to consult with them and their religious leaders when they choose to do so.[115]

In situations where the illness has compromised the competence of the patient to make a decision, the next of kin, or legally designated surrogate, should be given all the information to make an informed decision. However, it must be made clear that the surrogate's decision must be made in the patient's best interests or their clearly expressed

---

[114] SCHIAVO SCHINDLER v. SCHIAVO | https://caselaw.findlaw.com/us-11th-circuit/1360200.html
[115] Stamford Hospital vs. Vega, 674 A. 2d 821 (Conn., 1996)

wishes such as may have been expressed in a living will. Where religious beliefs are involved it must be made clear that a surrogate should not impose their own religious beliefs but should act in the best interests of the patient. If it is determined that a surrogate is not acting in the best interest of the patient, the physician may petition the court to overrule the surrogate's decision. In some instances, a court has been asked to overrule the decision of a mentally competent patient, but seldom does so.

In the case reported, the patient while mentally competent made a clear decision that he would not accept a blood transfusion. The decision was made after an unsolicited declaration from his spouse that he would not accept blood transfusion. Alternatives had not been discussed, including whether he would rather die than have a blood transfusion. When his condition deteriorated, the anaesthetist who saw him noted that he was disorientated, and wrote that the operation could not be done without the availability of a blood transfusion.

Determined to operate to save the patient's life, the consultant surgeon asks for the patient's son to come and make the decision. The spouse is the next of kin and should not have been bypassed; this was probably done believing that she would have refused the blood transfusion. The patient's son, having promised to come and speak to his father, is pre-empted by the surgeon who speaks with the patient and declares that he finds the patient lucid and competent to sign the consent form for operation and a blood transfusion. The operation is an initial success, and the son on arriving to speak with his father is surprised that the operation has been carried out and that blood is being transfused. He is shown a consent form with a mark, which he says bears no resemblance to his father's signature.

- ***Is saving a life justifiable by any means?***

Doctors, nurses and other health care workers are trained and licensed to treat patients and alleviate their suffering. Saving and preserving lives is a vital part of the function of health workers and in life-threatening emergencies treatment should be administered without waiting for consent to do so. However, emergency treatment must conform to the accepted standards of treatment, and should not be carried out against the legally expressed wishes of the patient.

Patients may legally express their wishes against specific emergency life-saving treatment measures in the form of a living will. Such declarations are not necessarily valid when the patient's life has been endangered by their own actions or that of others; e.g. attempted suicide, or assaults, and physicians would have to determine how explicit the instructions were in such cases.

In the situation described, the patient's life is threatened and in the opinion of the doctors his life could only be saved by a blood transfusion. However, the patient had previously declared that he did not want to be transfused. If this had been made clear in writing that this applied even if his life were threatened, then his wishes should have been respected.

• *Blood transfusion*

The transfusion of oxygen-carrying red blood cells, and blood coagulation products is essential in the management of some acute bleeding disorders. There are at present no good synthetic alternatives to blood and its products in dealing with some bleeding disorders. On the other hand, blood transfusion has many complications, and should be avoided unless absolutely necessary.

In order to avoid the use of blood transfusion, operative or other less invasive means that can stop bleeding should be employed as soon as possible. This has implications for the management of Jehovah's Witnesses as well as others, where there may be issues of blood supply or fear of spread of infections such as hepatitis and HIV.

In the case described, once the unpredictability of further bleeding was realized and that the patient was objecting to blood transfusion, the use of an operation to prevent further bleeding should have been considered and put to the patient. The risks would be increased but would not be as great as if the patient bled further and continued to refuse blood transfusion.

• *The Jehovah's Witness*

A Jehovah's Witness will not accept blood or blood products as a matter of faith; their beliefs should be respected.[116] However, it cannot be assumed that patients will follow this belief under all circumstances. Therefore, the advantages, alternatives and risks of a blood transfusion should be explained and the patient asked to sign a declaration on the decision they make.

There will be others of their faith who will wish to persuade the doctor against the use of blood transfusion. The patient should be given the opportunity to make their own decision and to request further advice; however, they should not be placed in a position of being coerced by anyone. Parents or surrogates should be cautioned about imposing their own beliefs on their charges. If the doctor believes that the decision of a parent or a surrogate is not in the best interests of the patient, particularly

---

[116] Two Christian groups that oppose medical care; http://www.religioustolerance.org/medical2.htm

when the patient's life is at stake, the doctor can petition the court to take over the guardianship of the patient.[117]

The health care worker, who is a Jehovah's Witness, has the right to their belief when they become a patient, but they have no right to impose their beliefs on others, including other Jehovah's Witnesses. While the transfusion of blood and blood products remains the accepted standard of care for some conditions, the health care worker who is a Jehovah's Witness would be negligent if blood transfusion was not appropriately offered to the affected patient, whether the patient were a Jehovah's Witness or not. As with any other religious belief, the health care worker can exercise the right of a conscientious objection, but such objection can only be exercised when the patient's life is not in danger and the patient has been placed in the care of a competent doctor who has no such conscientious objection.[118]

- ***Competence to consent***

All legally and mentally competent adults, irrespective of their age; minors under precedent or law depending on the jurisdiction;[119] parents, legal guardians, next of kin and legally appointed surrogates when the adult or minor is not competent to do so, have the right to consent for treatment.

A patient may be mentally incompetent because of mental or organic illness and that incompetence may be temporary. A common cause of temporary mental incompetence is hypoxia in a shocked patient. Attending doctors will make judgments about the mental competence of their patients and when in doubt refer the patient to the psychiatric service for an opinion. There is also available a rapid mental assessment tool which can be used to make the assessment.[120]

From the description given it is unlikely that the patient was mentally competent at the time he made his mark to assent to operation and blood transfusion.

---

[117] Jehovah's Witness children: when religion and the law collide P Wilson - 2005 www.health.bcu.ac.uk/webmodules/gm607D/.../
[118] Conscientious objection in medicine, J Savulescu BMJ 2006; 332; 294-297
[119] Family Law Reform Act; UK 1969; c.46
[120] Functional assessment staging (FAST). B Reisberg - Psychopharmacology bulletin, 1988; 24(4): 653-9

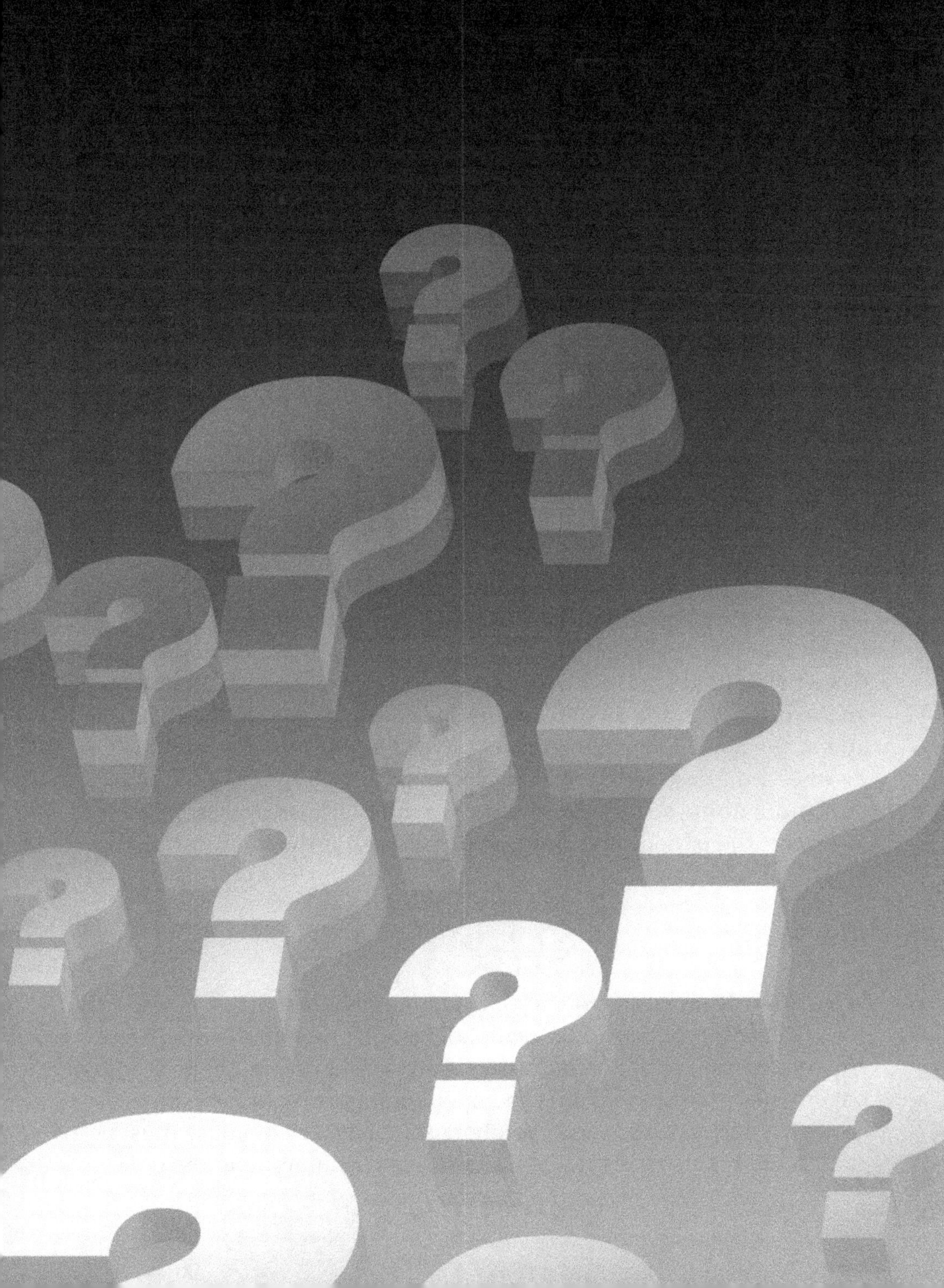

CONFIDENTIALITY

Reporting Domestic Abuse

Case report:
A 35-year-old woman consulted a psychiatrist and described daily altercations between her husband and her eldest son, who was 10 years old. She said her husband would drag her son by his arm, lift and shake him violently untill she tried to stop him. He hit the boy excessively when disciplining him. Some of this occurred when her son tried to intervene when he was hitting her. She said that her son was not doing well at school, and was reported as "acting out for attention".

The patient gave account of severe physical, emotional and sexual abuse, more so on weekends. The three younger children have witnessed the beatings but were never abused. The patient refused any intervention by the police, or to leave home for a crisis centre, making the point that she owned the house and was the main contributor in the family. She declined disclosure to her family, stating they would not believe her as her husband was loved by all of them, who viewed him as having saved her from the shame of having her first child out of wedlock with a very black man. She said that the colour issue also played out at school with remarks made to her eldest son about his being so dark.

She stated that she was afraid to even let him or her children know she was seeing a psychiatrist. The psychiatrist considered reporting the situation to the Child Care Board over the objections of the patient. Once the patient was aware of this she started talking about suicide and expressed grave anxiety about the safety of herself, the children and of the psychiatrist when her husband found out. The psychiatrist discussed the case with colleagues who advised reporting to the police; but before doing so she consulted with the police as to their capacity to protect the patient, the children and herself if the husband did react violently.

Issues raised

• *What is expected from a psychiatric consultation?*
A psychiatrist is expected to treat patients with mental disorders and any information obtained in consultation should be used to benefit the patient. In the absence of a law compelling reporting to the police, the issues of confidentiality and corroboration of a story of abuse must be considered before referring issues raised in consultation to the police.

A patient's confidentiality must be respected unless the confidential information has mortal consequences for a third party.[121]

Psychiatric referrals with all the public perception issues involved may be necessary for all of the persons involved as perpetrators or facilitators of abuse and this may involve parents, guardians and siblings. In jurisdictions where there is law compelling reporting of abuse, the state promises to ensure the confidentiality of the informant.[122]

In the situation reported it appears as if the patient would wish to have relief of her abusive situation, but is afraid of the consequences of it coming to light. The psychiatrists consulted think that the abuse should be reported to the police in spite of the objections of the patient, and this precipitates suicidal ideation.

- ***Confidentiality of the abused***

Confidentiality is crucial to the abused and may become a matter of life and death. When an abused person is removed from the abusive situation, the abuser will often seek them out in order to regain control. Therefore, seemingly simple solutions such as removal from the home may need to be done in secrecy. Even electronic databases of one's whereabouts such as bank and insurance records may have to be avoided.[123]

When children are taken into care and protection, it may not be possible to keep that information confidential at school, but the reasons should be. In all situations where abuse is reported, there should be safeguards to respect the confidentiality of the abused person as well as the informant.[124] Such safeguards increase the number of reports made, although it provides no guarantee as to the accuracy of the reports. The reports of abuse need to be investigated and are best done by a specially trained unit which understands the importance of the confidentiality of the abused persons and of the accused whilst the allegations are being investigated.[125] Investigations may be made by social services professionals or by the police, preferably by specially trained police units.

In the instance under consideration it is not clear if there are any confidentiality mechanisms in place, if a report is made to the police. The patient is terrified that her confidentiality will be broken and expresses suicidal intent.

---

[121] Tarasoff v. Regents of the University of California, 17 Cal. 3d 425, 551 P.2d 334, 131 Cal. Rptr. 14 (Cal. 1976)
[122] Child Care and Protection Act 2004 http://moj.gov.jm/laws/child-care-and-protection-act
[123] Why Privacy and Confidentiality Matters for Victims of Domestic ... https://www.techsafety.org/privacymatters/
[124] Disclosure of Confidential Child Abuse and Neglect Records - Child ... https://www.childwelfare.gov/topics/systemwide/laws-policies/statutes/confide
[125] Report Sexual Abuse of Children – CISOCA - jis.gov.jm/report-sexual-abuse-children-cisoca/

- *What is the health worker's role in pursuing a situation of childhood abuse?*

Health workers should act in the best interest of the patient in alleviating their condition. In abusive situations part of the aims of treatment would be to stop the abuse and this may involve the use of legal mechanisms and possible prosecution of the abuser. To be successful in any prosecution the health workers should collect any forensic evidence of the abuse as soon as possible.

In some instances of child abuse, it is the parents who are the agents of such abuse and given the opportunity they will try and prevent enquiries into the matter. Therefore, enough information should be sought in emergency situations before having to involve suspected parents in any situation requiring their consent, and to be prepared to have the child placed under protection from their parents if necessary.

In the case reported there is a complaint of both child and adult physical abuse, but there is no account of physical injuries. A lack of documented injury is likely to dampen the response of the police.

- *What responsibility does the health worker have in reporting a felony?*

In the absence of a mandatory requirement of reporting, the health care worker or any other responsible person should act in the best interest of a child and not that of the parents or even themselves in not wanting to be part of a court proceeding.

All citizens should report felonies to the police; the same duty applies to health care workers, taking into account the confidentiality of the patient and their wishes. Felonies may go unreported for fear of getting involved in the judicial system as a witness and sometimes the threat or feeling of a threat from the party reported as having committed the felony. In some jurisdictions, the system is very wasteful of the participants' time, and persons who get involved as witnesses may feel that their livelihood is jeopardised in one way or the other. Court appearances for health care workers as witnesses, are further complicated by the fact that they may be called upon to interpret the testimony they give, and to be cross-examined on their testimony.

Reporting of sexual abuse cases has been further complicated for health workers by some of the accused persons having brought civil suits, claiming that the evidence with which they were accused has been wrongfully obtained or maliciously given.[126] Nevertheless, health

---

[126] Ridicule or recourse: parents falsely accused of past sexual abuse fight back, J.M Whitesell, J Law & Health, 1996; 303

care workers should not choose to 'hear no evil, see no evil or speak no evil', for in doing so they would have abrogated their duty of care to the patient. Health care workers also have a duty of confidentiality to their patients, including those who are minors, and in proceeding along the prosecution path should always take into account what is in the best interest of the patient, both in the short and long term.

To determine what is in the best interest of the patient, the forensic evidence of history, physical, psychological and social must be obtained in the most thorough manner. Evidence may not be obtained in its entirety when premature reports are made to the police against the patient's wishes. Therefore, the timing of a report to the police should be carefully considered but not rejected, and may under appropriate circumstances be left to the child protection services.

The fact that not all cases of abuse are reported to the police has called for mandatory reporting where it does not exist.[127] Mandatory reporting may lead those who are reluctant to do so to 'hear and see no evil'; particularly if there are no mechanisms put in place to alleviate the fears of reporting that already exist.[128] Although this could be considered a negligent breach of duty on the part of a health care worker, those reluctant to report will balance the risks of not reporting to the consequences of reporting.

Consent from a minor. In general, a minor has no legal capacity to consent to medical treatment unless specific provisions have been made in law or judicial precedent.

Except in a life-saving emergency, parents have the legal power to consent to the treatment of their minor child including their further investigation and referral. Parents may disagree with health care workers about the course to be taken where there is child abuse and the parents or other siblings are thought to be involved. With active obstruction by the parents it may be difficult to obtain the evidence for a successful prosecution.

When a dispute with the parents cannot be resolved about the course to be taken, a child can be taken into care under the provisions of an act such as the Prevention of Cruelty to Children Act. This allows the child to be treated without the parent's consent. Such legal provisions are crucial in investigating instances of child abuse that involve parents.

---

[127] Perceptions of, Attitudes to, and Opinions on Child Sexual Abuse in the Eastern Caribbean. Research Team A D. Jones, E Trotman Jemmott et al UNICEF/Governments of the Eastern Caribbean 2008-2011; http://www.actionforchildren.org.uk/media/143143/child_sexual_abuse_in_the_eastern_caribbean.pdf
[128] Child Abuse: A Guide for Mandatory Reporters; 2011; http://www.dhs.state.ia.us/policyanalysis/policymanualpages/Manual_Documents/Master/comm164.pdf

Confidentiality of a minor. The right to confidentiality of a minor is like that of any other person, and is considered more precious than that of adults by protecting the child's identity in legal actions. This is done through a prohibition on the publication of the minor's name or any other identifiers. However, the legal capacity of a minor to maintain their confidentiality in medical matters is curtailed by the limitations on their capacity to make medical decisions for themselves. In the circumstance of childhood abuse, the risk of loss of confidentiality by removing a child from parental control has to be balanced against the risk of continued abuse.

In the report under consideration, the psychiatrist is faced with the dilemma of abuse of both a child and his mother. The mother wishes confidentiality to be maintained and rejects voluntary separation from the abuser. In the absence of a mandatory reporting requirement in the law, the suggestion of bringing in the police to deal with the abuser precipitates a medical crisis where the patient expresses suicidal intent.

- ### *Social worker/services enquiries*

Social services personnel should have the training to enquire into the social circumstances of a patient that may not have been elicited in a doctor's consultation. In accusations of abuse the domestic arrangements, including income and apparent expenditures, should be checked. Social services do not have the powers of the police in investigating a crime, but should have the ability to gather information that can guide and influence how a patient's case should be handled. Medical practitioners should use the information obtained by social services to assist in their therapeutic objectives, including determining what route of reporting should be employed.[129]

In the report given, social service workers are not deployed, presumably because of the ambiguity the patient shows in dealing with the situation.

- ### *The abuse victim*

The abuse victim may exhibit behaviours that bring them to attention for antisocial or criminal acts, including committing abusive acts themselves.[130] In children, such acts may be manifest in school as well as by learning disabilities.[131] Such acts can complicate any enquiry that

---

[129] The role of social workers in responding effectively to domestic abuse ...
www.safelives.org.uk/.../role-social-workers-responding-effectively-domestic-abuse
[130] Long-term consequences of childhood physical abuse. Malinosky-Rummell, R. R, and Hansen, D. J. (1993). Psychol. Bull. 114: 68–79
[131] Childhood sexual abuse, K L. Kinnear; ABC-CLIO; 2007

is being made including preserving confidentiality when third parties
are involved.

*In the situation described the patient complains of abuse of herself as well
as of her child. However, when reporting of the abuse to the police or the
child protection agency is raised, her mental distress increases to the point of
threatening suicide.*

- *Abuser's profile*

In ninety per cent of child sexual abuse cases, the offenders are male and
are often described as being unassertive, withdrawn, and emotionless.
Other common characteristics include a history of being themselves
abused (either physically or sexually), alcohol or drug abuse, little
satisfaction with sexual relationships with adults, lack of control over
their emotions, and occasionally mental illness.[132] In situations of physical
abuse the behaviour of the abusers may be similarly secretive to that of
sexual abusers; on the other hand the perpretrator may be more open,
particularly in societies that value the infliction of physical pain as
discipline. In many instances of physical abuse trying to discern the intent
of the abuser is the only dividing line that can be used.[133]

*In the case reported the abuser is described as being very well liked by the
patient's family, and is seen as the saviour from a relationship that had produced
the child that is being abused. This complicates the avenues of support for the
patient and raises the question as to whether the patient had been abused in
the family.*

- *The role of priests and other community leaders*

Priests and community leaders have an acknowledged role as spiritual
advisors, confidential counsellors and confidants. These roles become
somewhat ambiguous where crimes have been committed and are
hidden in the process. When priests are complicit in hiding crimes, they
could be viewed as facilitators of such crimes, but are seldom treated as
such. Unfortunately, the trust placed in priests and other leaders such
as teachers by communities is not always reciprocated, for some have
become opportunistic perpetrators of sexual abuse of children, both
girls and boys. In some jurisdictions, priests and teachers, along with
health care workers, have been listed as having to mandatorily report
childhood abuse.

---

[132] Synopsis of Psychiatry Behavioural Sciences in Clinical Psychiatry, 7th Ed. A Kaplan, B Sadock, J
Grebb, Williams&Wilkins 1999
[133] Discipline Versus Abuse - Child Welfare Information Gateway
https://www.childwelfare.gov/topics/can/defining/disc-abuse/

In the reported case, the teaching staff have recommended assessment of the child for a learning disability. However, there has been nothing said about any suspected abuse.

- ### Child protection
Many jurisdictions have a child protection agency that is responsible for protecting children from harm. Such agencies have the power to remove children to a place of safety, and to protect them from others, including their parents. These agencies should be equipped with professional staff capable of investigating abusive situations, and, in the best interests of the child and of the community, report crimes to the police.

In the situation described, none of the suggestions for removing the patient or the abused child from the home is acceptable to the patient. Reporting the abusing husband to the police is also resisted and precipitates threats of suicide.

- ### The police
The police have the responsibility to apprehend people suspected of criminal activity, and gather enough credible evidence that the person can be successfully prosecuted in a court of law. In accusations of abuse, forensic evidence collected medically may be of critical importance, and should be collected as soon as possible. Witness statements are likely to be conflicting and are best collected before accusations are made. Police should have specially trained officers to investigate accusations of abuse.

In the report given, the professionals consulted appear to be strongly of the opinion that the reported abuse should be reported to the police. Unfortunately, in the jurisdiction involved there is no specially trained unit in the police force to handle such cases, and it is not known what the response time would be should there be an worsening of the violence in the home.

- ### Legal issues
Parents, members of the family or household are most often the perpetrators of childhood abuse. Sexual abuse occurs mostly at home by a family member or someone well known to them. Adults who abuse children or condone such abuse may have been abused as children, and may see abuse as a right in return for financial support of the child. When financial benefit plays a definitive role in the sexual abuse of girls, the mother of the child may be competing with her daughter, expressed in jealousy or even fights.

In some instances, mothers condone the sexual abuse of their minor children for fear of losing material support from a man. This may be classified as a misdemeanour by the mother as contributing to the

delinquency of a minor, and is often not prosecuted because it is difficult
to obtain the appropriate witness statements. This situation often only
comes to light when there is domestic violence and the police are called
when injuries occur, usually in a fight between the mother and daughter.
In other instances, there has been a period of grooming by the abusers,
the parents and other children in institutional care.[134]

*In the report presented, the abused patient is frustrating the legal remedy
of the abusive situation. It suggests a long history of abuse that may only be
brought to light with severe injury. The suggestion of breaking the confidentiality
of the patient has precipitated suicidal expressions.*

[134] Setting 'Dem UP'; Personal, Familial and Institutional Grooming; A-M Mc Alinden; Social Legal
Studies, 2006 vol. 15 no. 3; 339-362

Social Media and the Profession

Case report:
A consultant/staff surgeon was approached by a concerned relative via an internet messenger platform on social media. The surgical team was in frequent face-to-face communication with the patient's next of kin and other relatives up to the receipt of this message.

Despite being invited to come for a consultation with the surgeon, the relative continued to communicate on-line, attempting to initiate discussion on their relative's condition. The attempts to establish an on-line relationship with the surgeon included issuing an invitation to dinner to discuss the patient's problem. The surgeon felt uneasy about the relative's approach and declined the dinner invitation. The patient's condition improved and further attempts at communication via social media stopped. No attempt was made by the relative to attend for the offered consultation.

The surgeon felt unease that he might have caused offence to a prominent member of the local community and asked advice as to whether he had handled the situation correctly.

Issues raised

- *Social media*

Social media embrace a number of forms of electronic communication where ideas and information are shared with groups of people who may or may not have been chosen by the individual. Messages, which can include pictures and videos, can be widely shared with or without the intention of the person sending the original message. The greatest but by no means the only problem in using such media in medical practice is patient confidentiality.

In the scenario presented the surgeon involved is contacted via a publicly available social media platform, and is cognisant of the danger of the breach of confidentiality that could occur in discussing a patient's problem by this means. Although declining to discuss the patient over this platform, the reason why is not made explicit and the overtures continued in trying to use this means of communication

- *Confidentiality and social media*

When using 'social media' medical professionals must consider the impact the communication may have on patients and on the wider public that may be reached. Any communication by public media that is intended for a patient, or any person that the patient has agreed to share the information with, should be marked CONFIDENTIAL and the recipients must have consented to this means of communication in advance.

In making any communication that is intended for or may reach a wider audience, all personalised patient information, including distinctive physical features, must be removed [facial features may not be the only distinctive feature]. In addition, the content must be professionally worded, accurate and up to date, for poor content not only reflects on the author but on the entire profession.

Medical and other health personnel may have to work under extremely stressful conditions and some distasteful postings have been made in such situations, such as posing with corpses in disaster situations. Such postings intended for a limited number of friends often go 'viral' and reach a much wider audience than was intended.

- *Professional use of social media*

Advertising, where allowed, is an area where medical professionals can properly use social media. It reaches a wider audience but one must be careful to stick to factual matters, avoid any exaggeration, and keep within any guidelines published by one's local regulatory body or professional representative group.

Another widely used purpose is group discussion and consultation; this has its challenges, for it is easy to concentrate on a disease process and not take into account the nuances of an individual patient's needs.

Social media are being used in some health care systems for patient and relative communication, both general and individual. A look at what was advocated as an advanced system although intended to show the doctor-patient relationship at the controlling centre of a network of media platforms, could also be interpreted as their being at risk of being overpowered and devoured by a complex network of information and health professionals.[135]

- *Professional hazards and social media*

The primary professional hazard in using social media for patient care is the unintended breach of confidentiality. This can be brought about by the wider dissemination of the communication by the recipient, and any such communication should only be done after the explicit

---

[135] Doctor-patient communication in the e-health era; Jonathan P Weiner; Israel Journal of Health Policy Research20121:33; https://ijhpr.biomedcentral.com/articles/10.1186/2045-4015-1-33

warning and informed consent of the patient and the person receiving the communication. Confidentiality may also be compromised by the use of identifiers other than a name, an address or a face, for there may be other distinctive physical features that can be a marker, particularly in small communities.

Opinions on a professional matter may not remain with the original person but may be shared more widely without the specific evidence used to form the opinion.

Dissatisfied patients, relatives, colleagues or 'friends' may use such platforms to voice anonymous complaints and make slanderous postings that may be difficult to trace. Infatuated patients or relatives may use the social media platform originally used for patient communication and stalk the professional; succumbing to what initially seems socially innocent can turn into a nightmare. Unfortunately, it is not advisable, nor is it sustainable, to create split professional and personal beings.

The only way to minimize such calamities is summarized by the GMC's and AMA's advice, which really reminds one to adhere to the other principles of good conduct in using the media.[136] [137] On the other hand, the American College of Surgeons bluntly advises not to use them at all.[138] Professional regulatory bodies should issue guidelines related to advertising of professional services and products using social media, and the application of any data controlling act within their jurisdiction.

---

[136] Doctors' use of social media; GMC 2013, https://www.gmc-uk.org/ethical-guidance/ethical-guidance-for-doctors/doctors-use-of-so
[137] Professionalism in the Use of Social Media https://www.ama-assn.org/delivering-care/ethics/professionalism-use-social-media
[138] Statement on Guidelines for the Ethical Use of Social Media ... bulletin.facs.org/2019/05/statement-on-guidelines-for-the-ethical-use-of-social-media-by-su

COUNSELLING

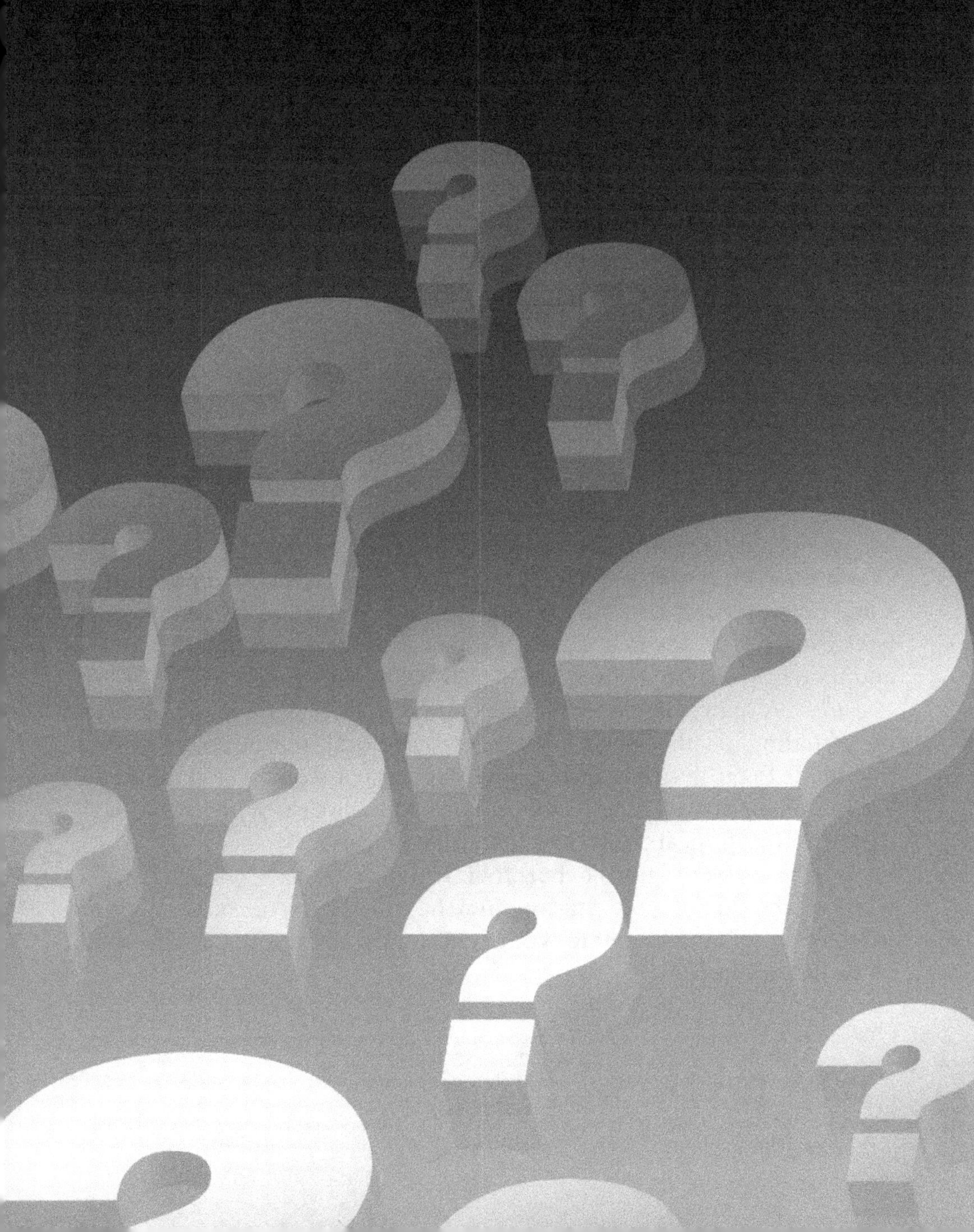

Case report:
A 45-year-old woman, who has had several miscarriages in the last ten years, whilst under the care of the obstetric department, was found to be pregnant again. She is admitted to hospital for complications of her pregnancy and an ultrasound done at 22 weeks gestation showed that the foetus has a significant abnormality. A consultation was held with the paediatricians, and the mother is told that the child's abnormality could be treated by surgery after birth. The proposed surgery would not correct the underlying genetic abnormality but would improve the chances of the child surviving. After being advised of the other options, the woman states that she would continue with the pregnancy and 'then see what happens'. The obstetrician then asked the nurse to make arrangements for him to speak to the woman's husband about the decision made.

Issues raised:

• *Precious pregnancies*
Pregnancies are always precious, but they may be more precious under any number of circumstances related to the mother or father, religious values or culture. The state may also have an interest in a 'precious' pregnancy when population growth is encouraged.

Mother. Most women respond to an innate reproductive drive and at some time may feel that their biological clock is running out and seek to have a child. The desire to have a child carries increased risks for mother and foetus when the woman reaches 35-years old.[139]

Father. A man's desire to father a child is driven by an innate desire of perpetuating his lineage, as distinct from a sexual/reproductive drive, that tends to outlive the reproductive capacity of women of similar age.[140] There is some risk of genetic abnormality to the foetus with the older male, but this appears to be less than in females.[141]

Religion. Most religions exhort their followers to have children and women who do not have children may be called barren. Some religions try to bar any impediment to women becoming pregnant, outside of, or within marriage.[142]

---

[139] Elevated risks of pregnancy complications and adverse outcomes with increasing maternal age; B. Luke, and M. B. Brown; Hum. Reprod. 2007 22 (5): 1264-1272
[140] Why Men Matter: Mating Patterns Drive Evolution of Human Lifespan. S D. Tuljapurkar, TSD, Puleston CO, Gurven 2007, PLoS ONE 2(8): e785. doi: 10.1371/journal.pone.0000785
[141] Genetic Disease in the Offspring of Older Fathers, JM Friedman, Obst & Gynae; 1981 Vol 57[6]
[142] Religion and Reproductive Health and Rights; T A Obaid J Am Acad Relig 2005 73 (4): 1155-1173

Culture. Many cultures have a view that womanhood and manhood are only attained when a child has been produced. Women who do not have children may be stigmatised and be called names such as 'mules'; and both men and women may be characterised as homosexuals and stigmatised in that way.[143] The stigmatisation of men as homosexuals may lead some men to seek to father a child as a masquerade for their sexual preference. In some societies there is an emerging culture of normalising homosexual relationships into family units through marriage/civil unions and bringing up children, who may be adopted or carry the genetic linage of one of the partners through surrogacy.

Cultural beliefs about having children may involve obtaining economic support. A woman may have the view that a man would not support her and her household without her producing a child for him. Both men and women may see the rearing of children as a means of increasing the number of workers in the household and as a means of support for them when they are unable to work.

This view of children as future workers may be combined in some cultures with value judgments of the child's gender, where most often females are devalued and may be aborted on those grounds. Some states have passed laws forbidding abortion on the grounds of gender.[144]

The State. Outside of theocratic direction, the state may have an interest in the number of babies produced, depending on the economic policy that is adopted. Incentives/sanctions for or against having children may be put in place. In those places where the state intervenes vigorously against having children, gender choice may become a dominant factor in bearing children.[145]

- *Foetal abnormalities*

Before making an examination for foetal abnormalities, one should make clear to the parents why it is being done, what one is looking for, and when such an examination should be made.[146] There should also be a plan established as to what will or should be done with the information obtained. Foetal examinations are made with a view to assessing obstetric progress, to diagnose maternal and foetal abnormalities, and to determine

[143] The Stigma of Involuntary Childlessness; Miall, C E; Soc. Probs. 1986; 33, 4. 268

[144] Sex-Selective Abortions in India; F Arnold, S Kishor, T. K. Roy, Population and Development Review; 2004; Vol 28, Iss 4, pgs. 759–785, DOI: 10.1111/j.1728-4457.2002.00759.x

[145] The ethics of sex selection: a comparison of the attitudes and experiences of primary care physicians and physician providers of clinical sex selection services. Puri S, Nachtigall RD, Fertil. Steril. 2010,93 (7): 2107–14.

[146] First- and second-trimester evaluation of risk for Down Syndrome Ball RH, Caughey AB, Malone FD, et al Obstet Gynecol 2007; 110 (1): 10–7..

the gender of the child. The examination method most commonly used is ultrasound, with some genetic testing by amniocentesis.[147] Progress of the pregnancy and defining the obstetric risks are crucial to the safety of both mother and child. The diagnosis of a foetal abnormality is of prime importance to the parents and they should be counselled before any investigation is done that the possibility of finding an abnormal foetus exists. The risks of tests such as amniocentesis must be explained to the parents before the procedure. An exploration of what can be done in the event an abnormality is detected can be left at a general level, and should include the option of termination of the pregnancy within the limits of the law in the jurisdiction.[148]

Some determination should be made of the attitude of the parents to the gender of the child, particularly in those societies where a termination of a pregnancy may be sought depending on the child's gender. It is unethical and illegal to terminate a pregnancy because of the gender of the foetus, even in countries where it is a widely accepted practice.[149] Counselling may be the only opportunity to influence the thoughts or actions of parents; for example, on illegal abortion, abandonment of the infant or even infanticide.

The timing of foetal diagnostic investigations should relate to determining obstetric decisions; decisions regarding possible termination of the pregnancy; and the possibilities of the treatment of any foetal abnormalities. The treatment of foetal abnormalities may be done intra-partum or post-partum depending on the facilities and expertise available.[150]

In the case described, an autopsy had not been done on any of the previous aborted foetuses to establish why they failed to reach term. There was also no record of the mother having been counselled about any risks to herself, or the possibility of the baby having Down Syndrome, and the requirements that may be needed to bring up such a child.

- ### *Costs - human and financial*

The immediate and long-term costs should be considered in relation to the mother, the family, and the medical and support services available.

---

[147] Prenatal Screen Detects Foetal Abnormalities; C O'Connor, 2008 Nature Education 1(1)

[148] Second-Trimester Abortion for Foetal Anomalies or Fetal Death: Labor Induction Compared With Dilation and Evacuation; Bryant, A G.; Grimes, D A.; Garrett, J M.; Stuart, G S; Obstetrics & Gynaecology: 2011 - Volume 117 - Issue 4 - pgs. 788-792

[149] The Pre-natal Diagnostic Techniques (Regulation and Prevention of Misuse) Act, No. 57 of 1994, and the Pre-natal Diagnostic Technologies (Regulation and Prevention of Misuse) Amendment Act, No. 2002, No. 14 of 2003; India

[150] A Surgical Approach to the Treatment of Foetal Hydrocephalus; W H. Clewell, M L. Johnson, P R. Meier, et al N Eng. J Med 1982; 306:1320-1325

The costs to the mother of a high-risk pregnancy may be measured in her emotional and physical health. In addition, the time that may have to be devoted to a child with disabilities may affect other opportunities that the woman and the family may have.

The emotional and family support that is required to deal with a high-risk pregnancy is heightened by the additional impact of having a child that requires extra support. The relationship between mother and father may be broken by the increased demands on the relationship. There is often a loss of earnings either directly by the mother during the pregnancy, or in looking after the child, and indirectly by a supportive father. However, it should be noted that families might remain stable in these situations where there is additional family or social services support. or additional financial inputs.

Medical costs. The costs incurred in looking after a high-risk pregnancy can be considerable, taking into account professional fees, hospitalisation and medication. These costs increase if there is an abnormal, premature or sick child born.[151] These costs have to be borne by the patient/family directly, by the state, or by insurance. The likely costs can only be borne individually by the very wealthy. State funded services are often limited and insufficient to meet all of the demands of high-quality care. Insurance services usually have limitations, either in terms of the quantity of funds that the company will disburse on any one illness, on the types of illness that they will pay for, or the payment for third parties such as an infant.

High physician costs are also influenced by the fact that obstetrics is seen as a very high-risk area for malpractice claims, and, as a result, carries a very high medical malpractice insurance premium.[152]

Support services. Apart from the medical services that are required, there is a need for other services such as counselling and any special dietary needs during the pregnancy. In addition, social support services such as national insurance payments for previously employed mothers and special leave from employment may be required. After the birth of an infant with abnormalities other support services from both state and NGO agencies may be required in order to look after the needs of the infant, and, where necessary, its growth through childhood and into adult life.

---

[151] Telemedicine: cost-effective management of high-risk pregnancy. Morrison J, Bergauer NK, Jacques D, Coleman SK, Stanziano GJ. Manag Care. 2001; 10(11): 42-6, 48-9
[152] Medical Professional Liability and the Delivery of Obstetrical Care: Volume I (1989) Institute of Medicine (IOM); http://www.nap.edu/openbook.php?record_id=1206&page=92

In the case described there are deficiencies in good care; beyond meeting the obstetric challenges there appears to have been no thought given to the counselling needs of the mother or father in relation to the risks of the pregnancy, or the possibility of an abnormal infant. Once the diagnosis of an abnormal foetus is made the paediatricians are brought into the picture; however, there is no indication that the ability of the mother/family to support an abnormal child has been explored. There was a clear need for counselling and the exploration of social support services to be added to the physician/medical services in the management of the high-risk pregnancy.

Case report 1:
An 18-year-old was admitted to hospital at 26 weeks gestation with a seizure episode. She is HIV positive. A previous pregnancy, while she was in school, had been terminated. This pregnancy had been uneventful until the seizure occurred, and she was on the Nevaripine protocol for prevention of mother-to-child transmission of HIV.

She was diagnosed as having eclampsia and was treated as such. Induction of labour was attempted but failed four times. A caesarean section was arranged. A long time was taken for delivery of the baby, which required 20 minutes of resuscitative efforts before it was transferred to the neonatal intensive care unit. The infant was assessed as 29 weeks gestation, weighing 900 Gms, and was treated intensively for hyaline membrane disease and sepsis. The infant was discharged after eight weeks on Vidaylin, Galfer and Eprex weighing 1590 Gms.

Case report 2:
A 20-year-old woman presented to the antenatal clinic stating that she had several months of missing periods. She was living with her boyfriend, her three-year-old child and his three children. Her pregnancy was confirmed and she had 'booking' tests done, including an HIV test. On her next visit she was told that the baby was 20 weeks gestation, and that she was HIV positive. Her reaction was one of disbelief. When she was told that her boyfriend should be told about her HIV test, she insisted that she did not want him to know. When asked why, she repeated that she did not believe that she had HIV and if she carried home that news she didn't know what would happen to her.

The doctor reiterated that she was HIV positive citing the reliability of the tests but said the test could be repeated if she insisted on it. He then asked her if she was not going to tell her boyfriend, was she going to stop having sex with him? She said she couldn't do that, but would ask him to use a condom as they were doing before. In response to a question as to whether she had any other boyfriends, she said she had another boyfriend a year ago, but when asked who he was she said she was not going to give his name. The doctor expressed particular concern that she was not going to disclose her status to her boyfriend, and said that she was going to talk to some other people about that. Meanwhile, a decision had to be made to stop the baby becoming infected, and a referral would be made to the HIV/AIDS centre for medication. The patient responded that she did not want to go to the AIDS centre and she would rather get rid of the baby. The doctor responded that to get rid of the baby at this stage she would have to get another opinion and she was going to send her to see a psychiatrist.

Case report 3:

A 40-year-old woman was admitted to hospital with a history of headaches for several weeks, increasing confusion and diminishing responsiveness over several days. Her husband said that there was no previous illness, but said that they were under stress after having had to seek shelter with the patient's sister after the loss of their home.

On examination, she was cachectic, dehydrated, and in cardiopulmonary distress; generalized lymphadenopathy and a pustular rash were observed. An encephalitis with an immunodeficiency state was diagnosed. Additional information sought from the husband was not useful, but the patient's best friend stated that she had an extra-marital relationship with another man. An HIV test was positive, but was not recorded in the notes as one of the tests ordered. In spite of intensive antibiotic and supportive treatment, she died. Her husband and family were not informed of the diagnosis of AIDS.

Issues raised

- ### The first pregnancy

The age of consent to sexual intercourse is important to determine whether a pregnant adolescent was subjected to any criminal action such as statutory rape.[153] The age of consent varies in jurisdictions from 12 years old to 20 years and may vary between boys and girls.[154] It is also important to know what law exists in relation to termination of pregnancies in the jurisdiction. In one jurisdiction a 16-year-old can take the decision to terminate a pregnancy under 12 weeks gestation without the permission of her parents.[155] In addition, a child who has been pregnant, could be treated as a liberated minor and be given contraceptives without the knowledge or consent of the parents, if the child requested that confidentiality be kept, and the doctor felt that it was in the best interest of the minor to do so.[156]

In the first case reported, the patient is 18 years old, the age of majority; it is possible that she was under the age of 16 when she was pregnant for the first time

---

[153] Definition of Statutory Rape; http://legal-dictionary.thefreedictionary.com/Statutory+Rape
[154] Worldwide Ages of Consent; http://www.avert.org/age-of-consent.htm
[155] Laws of Barbados; Medical Termination of Pregnancy Act 1983; Cap 44A
[156] Gillick v West Norfolk Area Health Authority 1985-3 A.E.R. 402

and still attending school. There is nothing in the narrative to state under whose authority the termination of pregnancy was done, whether an HIV test was done, and if any enquiry was made as to the identity of the father.

In the second case report, the woman would have been 17 years old and still under the age of majority when she had her first child. There is no account given as to whether HIV testing was done during the first pregnancy, or any information about the father.

• ***Was the termination of the pregnancy within the provisions of the law?***

The Termination of Pregnancy Act in the jurisdiction concerned calls for the patient to be counselled at the time of consultation on the termination; depending on the time of gestation there are other provisions in relation to second opinions and hospitalisation. Counselling should include counselling about HIV as well as contraceptive advice, and should not be seen as simply satisfying the terms of the act but should be aimed at preventing further problems such as preventing HIV infection through safer sex practice.

In the first case reported there is not sufficient information given to determine whether the termination of the patient's first pregnancy was within the provisions in law. In the second case reported the provisions in law are being followed for the stage of the gestation.

There was no information in either of the first two case reports to determine whether HIV testing was done during the first pregnancies. If so there does not appear to have been any effective counselling that prevented the acquisition or spread of HIV infection between pregnancies.

• ***Who is the father in pregnancies?***

Identification of the father is of importance in relation to the age of the father and the age of the minor, if she is under the age of consent. The father may also be the person who passed on HIV infection to the pregnant minor/woman and it is important to diagnose the HIV status of the father or other sexual partners and provide the education and counselling necessary to prevent further spread of HIV. If it is discovered that the sexual partner knew himself to be HIV positive, consideration may have to be given to prosecution under the Offences Against the Person Act, which in the jurisdiction states: "Any person who unlawfully and maliciously or recklessly engages in conduct which places, or may place, another person in danger of death or serious bodily harm is guilty of an offence and is liable on conviction on indictment to imprisonment for life".[157]

In the first case reported there is no mention of any enquiries into who the father was. In the second report there is an assumption that the live-in boyfriend is the father, but the patient is reluctant to inform him or her previous sexual partners of her HIV status.

• *The rights of a father*

Maternity is a fact; paternity is an act of faith.[158] The father is the person that the mother states he is and who acknowledges it. Legally he is the spouse, the adopted parent or the person who registers his name on the birth certificate of a child. In cases of dispute as to who is the biological father, DNA testing can be done.

Does the father have the right to know of the mother's HIV status? A mother has the right to confidentiality. However, through supportive counselling she should be encouraged to let her sexual partners know her HIV status. This would also involve counselling of the partner before he is tested. Such counselling would need to stress the man's responsibility to any other sexual partners he may have. If the mother's HIV positive status was detected before the particular pregnancy and she did not let her sexual partner know of her status, then there is legal precedent to break her confidentiality and let the partner know without her consent.[159]

However, one must always be conscious of the complex relationships that may exist between partners and in particular as they relate to economic support when making decisions on these delicate matters.[160]

What role should the health staff play in protecting the father's health? Staff have an obligation to look at the HIV status of all the sexual contacts of an HIV positive patient. This is best done with confidentiality and the cooperation of the HIV positive person. Staff have the right to warn any sexual contact that has been knowingly put at risk by a patient. It is therefore vital to know when the HIV status was known and if the risk behaviour continued after the status was known.

What rights does the father have to information about the baby? A father has the legal right to all information about his child. Therefore, in situations where there is an HIV positive baby the father should be told irrespective of the indirect breach of the confidentiality of the mother's status.

---

[157] Laws of Barbados; Offences Against the Person Act Cap 141 section 19
[158] St. Joseph, a Father of Fathers; http://www.kofc.org/en/columbia/detail/2012_03_st_joseph.html
[159] Non-disclosure of HIV status [2006] 2 FLR 50 FD; UK law; Bodey J
[160] Non-disclosure of maternal HIV status to the father during pregnancy: risk factors and consequences; C Jasseron, L Mandelbrot et al; 17th Conference on Retroviruses and Opportunistic Infections CROI 2010; http://retroconference.org/2010/PDFs/894.pdf

In the first case report there is no record of any enquiry as to who the father might be. It could be argued that the father's right to know outweighs that of the mother's right to confidentiality on this occasion, since she should have informed him about her status.

In the second case report the woman is adamant about not wanting to identify or inform her sexual partners about her HIV status, and even proposes that she terminates her pregnancy to avoid being referred to the HIV clinic. Health staff must weigh the patient's desire for confidentiality against the rights of her sexual partners who may be at mortal risk from untreated HIV infection.

- ### The HIV positive woman and pregnancy

Should HIV positive women be allowed to have a baby? There is
a basic right of a woman to autonomy and to consent to sexual
intercourse once she reaches the legal age of consent and presumably
thereby to reproduce. However, being able to reproduce also involves
responsibilities for the father and responsibilities of both parents to the
baby; these responsibilities must be taken into account when conflict
arises. The autonomy of persons can be proscribed in law but in most
jurisdictions there is nothing in the law against a woman's right to
reproduce.[161] However, when a woman is HIV positive she needs to
be counselled in relation to all of the problems the child will face, as
well as the risks to which she exposes her sexual partner. A woman
expressing such a desire should be encouraged to reveal her HIV status
to her partner, and if she does not there is a strong case for breaking her
confidentiality and warning the third party if that party is known. The
alternative to becoming pregnant and not risking transmission to a HIV
negative sexual partner is to use artificial insemination.

Should a complication during a pregnancy be treated differently? The
pregnant woman should be treated with the same standard of care
whether she is HIV positive or not. All of the infants will not be infected
with HIV and therefore should have the opportunity of any other child.
The use of antiretroviral therapy in the perinatal period has reduced the
rate of transmission of HIV from mother to infant.[162]

Should an HIV positive woman be offered Caesarean Section? The
use of a C-section to reduce the risk of transmission in the absence
of perinatal antiretroviral therapy is often a moot point, for in those
countries which cannot afford perinatal therapy an increase in the

---

[161] WHO Sexual and reproductive health; http://who.int/reproductivehealth/en/
[162] Reduction of maternal to child transmission of HIV with AZT, St. John, Kumar, Cave 1999; WIMJ Vol 48; suppl 2; 33

number of elective caesarean sections cannot be afforded either.[163] Therefore, the decision to do a C- section should be made as for any other pregnancy.

What about a second pregnancy? Similar issues arise as with the first pregnancy; however, if HIV was discovered during the first pregnancy, one has to consider whether the sexual partner in the second pregnancy has been unlawfully put at risk. One should also consider what effect the availability of antiretroviral drug therapy only for the reduction of mother to child transmission, may have on the mother who has no other opportunity of getting such treatment.

In one study, 27 or 44% of HIV positive women who had a second or more pregnancies while they were known to be HIV positive were reported; it was reported that a third of the women did not know of the risk of transmission to the baby or that the AZT that they were given was to reduce the risk of transmission. Those figures suggest that either the women are lying to the investigators. or that the counselling that they received was particularly ineffective.[164]

In the first two case reports the HIV status during the mothers' first pregnancies it is not known. Whilst it appears that the obstetric care is beyond reproach, the handling of the at-risk sexual partners needs to be improved.

• *The Infant*

Should an HIV positive premature infant be treated the same as any other? All infants should be treated in the same manner. One does not know if the infant is infected, particularly when antiretroviral treatment is being given to reduce the transmission of the virus. The right of the child to live in spite of the level of disability has been established in case law even in cases of severe disability such an anencephalic infant.[165] Closing the door on the infants of HIV positive mothers not only ignores the fact that they may not be infected but also denies them the opportunity to benefit from advances in care. It also denies the parents of the child what they may have ardently desired.

Should the infant be ventilated if ventilators are scarce? All infants should be treated equally and in situations where ventilation facilities are limited, protocols should be formulated for the guidance of staff.

---

[163] Elective caesarean-section versus vaginal delivery in prevention of vertical HIV-1 transmission: a randomised clinical trial. Parazzini, F, Ricci, E et al; LANCET 1999, 353 (9158) 1035 - 1039
[164] KAP among HIV infected women with repeated childbirths in Barbados; Kumar and St. John WIMJ 2001 Vol 50 supp 2; 16
[165] One advocate's viewpoint: conflict and tensions in the Baby K case; Flannery, J. The Journal of Law, Medicine & Ethics 1995; 23 (1): 7–12

What happens to the infant if the mother dies? The father or other relatives will be responsible for looking after the child. If there are no relatives willing to undertake the child's care, the responsibility lies with the child protection services which would be responsible for arranging adoption or finding foster parents.

In the first case report, the infant was treated with all the facilities available and was able to be discharged from hospital doing well.

In the second case report, the patient is caught up in a maelstrom of denial of her HIV infection and even proposes to 'get rid of the baby' to avoid attending the HIV clinic for therapy to prevent mother to child transmission.

- ### *Did the patient/surrogate know that an HIV test was done?*

A patient should consent to anything including tests that are done on them. An HIV test carries a lot of implications for the patient and they should be warned of the consequences through pre-test counselling. The implications involve knowledge about the testing process including the window period; the ways of transmission of the virus and responsibilities in preventing its spread; preparation for the stigma and discrimination that exists; and the options available for treatment.

A policy of 'routine' testing for HIV has been advocated for persons attending health care settings, based on the argument that early detection of HIV gives a better chance of effective HIV treatment. When challenged about the propriety of 'secretly' testing persons for HIV, proponents of the policy have argued that patients would be able to 'opt-out' of such testing if they wish.[166] However, the question remains how does a patient opt-out if they are not told that the 'routine' test is being done.

In the first two case reports it was not clear if the patients knew they were being tested, and in the third case the patient is not mentally competent and the patient's husband is kept in the dark about the testing and its result. It appears as if there is a policy of 'routine' testing in the institution and the lack of effective counselling shows up in the reaction of the patient in the second case report.

In the third case report, the HIV testing was kept secret presumably on the basis of patient confidentiality. However, with the death of the patient, the husband should be considered at possible mortal risk and undergo counselling and HIV testing.

- ### *Has the patient been tested before?*

One of the pieces of information required prior to testing for HIV is to

---

[166] HIV Testing in Clinical Settings | HIV Testing | HIV/AIDS | CDC www.cdc.gov/hiv/t...United States Centers for Disease Control and Prevention...2015

find out if testing has been done before and what was the result. If the result was negative and is now positive, there are clear implications for contact tracing of any sexual partners. If testing was positive before, there are clear implications for the attitude of the patient to the risks of transmission to the father and infant in pregnant patients, and to sexual partners in general. There are policies advocating 'routine' testing where all persons attending health care facilities are offered HIV testing and this implies that no queries need be made of previous testing.[167]

In the case reports given there was no mention of enquiry or a record of HIV testing being done previously. In the third case report it is specifically noted that the positive HIV test was not placed in the patient's notes. This suggests that the policy for testing for HIV is that of secrecy with no regard for responsibility in relation to the patient's sexual contacts. The deliberate lack of recording of test results can have serious legal implications should there be any enquiry into the transmission of HIV to others.

- ***Is confirmatory testing done before a positive test result is sent out?***

HIV testing is done on the presence of antibodies to the virus and may have both false negative and false positive results. The false negative test is related to recent transmission and this can be suspected on the basis of the history, and further testing at a later date. A false positive test is detected by repeating the test and getting a negative result, as well as by testing using a different test method.[168] The possibility that the test result is that of another person depends on the integrity of the identification system in the laboratory, and if there is doubt another sample should be submitted and tested.

In the 2nd case reported the patient has challenged the validity of the positive test result.

Attempts at reassurance including suggesting the test be repeated have not swayed her.

- ***VCT vs. Mandatory vs. 'Routine' testing.***

Given the fear and stigma generated with the advent of AIDS in 1981 and the tests developed between 1983 and 1985, voluntary counselling and testing [VCT] emerged as the preferred method of testing for HIV. Pre-test counselling gave the opportunity for the patient to prepare mentally, and

---

[167] Revised Recommendations for HIV Testing of Adults, Adolescents, and Pregnant Women in Health-Care Settings; B M. Branson, H. Hunter Handsfield, et al, CDC MMWR reports 2006 / 55(RR14); 1-17; http://www.cdc.gov/mmwr/preview/mmwrhtml/rr5514a1.htm
[168] HIV Antibody Confirmation Tests; http://hivinsite.ucsf.edu/insite?page=basics-01-01

to fully participate in the decision for testing and the subsequent actions that should be taken. In the absence of treatment at that time, there were calls for isolation, imprisonment, and exclusion from the workplace and living accommodation. This placed a big burden on the patient to even agree to be tested, and it could not be effectively done without the support of good counselling. Knowledge of the test result. with counselling. results in the prevention of spread of HIV by a better appreciation of protecting oneself, and seeking earlier treatment measures.[169]

The use of VCT was counter-balanced by the call for mandatory testing. This was advocated with a view to excluding persons from a variety of activities, including health care itself.[170] As effective antiretroviral treatment became available, the call was made for routine testing – i.e. all persons attending health care facilities would be tested for HIV, unless they specifically refused to be tested [CDC 2006].

These various forms of testing were more easily described than practised, depending on the attitude of the providers of care and their willingness, or lack thereof, to counsel patients and obtain their explicit consent to being tested. What is often practised is testing without the explicit knowledge of the patient and only 'facing up to the issues' if the tests come back positive. Facing up to the issues usually means referring them to other services where others handle the problems.

Sometimes the discussion centres on whether there should be provider or client- initiated testing;[171] this should never be an either/or situation and really masks the issue of how informed the consent for testing should be. Informed consent depends on the quality of pre-test counselling.

Pre-test counselling – should be sufficiently thorough to prepare the patient for the psychosocial issues that may arise, as well as the possible defects in the testing procedures. Counselling at its best will not prevent all of the problems that arise; patients may still go into denial, fear the stigmatization that may occur, and may not wish to warn their vulnerable intimate contacts. This means that counselling has to continue and build on what has gone before. Pre-test counselling can be less intensive depending on the individual and general community knowledge about HIV/AIDS, and the knowledge among the professionals responsible for the diagnosis and care of patients.

---

[169] Voluntary Counselling and Testing (VCT) for HIV Prevention; http://www.unfpa.org/hiv/prevention/hivprev5b.htm
[170] AIDS, Privacy & the Community: The Ethics of Mandatory AIDS Testing and Disclosure; Issues in Ethics - V. 3, N. 3; 1990; http://www.scu.edu/ethics/publications/iie/v3n3/AIDS.html
[171] GUIDANCE ON PROVIDER-INITIATED HIV TESTING AND COUNSELLING IN HEALTH FACILITIES; WHO/UNAIDS 2007;http://www.who.int/hiv/pub/guidelines/9789241595568_en.pdf

Stigmatization and discrimination in relation to STDs has been present for generations and had led to laws ensuring the confidentiality of patients and their sexual contacts; establishment of special clinics;[172] but also to repressive laws related to job availability, particularly in the government sectors. Historically persons infected with STDs, and especially syphilis, were the main targets of these repressive measures. These regulations persisted in large measure even after treatment with antibiotics became available. In the case of HIV/AIDS the historical situation was overlaid by the fact that AIDS had emerged as a highly fatal disease among male homosexuals.[173] Therefore, all of the old stigmatization of STDs was enhanced by the societal and religious condemnation of homosexuals. In fact, AIDS was called the Wrath of God in most religions and there were calls for and enactment of repressive laws for those affected by HIV/AIDS.[174]

The adverse societal, business and health professionals reaction to patients and families affected by HIV was inevitable given the reaction of the community and religious leaders. Inevitably there were calls for more coercive measures towards those who were ill or thought to be at risk, and questioning of how informed consent for testing should be. Advocacy for the rights of patients as an indispensable tool in containing the spread of the disease in 'free' societies, led to the retention of counselling even if pre-test counselling was abandoned in the pressure generated for mandatory and 'routine' testing.[175] Advocacy for the rights of HIV affected persons did not stem the tide of discrimination, for in many places criminalization statutes for HIV were passed; jobs were lost or denied; health and other insurance denied, and travel denied.[176] As time has passed and the fear of contagion has regressed, many of the issues of counselling patients have remained.

Post-test counselling – by whom? Once the discipline and constraints of pre-test counselling was abandoned by those who order the patient to be tested. The result was that, without the benefit of counselling, many persons were unequipped to deal with issues such as the fear of death; the feeling of rejection and ostracism by partners, family, community, and the work place; the fear of life-long loss of intimate relationships; and the

---

[172] Stigmatization, scapegoating and discrimination in sexually transmitted diseases: Overcoming 'them' and 'us'; N Gilmore, M A. Somerville; Social Science & Medicine, 1994, 39, [9,] 1339-1358
[173] CDC. Pneumocystis pneumonia --- Los Angeles. MMWR 1981; 30:250--2
[174] Baggett, D J., "AIDS and the Wrath of God" (1994); http://digitalcommons.liberty.edu/sor_fac_pubs/157
[175] CDC Hints at HIV Testing Without Consent; M Cichocki, About.com Guide, 2009; http://aids.about.com/b/2009/08/17/cdc-recommends-mandatory-hiv-testing-without-consent.htm
[176] Discriminatory laws contribute to spread of HIV/AIDS: report D Singer; Jurist 2010; http://jurist.org/paperchase/2010/07/discriminatory-laws-contribute-to-spread-of-hiv-aids-report.php

fear of violence within the home and in the community. All of these result in responses of denial, anger, suicidal ideation, and revenge. The patient may therefore be left in a worse situation than where they started, and have to start establishing new relationships with other practitioners, who depending on the prevalence of HIV may themselves be overwhelmed.[177]

In the first case report, the emphasis is on handling the obstetric complication, and so the efficacy of HIV counselling cannot be judged, although there is a notable absence of any mention of a father in the care that is required.

In the second case report, in the apparent absence of any pre-test counselling of the patient, dealing with the implications of a positive test became challenging.

In the third case report, the physicians caring for the patient have chosen to keep the testing of the patient, and even the possibility of the diagnosis, secret, leaving the sexual contacts of the patient unaware and vulnerable to the same late presentation with AIDS as the patient did.

- ***The reactions of health professionals to HIV infected patients***
Health professionals' reactions to HIV/AIDS patients have included fear of transmission; resistance to providing counselling; avoidance of explicit consent to testing; the suppression / expression of prejudices; evasion of care; and impatience with ethical and legal constraints.[178] These reactions lead to defective care and compromise the cooperation of patients with important aspects of care such as contact tracing.

In the first two case reports there is a possible lack of focus on HIV counselling and prevention during the first pregnancies. The professionals' direct avoidance of counselling in the second case report has almost certainly contributed to the denial and general lack of co-operation of the patient.

In the third case report the secrecy and lack of candour with the surrogate of the incapacitated patient, lead the professionals into a dilemma as to how sexual contacts of the dead patient should be warned; they opt to do nothing.

- ***Legal status of contact tracing.***
In tracing intimate sexual contacts it is necessary to get the cooperation of patients and their relations. In the absence of an accusation of a crime, the law cannot achieve contact tracing without the willing cooperation of a patient, or breaking their confidentiality.[179] Making assumptions about sexual contacts can lead to mistakes that can have deadly social and

---

[177] Posttraumatic stress disorder in response to HIV infection; B Kelly, B. Raphael, et al; General Hospital Psychiatry; 1998; 20, 6, 345-352

[178] Health Professions, Codes, and the Right to Refuse to Treat HIV-Infectious Patients; B Freedman, The Hastings Center Report, 1988, 18, 2, 20-25

[179] AIDS and Confidentiality; Contact Tracing and "Duty to inform" http://students.washington.edu/aed/archivemidget/980303.htm

domestic consequences. Similar pitfalls can arise in determining when a third party at risk should be warned.

Warning third parties at mortal risk has been established by judicial precedent in several jurisdictions. In relation to HIV/AIDS the principle was an easy one to argue when AIDS was a highly fatal disease without effective treatment for it. The availability of effective antiretroviral treatment for HIV and the absence of specific law to warn third parties do not compel the health professional to warn third parties at risk for HIV infection any more than their professional duty of contact tracing of any other sexually transmitted disease.[180]

Legislative and other impediments in handling HIV. Other impediments for health professionals working in the area of HIV / AIDS include:
- the confidentiality and consent restraints in minors, particularly so for those between the age for consent to sexual intercourse and the age when they reach a majority, and can consent to medical treatment.
- lack of confidence in relying on judicial / professional precedent related to contact tracing, partner notification, and warning of third parties.
- lack of a clear legal/ethical framework in many jurisdictions in dealing with high-risk persons such as HIV positives; prostitutes; men who have sex with men [MSM]; prisoners; and IV drug abusers.

In the cases described there are issues on which the professionals concerned lack clear direction. In each case there is a defect in the tracing of the sexual contacts of the patients.

In the first case report there is nothing to suggest that sexual contact tracing is a priority in the current pregnancy or the first. In the second report the professionals do not appear to be able to cope with the patient's denial of her status and sexual contacts.

In the third case report the doctors set out to hide the diagnosis from possible sexual contacts of the patient, even after death.

---

[180] Duty to warn: when should confidentiality be breached? Oppenheimer K, Swanson G. J Fam Pract. 1990; 30(2): 179-84

Case report 1:
A young man is brought by ambulance from the scene of an accident to the Accident and Emergency Department where he is assessed as having major abdominal and chest injuries. Basic life support measures are instituted and the surgical team on call is summoned to the department urgently. The surgical team decides that the patient should be transferred to the operating theatre urgently, via the X-ray Department.

The young man's family arrive at the Accident and Emergency Department, and are told that he is seriously injured, and that it has been decided that he needs to be operated on. They ask if they can see the young man and are told no. They ask to speak to the doctor and they receive a message that the doctor cannot speak to them now, but they should go up to the operating theatre and the doctor will speak to them when it becomes possible.

A consultant surgeon who is not on duty sees the patient being hurried out of the X-ray Department by the junior staff on duty and is told by one of them that the patient is on the way to the operating theatre for immediate laparotomy. The consultant decides to go up to the operating theatre to see if he can be of any assistance. On reaching there he is told that the senior resident is in the operating theatre and the patient is in the recovery room awaiting transfer as soon as the anaesthetist arrives. The consultant opines that the patient should go to the operating theatre and resuscitation efforts continued there whilst the anaesthetist arrives. This is done at the same time the anaesthetist is arriving.

The consultant decides to put on a white coat and overshoes and goes to the operating room to see if he can offer any advice or help. In the operating room, the patient has had a cardiac arrest and vigorous resuscitative efforts are undertaken for 45 minutes before giving up.

The surgeon on leaving the operating theatre passes by the anxious relatives one of whom asks what has been happening to their relative. The surgeon stops and tells the relatives that he is very sorry but their relative did not make it. He further states that all efforts were made for much longer than the usual time for cardiac resuscitation. He then extends his condolences and adds that the other doctors will be able to give them more details about the injuries sustained.

The next day the hospital receives a letter of complaint calling the surgeon by name and saying that little was done to save their relative's life, for they could see that the surgeon who spoke to them was neatly clothed and could not have been making any effort to save their relative's life.

Case report 2:

A 68-year-old woman presented to the Emergency Department. She was a visitor from Britain and gave a ten-day history of abdominal pain, which was now located in the right lower quadrant. Her examination at the time revealed generalized peritonitis. She had a CT scan of the abdomen and pelvis, which showed a thickened caecum and appendix with evidence of intra-abdominal collections.

The patient consented for laparotomy, the base of appendix was perforated and the caecum and appendix inflamed and thickened. There were multiple intra-abdominal collections of pus. A limited right hemi-colectomy was performed. The patient made a steady recovery and was discharged from hospital on the ninth day post-op. The histology report showed a caecal adenocarcinoma.

The patient was asked if she wanted to know the findings of her histology and she advised that she would rather have that information when she returned home and had her family around her, given the possibility of adverse news. She was subsequently discharged and the documentation sent to her son at the patient's request for revealing on her return to England.

Issues raised

- ### *Communicating – what and to whom*

The message. Bad news comes in many forms; it may be a diagnosis of a terminal illness, cancer, complications of treatment or the delay or cancellation of anticipated therapy such as an operation. Death is often the most devastating news but it is not the patient who receives it.

The recipient. As with death, the recipient of bad news is not always the patient, it may be relatives, or other relations of the patient. The recipient may be of any age and level of education, and these must be taken into account, as well as the previous experiences of the person/s receiving the news.

In the first case report, the bad news of death is delivered to relatives who are unprepared for such news. A doctor who was not directly involved in the care of the patient has also delivered the bad news.

In the second case report, the bad news is not delivered to the patient on the basis that they are not ready to receive it, and it is left to a relative in a remote situation. Control over the message has been lost and the patient's further consultation for necessary treatment is left in the hands of an untrained and inexperienced relative.

The messenger. The effective communication of any message depends on who delivers the message; with bad news this may best be the done by the most senior person or by the person who has been most involved with and knowledgeable about the patient. Sometimes age and age difference matter, and an elderly patient may not see a very young-looking person as a credible professional.

Experience is invaluable in delivering a message, for one should have learnt to deal with a variety of situations, patients and reactions. Experience should also illustrate the important role that attitudes and knowledge of both parties will play in effective communication.

In the first case report the doctor imparting the bad news has not been directly involved, but appeared to be acting in good faith as a good Samaritan.

In the second report the doctor has been guided by the anxiety of the patient, and rather than dealing with that chooses to lose control of the message by putting the responsibility on a relative who is in communication from another country over the phone.

- ***Communicating is a process***

The method. The location in which the news is given and the demeanour of the person giving the message is very important. Privacy should be assured so that confidentiality can be maintained. Delivering a message in the presence of family members is not always appropriate and guidance should be obtained from the patient as to when they need the presence of relatives, friends or others such as priests or other professionals.[181]

The demeanour and appearance of the messenger can distort a message and bring great distress to the recipient of the message. A fresh and neatly dressed doctor who brings a message of a patient being dealt with as a serious emergency could suggest to those receiving the news that little was being done. Therefore, as an integral part of the message any anomaly in appearance should be addressed by the messenger. A messenger towering over the recipient of a message conveys a quite different impression and level of involvement to the one who gets to the same level of eye contact. A broad smile from the messenger is as inappropriate as the one who is totally grim and may not give the hope that it is intended to convey.

In the first case report, the messenger is responding to an enquiry from very anxious relatives, and delivers an accurate and compassionate response. However, the doctor does not explain his role or lack thereof in the care of the patient and the message becomes distorted as a result.

---

[181] SPIKES — A Six-Step Protocol for Delivering Bad News: Application to the patient with cancer: WF Baile et al The Oncologist August 2000 vol. 5 no. 4 302-311 theoncologist.alphamedpress.org/content/5/4/302

In the second case report the patient's anxiety on being away from her home country is accepted as a good reason for not imparting the bad news and the decision is made to lose control of the message to a relative whose capacity to handle the situation is unknown.

Timing. The timing of a message is important when bad news is being delivered. A judgment must be made about delivering the news immediately, or allowing the recipients of the news time to prepare themselves. Unexpected sudden deaths are best communicated right away, as are those that have been anticipated; however, there should be a commitment given to communicate further if necessary. Deaths that have not been anticipated and other bad news should be communicated giving sufficient time for the recipient to compose himself or herself and, if necessary, to gather any support they need.

The timing of the doctor involved in the first case reported seems appropriate from a humanitarian point of view, and the reaction of the relatives could not be readily anticipated. In the second case report one does not know what the outcome will be of delivering the bad news if it is delivered at all. Control over the message by a professional has been given up on the grounds of letting the patient and their relatives choose the timing. Unfortunately, the nature of the disease and the need for further treatment do not allow for a relaxed schedule that may never come.

Finding the time to deliver the news is most important; the messenger should not appear as if they are in a hurry, and must give enough time for the person to reflect and to ask any questions.

Repetition of the news or message may be necessary at the time or at a subsequent time, for denial is a powerful state of mind on receiving bad news.

A plan of action should be formulated to deal with the situation, even if it has to be refined later. Where necessary the plan should involve the family and other professions.

- *Consultation or second opinions* should be offered and be prepared to refine the treatment plan that was offered.
- *Response and feedback* from the person is very important in resolving any situation at hand. One should listen carefully, even to silence, for it may be a prelude to the emotions that often accompany the receipt of bad news. One should ask what the person has heard and give time for reflection. Patients or other recipients of bad news may go through the stages of denial, anger, depression and resignation, and may require help from a trained counsellor.
- *Denial* is often seen in patients who have received a diagnosis of cancer or HIV. They may report to others a completely different

diagnosis and will seek other opinions or further advice and tests to try and disprove the diagnosis. This may result in delay in carrying out treatment and may need to be handled by psychological counselling and the involvement of relatives within the bounds of the patient's confidentiality.

- *Anger* at themselves or others may follow or precede denial. It comes particularly when there has been a delay in diagnosis or at the news of an incurable disorder, such as HIV or some cancers, which could have been avoided by the action of others. The anger may be intense enough to formulate thoughts of harming others and undertaking legal action.
- *Depression* is a natural consequence of receiving bad news; it is usually transient, particularly when a credible plan of action is presented to deal with the problem. However, it may be severe enough to require medication.
- *Resignation* may be one of the manifestations of depression although couched in terms of acceptance of the situation. It may manifest itself by refusing treatment or accepting treatment with the minimum of participation in decision-making.

Be Prepared. Like any other situation being prepared for having to deal with bad news is most likely to have a good outcome. Begin preparing oneself and the patient from the first visit, taking notes of personal and family history and establishing who the patient will or will not trust. Determine if there are dominant persons in the family who may be making the decisions and establish with the patient who, if anyone, they wish to be involved in making their decisions.

When dealing with relatives, be warned that health care worker relatives from metropolitan countries often assume that that those working in a 'third world country' are not up to date. Try to tolerate the attitude rather than resent the person, and have a researched plan of action ready.

The relatives in the first case report are clearly suspicious of the standard of care in the hospital concerned, and have seized on the appearance of the doctor who first spoke to them to cast aspersions on the standard of care delivered to their deceased relative.

In the second case report, the doctors have used the natural anxiety of the patient to avoid delivering the message and have left it 'at the patient's wishes' to her son. They have lost control of the message, and could have deputed the responsibility to a designated doctor in the patient's country.

- *Consenting to treatment in difficult situations*

Reveal all of the possibilities early and before operation during the consenting process. Remember that in obtaining informed consent the patient should be told the *'material facts, risks, complications and alternatives to the procedure that a reasonable person in the patient's situation could consider significant in deciding whether to* consent'.[182] Critical risks specific to an operation, no matter how rare, should be revealed to the patient.[183] It is important to ensure that the message has been received accurately, even if it means asking what was understood. It is also important where necessary to give time for reflection and consultation with family and to find the time to come back to the matter. Where further action and consultation is required these must be detailed and one must be prepared to refine one's course of action, including offering the patient second opinions.

In the second case report, it was anticipated that there would be an adverse reaction to the news, but there was also the need to explain that further treatment with chemotherapy is recommended. This is a task that should be undertaken by an experienced professional, but it was decided to leave it to the judgment of her son when she returns to her country of origin.

- *Remote situations*

Emergencies may arise with patients who are travelling on business or holiday, and they may be anxious to get back to their country before the situation is fully resolved. In such situations a detailed report should be made, and should be transmitted to a doctor who will undertake responsibility if that is known. When it is not known who will be undertaking responsibility, the report should be made available to the patient or other responsible person for transmission to the doctor who does undertake responsibility.

In the second case report there is no attempt to identify and communicate with a doctor who will be responsible for the continuing care and referral for further treatment that is necessary.

---

[182] Gouse v. Cassell (615 A.2d 331) 1992
[183] Chester v Afshar [2004] UKHL 41; [2005] 1 A.C. 134; [2004] 3 W.L.R. 927; [2004] 4 All E.R. 587

ALTERNATIVES IN MEDICINE

Case history:

A 75-year-old woman was referred to a surgeon with a diagnosis of carcinoma of the caecum. Eighteen months previously she had seen an alternative medicine practitioner who diagnosed anaemia and recommended a course of therapy. After six months she was feeling worse and she saw a medical practitioner who investigated her and treated her anaemia, with some improvement. She continued to lose weight and consulted another practitioner a year later. Further investigations were done and showed a carcinoma of the caecum with no evidence of metastatic spread.

She was advised to have surgical treatment. Her daughter enquired about alternative medical treatment for the cancer, and the surgeon explained that this tumour was not amenable to radiotherapy or chemotherapy. She was given a date for surgery, but near to the date she rang to say that she would have to make a new date.

Two months later she rang and said that she had started therapy with an 'alternative' medicine doctor and asked to have an appointment to discuss the matter. At the appointment her daughter detailed the investigation and treatment her mother had gone through, asked the surgeon what his opinion was, and whether he would be prepared to consult with the 'doctor'. The patient when asked stated that she had had no improvement, that the regimen was very demanding and that was why she had lapsed and had a cup of tea. The patient returned two weeks later with a letter from her alternative practitioner stating that the patient had been improving until she digressed from the regimen, that the tumour was growing again and that the patient should have surgery at which the alternative practitioner was willing to assist. Surgery was scheduled shortly after and a large tumour infiltrating the adjacent small bowel was excised en bloc.

Issues raised

- *What is Alternative Medicine?*

Alternative medicine is the healing arts not taught in traditional western medical schools; it promotes options to conventional medicine. An example of an alternative therapy is using a special diet to treat cancer instead of undergoing surgery, radiation, or chemotherapy.

Complementary medicine is used together with conventional medicine;[184] alternative medicine is used in place of conventional medicine.

In the report presented, the patient and her daughter have sought a complementary approach to treatment, and have consulted an alternative medicine practitioner who had convinced the patient that his methods could treat the cancer. When it was clear that the patient was not satisfied with progress, the alternative practitioner wrote to suggest joint treatment.

• *What is the legal role of alternative practitioners in medical practice?*
Alternative medical practitioners are variously described and characterised in different jurisdictions.[185] The question is how proscribed is their area of practice in law and their training and ability to make diagnoses. The limits of practice of chiropractors and others registered under their professional regulatory act are described in those acts. For example, one Paramedical Professions Act recognises four categories of procedures which can be performed by a paramedical practitioner. These are chiropractic, diagnostic and therapeutic radiography, occupational therapy and physiotherapy.[186]

Although medical registration acts state that it is illegal to practise medicine without being a registered medical practitioner, the practice of medicine is not well defined and the law cannot prevent the application of home remedies.[187] Professional conduct regulations for registered health professionals other than doctors are described in very similar terms to those of medical practitioners, but in jurisdictions where doctors are prohibited from advertising, there is no such prohibition for alternative practitioners.

• *Was the patient properly investigated by the medical practitioners?*
Patients may have to be investigated to come to a conclusive diagnosis, investigations may be curtailed for economic or other reasons; where this occurs, it should be made clear to the patient the reasons why the investigation has been curtailed and objectives should be set for the further pursuance of the diagnosis. It is unwise without firsthand information to make adverse comment on a physician's course of action; this could lead patients to take legal action that may or may not prove to

---

[184] Complementary and Alternative Medicine; info@nccam.nih.gov
[185] Legal Status of Traditional Medicine and Complementary/Alternative Medicine: A Worldwide Review; WHO/EDM/TRM/2001
[186] Laws of Barbados; Paramedical Professions Act 1975.CAP 372C
[187] Laws of Barbados; Medical Registration Act LRO 1978; CAP 371;sect 17

be justified. However, the provision of expert opinion on the facts given in a legal enquiry is another matter and is both legally and ethically defensible.[188]

In the case reported it appears as if the first medical practitioner and the endoscopist inadequately investigated the patient's anaemia. The lack of a diagnosis or relief of symptoms will lead patients to seek other opinions.

- *Weighing a relative's intervention about a competent patient.*
Caution should be exercised in responding to the intervention of relatives without clear direction from a competent patient. This must be kept in mind particularly in elderly patients where the relative may feel they have to assume control. Responding to a relative should be done with the greatest of caution in the absence of the patient. Such interactions may lead to decisions that the patient might not desire but feel compelled to accept. The doctor should try to get the patient to make their own decision and intervene when they consider the advice given by the relative to be wrong. When the patient is not competent to make decisions, it is the responsibility of the established next of kin to make the decision. One should be cautious about responding to relatives other than the next of kin, particularly since one may not be aware of what factors may be impinging on the decisions being made.

In the instance described there is no clear indication that the dominant interventions of the patient's daughter are not wanted by the patient, but cannot be discounted.

- *How should an enquiry about delaying treatment be handled?*
The facts about the natural history of the condition and the treatment alternatives and timing should be given to patients when dealing with diagnosed cancers, and other progressive disease and the patient allowed to come to their own decision about the treatment options. Patients should be given enough time to reflect and to talk with their relatives before they are required to make a decision. Patients are often confused and in denial when a diagnosis of cancer or HIV disease is made, and counselling and support groups may provide an invaluable service in helping the patient to come to grips with their fears. Since the progression of disease is variable in individuals, no categorical predictions should be given about the disease or the results of therapy.

In the report given there is no account given of any discussion that the surgeon may have had with the patient about the issues of delay. A clear bond

---

[188] The Medical Expert Witness I. S. Trostler, Radiology, 1931; 17, 807-815

*of trust has not been established with the surgeon, or in the surgeon's views on
alternative approaches.*

• **What is the responsibility to pursue patients with life-threatening
illness?**
Practitioners have a responsibility to pursue or follow up patients under
their care whom they know have life-threatening illness. If the patient
has defaulted, an effort should be made to make sure that it is not a
misunderstanding on the patient's part. Patients may be in denial and
may get a totally different impression from that the doctor intended to
convey, or thought they had conveyed. This is a problem particularly
where there are time constraints in the consultation process.

*In the report given, it appears that the surgeon having heard from the patient
that they had consulted an alternative practitioner did not wish to be seen
as questioning the patient's choice. A passive approach to the patient's delay
appears to have been taken.*

• **Should physicians express 'views' on alternative medicine to
patients?**
In any area of practice there may be opinions and beliefs that should
be clearly separated from facts. Comment should not be made on what
one does not know except to state just that. Opinions that are not based
on fact should be clearly identified and where necessary alternative
investigations or opinions sought.

*From the report given it appears that the surgeon has avoided giving any view
on the alternative treatment that the patient sought. This approach could have led
the patient to strengthen their belief in the practice.*

• **Should doctors work with 'alternative' practitioners?**
It is unprofessional to associate with unlicensed persons in the treatment
of patients.[189] Medical practitioners normally work with and send patients
to physiotherapists, occupational therapists and others who are registered
under the appropriate health professions act. Most registered health
professionals other than medical practitioners have a limited diagnostic
role and the relationship between medical practitioners and other health
professionals who do diagnostic as well as therapeutic work is not clear.
Questions therefore arise as to the boundaries of practice of chiropractors,
chiropodists and other alternative medical practitioners, as in fact they
do among medical practitioners and their specialties. The boundaries of

---

[189] Laws of Barbados; Medical Registration Act, Regulations CAP 371; 1972; Pt. V, 21,2,i

practice of health professionals will either be contained in the appropriate registration legislation, or will be determined by the appropriate regulatory body.

There is no limit to the autonomy of a patient to choose who should treat them unless forbidden by law.

In the report given there was nothing to suggest that the alternative medicine practitioner, who was a registered health professional, was acting outside the law. However, the surgeon does not appear to have accepted the invitation to be in a professional relationship of joint treatment.

The Challenge of a Patient's Right

Case report:
A 29-year-old woman presented to an antenatal clinic with a history of a normal delivery 12 years ago, but two later miscarriages at nine and 10 weeks gestation. Booking investigations were normal with the ultrasound revealing twins at 10 weeks gestation; she was counselled re monitoring versus elective cerclage of the cervix. Cerclage was done at 14 weeks gestation and progress monitored by ultrasonography.

She requested a home birth in the squatting position and said she wished to leave the placentas attached until the babies "kick them off". She was counselled about the high-risks of her pregnancy and the adverse effect of delayed cord clamping on infants; but restated her preferred management although she understood the increased risks. At 33 weeks it was found that one twin had a footling breach and the other a transverse lie; the patient said she would employ natural herbs to deal with it. She reiterated her wish for a "controlled birthing environment" at home, and said she was considering a "water birth". She was encouraged to visit and meet with the midwives. A week later she had spontaneous rupture of the membranes, the cerclage was removed and she was further counselled about the risks involved. The paediatricians came and discussed with her the treatment she should expect for premature babies. In the following two weeks she refused the supplemental iron prescribed, and used merengue seeds and natural foods instead. At 36 weeks she declined induction of labour or a caesarean section and she reiterated her previous wishes, which were objected to by some staff as having special privileges. She eventually agreed to induction, and was allowed to set up an altar and put up posters and ornaments, but candles were not allowed. A smooth and uneventful labour and delivery occurred and mother and babies went home on day four.

Issues raised

* *Rights of the mother*

A pregnant woman has the rights of any competent adult to consent to or refuse treatment unless compelled to do otherwise by a court order. However, the treatment she may request or be offered is constrained by the law when such treatment directly affects the foetus to the point of termination of a pregnancy. The laws on termination/abortion vary widely in different jurisdictions. The variation is from a total prohibition or only in instances to save the woman's life, to a variety of circumstances that may involve how the pregnancy was conceived; e.g. rape or incest; the health or socio-economic circumstances of the woman; the possible viability of the foetus or serious or fatal abnormalities that are diagnosed or anticipated.[190]

Religious and cultural beliefs often determine how a woman will deal with a pregnancy, from not tolerating an abortion for any reason, to requesting a termination based on the gender of the foetus.[191]

In the case reported there is no suggestion that a termination of the pregnancy is contemplated, quite the opposite. Although she has asked to be treated in an unconventional manner the doctors found, after initial resistance on their part, that many of her requests can be accommodated within the normal standards of care.

- ### *Rights of the unborn*

The rights of the unborn cannot be separated from those of the woman who is pregnant. Therefore, any will to express a right to the unborn must be legislated to constrain the autonomy of the pregnant woman to control over her body.[192] These laws usually relate to proscribing a woman's wish for an abortion; and more recently to try and remove any control she may have over when she conceives. In most instances such rights of the unborn are not exercised when the life of the pregnant woman is at risk, or when an abnormality in the unborn is seen as a serious risk to its life or health.

Questions may arise when there is more than one foetus, when one is faring better than the other, and what should be done to ensure that one foetus does not end up with the serious problems of prematurity or endanger the other.

The question of the rights of the unborn arose when the mother refused to consider a caesarean section as a means of delivering her babies. Such refusal could have been a dangerous threat to the infants during delivery if there was foetal distress.

- ### *Rights of the father*

A father should have an interest in the pregnancy that he has fathered, but in most jurisdictions he has no rights to determine its outcome, although in some countries a husband is required to authorize an

---

[190] http://worldabortionlaws.com/map/
[191] The Pre-natal Diagnostic Techniques (Regulation and Prevention of Misuse) Act, No. 57 of 1994, and the Pre-natal Diagnostic Technologies (Regulation and Prevention of Misuse) Amendment Act, No. 2002, No. 14 of 2003. Gov. India
[192] Rights of the Unborn Child; http://www.life.org.nz/abortion/abortionlegalkeyissues/rightsunbornchild/

abortion.[193] During a pregnancy it is prudent to involve the father in the decision-making process, as long as it is seen as advisory and consensual and not overriding the decisions of the competent woman to make decisions about her life or health. A father can only seek to impose a decision contrary to that of the mother in relation to the unborn through an order of the court. Such an order is unlikely to be obtained unless it could be shown that the mother is being irrational or reckless towards the unborn infant.

When the child is born both parents have rights to make decisions about the child's health and treatment, although it may be a lot more difficult for the unwed father.[194]

In the case reported, the father's role is not described.

- ### *Rights of the doctor/health professionals*

Doctors and other health professionals have the rights of every citizen, but they also have the legal right to carry out treatments, which have a potential to do harm. The health professional also has responsibilities to their patients; for example, a patient cannot be abandoned no matter how difficult they may be, and they have to be treated when an emergency arises no matter if the problem was self-inflicted or the result of an illegal act. These responsibilities are set out in law regulating the professions, and in professional codes of conduct.[195, 196]

The health professional is also asked to respect a patient's religious and cultural values, and this must involve not proselytizing their own when it varies from that of the patient. However, the professional has a right to a conscientious objection to carrying out or taking part in procedures such as a lawful termination of a pregnancy.[197] The exercise of such a conscientious objection cannot be to the detriment of the patient who should be placed in competent hands to carry out any lawful treatment.

Health professionals have the right to refuse to treat a patient by means or with procedures that they consider dangerous, outside the normal standards of the profession or their own competence.[198]

---

[193] A Global Review of Laws on Induced Abortion, 1985-1997; A Rahman, L Katzive and S. K. Henshaw; International Family Planning Perspectives, 1998, Vol 24, 2

[194] Establishing the biological rights doctrine to protect unwed fathers in contested adoptions T. L. Craig ; http://www.law.fsu.edu/journals/lawreview/downloads/252/craig.pdf

[195] Medical Professions Act, 2011-1. Laws of Barbados

[196] WMA International Code of Medical Ethics 1949 and amended 2006; http://www.wma.net/en/30publications/10policies/c8/

[197] Conscientious objection in medicine; J Savulescu, BMJ. 2006 February 4; 332(7536): 294–297

[198] Refusing to Treat: Are There Limits to Physician "Conscience" Claims? B Patsner; http://www.law.uh.edu/healthlaw/perspectives/2008/(BP)%20conscience.pdf

However, in exercising that right the professional has the duty to offer alternatives to the patient or to refer the patient to an available competent professional.

In the case described some of the professionals appear to feel that their knowledge and authority is being challenged. To compound the challenge was the patient's insistence on 'naturalistic' treatment and the use of cultural/religious practices that were not familiar to the professionals. In the end continuing engagement allowed both conventional and unconventional practices, whilst excluding those considered dangerous.

- ***Competing rights***

Resolution of conflicting rights depends on the knowledge of contending parties of their own rights and those of others. Such information is frequently not available to patients and if something goes wrong during treatment and is not handled sensitively, a complaint of negligence may be laid.

Professionals must understand and exercise their responsibilities to their patients and to the community as expressed in the law in their jurisdiction. Of particular importance is obtaining informed consent to treatment; which involves the patient being made aware of and understanding the advantages and risks of the treatment proposed.[199]

When conflict occurs in a patient care setting, having written codes of conduct available to both staff and patients can assist in conflict resolution. Clinical guidelines, along with the assistance of independent knowledgeable persons in ethics and the particular clinical field, are particularly useful when professionals disagree.[200]

In the report given, a potential conflict between a strong-willed patient and the health professionals is diffused by the adoption of a non-judgmental approach, and allowing practices that are not standard but judged to be not dangerous. Furthermore, time is taken to explain the reasons every step in the complex treatment is undertaken. In the end both the patient and the professionals compromise on their views and the outcome was satisfactory to both parties.

---

[199] AMA Code of Ethics; http://www.ama-assn.org/ama/pub/physician-resources/legal-topics/patient-physician-relationship-topics/informed-consent.page
[200] Standards and ethics guidance for doctors. GMC; 2013; http://www.gmc-uk.org/publications/standards_guidance_for_doctors.asp

TO LIVE OR DIE

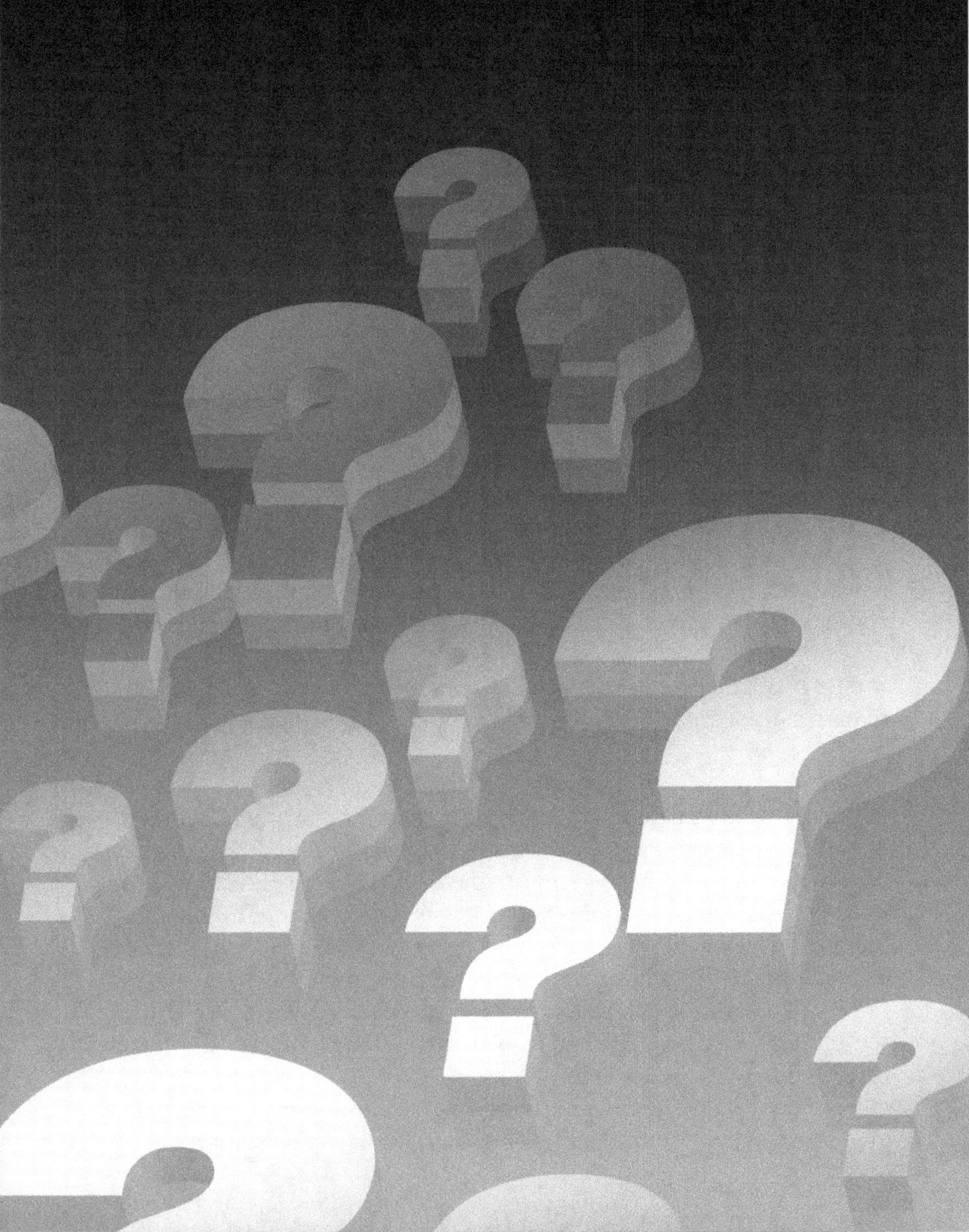

Do Not Resuscitate

Case report 1:

A 60-year-old woman was admitted having collapsed at home after complaining of severe headache and vomiting. She was comatose, Glasgow coma scale 3/15 and she was placed on ventilation. A diagnosis of acute sub-arachnoid haemorrhage was confirmed on CT scan. A neurosurgeon in consultation advised reassessment after 48 hours. On day five post-admission there was spontaneous eye-opening and a cerebral angiogram was done and an anterior communicating artery aneurysm was shown. Surgery was scheduled for the next operating list on day nine. On the day before surgery the patient spiked a temperature and became drowsier; re-bleeding was suspected and the surgery was postponed. A tracheostomy and gastrostomy were done.

On day 13 the aneurysm was clipped and the relatives were informed that neurological recovery would be prolonged and irreversible neurologic deficit was possible. The postoperative course was complicated by multiple problems including transient diabetes insipidus, antibiotic resistant infections at the gastrostomy site and in. tracheal aspirates. She developed a pneumonia and hydrocephalus was observed on a repeat CT scan. Oliguria developed and there was hypoproteinemia with generalized oedema, anaemia [requiring transfusions] and persistent pyrexia.

On day 65 after admission there was no improvement in the patient's neurological status with a GCS of 6/15. She could not be weaned off the ventilator, the pyrexia persisted, but there was some improvement in renal function.

Her husband who visited regularly and remained hopeful, requested that no extraordinary medical treatment should be given.

Case report 2:

An 80-year-old female attended the emergency department complaining of not eating or drinking for the last two weeks and vomiting twice during that period. She also complained of weakness and being unable to walk unaided. On examination she was pale and dehydrated but there were no other abnormal physical signs. Investigations confirmed an anaemia, Hb 7.8gm/dl, and dehydration with a blood urea of 26.4 mmols/l, creatinine 310mmols/l. After discussion with the medical service she was discharged on iron tablets, vitamins and oral fluids to be reviewed in one week's time.

Four days later she returns to the emergency department complaining of generalised abdominal pain. On examination she was distressed,

pale and there was tenderness around the umbilicus but no guarding
or rigidity and bowel sounds were present. Intestinal obstruction was
queried and she was referred to the surgical service.

The surgical notes recorded restlessness, dehydration, a pulse rate
of 110 / min and BP 80/57 mms.Hg. The abdomen was distended and
tender all over with guarding and rebound. An abdominal X-ray showed
air in the peritoneum. A diagnosis of perforated viscus was made and
resuscitation done in preparation for operation.

At surgery an inoperable perforated gastric carcinoma was found. She
was extubated on the operating table but required pressors to maintain
her blood pressure. She had a cardio-respiratory arrest in the recovery
room, was resuscitated and attached to a ventilator. Two days later it is
noted that she is unconscious and full support measures are continued.
One week later she is awake but has multi organ failure.

The decision is made that the minimum should be done and do not
resuscitate [DNR] orders should be discussed with her son. Two weeks
later she extubated in the early morning, had a cardio-respiratory arrest
and could not be resuscitated.

Case report 3:

A 17-year-old female with cerebral palsy, who suffers from seizures and
asthma, presented to the emergency department in severe respiratory
distress and was intubated in the department. She had been admitted
to hospital on numerous occasions with asthmatic attacks and seizures.
She was blind, did not talk, but according to her mother she heard well.
She was normally cared for at home by her mother and her family and
was confined to her bed or a wheel chair. She was normally fed a liquid
dietary supplement, but coughed whilst being fed. She had copious oral
secretions, which were handled by postural drainage.

She was admitted to an intensive care unit with a diagnosis of
aspiration pneumonitis. She was malnourished, had a scoliosis and severe
limb contractures, but no bedsores. In the following week ventilation
support continued and seizures and metabolic derangements were
treated. Attempts at weaning her from the ventilator proved futile. The
diagnosis of chronic aspiration syndrome was made and discontinuation
of ventilation support was discussed with her mother.

Issues raised

• *Should patients be offered surgery when the outlook is poor?*
When this question is posed a number of issues come into play, these

include that one should do no further harm, try to determine what is in the best interest of the patient along with the surrogate who is usually required to consent for the patient. These decisions include the fact that life support measures will almost certainly be required.

'Do no harm.' The decision on whether to advise surgery that carries serious risks of harm depends on the expert knowledge of the surgeon. There are situations where medical knowledge and practice are evolving and outcomes will depend on the skills and services available, or on the will to experiment to see if improvement in outcomes can be achieved. The perception of the harm that can be done may differ depending on whether it is the doctor, the patient, their relatives or even the society. Thus, a surgeon may have the attitude that given the patient's condition they are likely to die and no harm is done by carrying out a risky procedure, as long as it has a small possibility of success.

'The operation was a success but the patient died' has been most often quoted as a form of joke, but the underlying issue is that in the world of medicine the surgeon may be seen as meddlesome, experimenting or driven by profit. The attitude to slim chances is influenced by factors such as the age of the patient and their social characteristics. Younger patients are more likely to have interventions advised that would normally be considered futile or in short supply than in older patients.[201] There is no doubt that advanced age does influence outcomes but this is more dependent on other concurrent diseases than the age itself. It could be said that age discrimination is practised in decision making, and may be reflected in whether an older patient is admitted to hospital when ill, and if admitted may be characterised in terms such as 'elderly for care'.

Age discrimination is a reality in health care and the wider society. It is not only seen in the decisions that health professionals make, but also in the attitudes of relatives and the society in general to the value of a patient's life depending on the age of very ill. Therefore, making difficult decisions that may be seen as doing possible harm must be balanced by the other imperatives of beneficence, and obtaining informed consent.[202]

'Beneficence'. The anticipated good must be defined.[203] The four considerations that are usually taken into account are relief of symptoms, cure of disease, prolongation of life and improvement in the quality of

[201] Principles for allocation of scarce medical interventions; G Persad, A Wertheimer, E J Emanuel; Lancet 2009; 373: 423–31; http://www.ncpa.org/pdfs/PIIS0140673609601379.pdf
[202] Value judgments in the decision-making process for the elderly patient; J Ubachs-Moust, R Houtepen, R Vos, R ter Meulen J Med Ethics 2008;34:863-868
[203] Evaluating the Quality of Medical Care; A Donabedian; The Milbank Quarterly, Vol. 83, No. 4, 2005 (pp. 691–729) http://www.milbank.org/uploads/documents/QuarterlyCentennialEdition/Eval.%20Quality%20of%20Med.%20Care.pdf

life. These goals may coalesce but will not necessarily do so. When the goals of doing good do not converge, one or other may weigh heavily in the thinking of the patient or relative in giving consent to a procedure.

Quality of life is a judgment that must be individualized and can be measured.[204] Thus the quality of life of a patient who has a neurological deficit may appear to depend on the extent of the deficit. In reality the quality of life depends on a variety of factors such as the age of the patient, concurrent illness, the will of the patient, the health of the family that undertakes care, and the availability and costs of services for care. All of these factors should have a bearing on the decision-making process, not only of the doctor, but should be taken into account in the formation of institutional guidelines or protocols drawn up for difficult situations. These factors should also play a part in the judgment of the person/ surrogate called upon to provide consent for treatment.

'Informed surrogate consent'. Informed consent is one where the patient or their surrogate is made aware of all the significant risks and alternatives of the proposed procedure.[205] When the decision is to be made by a surrogate such as the next of kin, a parent or a guardian, the values and beliefs of that person will inevitably impinge on the decision making process. The surrogate's view of their level of responsibility will vary as they are called upon to make judgments about prolonging life versus the quality of life.

Coming to a decision about prolonging life as against the quality of life of another person is an awesome responsibility which no one person would wish to undertake by themself. In addition to family and other persons like the patient's priest, an institution should have readily available resources to assist a surrogate in coming to a decision. Unless there has been a prior determination, the decision time in an emergency is often too short for a surrogate to grapple with all the complexity involved and they will usually opt for prolonging life and face the other issues later.[206]

The role of religious beliefs as well as trust in the medical profession is crucial in making decisions about the prolongation of life. Thus, a Jehovah's Witness may decide, even for another, that life is not worth living, if a blood transfusion is to be administered; but for other persons of faith, blood transfusion is usually seen as an essential part of saving life. A

---

[204] The Lawton Instrumental Activities of Daily Living (IADL) Scale; AJN t 2008 t Vol. 108, No. 4

[205] Surrogate Decision-Making and Related Issues; Beck, C; Shue, V; Alzheimer Disease & Associated Disorders: 2003;Vol17, S12-S16

[206] Statistical methods that distinguish between attributes of assessment: prolongation of life versus quality of life; Loewy JW, Kapadia AS, Hsi B, Davis BR. Med Decis Making. 1992; 12(2): 83-92

Catholic may see the preservation of life as necessary even if it endangers the life of another. This is widely debated in relation to abortion but was also illustrated when the separation of Siamese twins involving the sacrifice of one of them was presented to Catholic parents.[207] Health care staff should be cautioned about proselytizing or projecting their own religious beliefs onto patients. On the other hand, a health professional's right of conscientious objection in treating patients seeking an abortion is to be respected, providing they place the care of the patient into other competent hands, and do not endanger a patient's life in an emergency situation.[208]

Complex determinations about life, death and quality of life cannot be made with 'perfection' and are best not made alone; even when one hears the statement "doctor you know best". That statement is not necessarily an expression of confidence but may be one of resignation in a situation where the burden of decision-making is too heavy to bear. When a surrogate makes a decision in an emergency situation that appears not to preserve life, it is based on religious belief or on distrust of the profession or the particular professional. In such cases a second opinion or further discussion may be required.

When strong and opposing views emerge, only a court can make the determination as to the course of action to be taken - a course that the court thinks should be in the best interest of the patient. Courts have repeatedly put stress on the autonomy of the mentally competent adult and will seek to discern what the patient would have wanted when they were competent - this is not always easily determined.[209] Some patients in anticipation of being unable to make a decision for themselves in some situations, have made advanced directives, sometimes called living wills, to express their views on treatment as their settled position.[210]

'Living wills' are made by persons who, having thought about the issues of their life versus the quality of their life, seek to legally bind the hand of the professionals to a course of action should they be unable to participate in the decision about their care. Living wills also seek to absolve the physician from the fear of legal action should they, in carrying out the patient's wishes, appear to stray from the accepted medical standard of practice of the day.[211] Like any other will there has

---

[207] Conjoined Twins and Catholic Moral Analysis: Extraordinary Means and Casuistical Consistency; M. C Kaveny; Kennedy Institute of Ethics Journal, 2002 Vol 12, No 2, pp. 115-140
[208] Conscientious objection in medicine; J Savulescu BMJ; 2006; 332; 294-297
[209] Supreme Court Orders 544 U.S. Order in pending case 04A825 Schiavo, ex rel. Schindler v. Schiavo, Michael, et al.2005
[210] Advance health care directive; Wikipedia.org
[211] Acting on a Living Will : a physician's dilemma. M Gordon and D Levitt, CMAJ. 1996; 155(7): 893–895

to be an executor, who when faced with the reality of a life or death decision, particularly in an emergency situation, will often opt for life thus giving an opportunity to correct or fine tune the previous decision.

In the first case reported, the surgeon may have been influenced to not offer the operation if the patient was as old [80 years] as the second reported patient. In the second case the physicians may have admitted a patient with anaemia and renal impairment who is vomiting if she were as young as the first patient [60 years].

In both cases the patient has survived a serious emergency event and the decision-makers have decided that although surgery is risky it is worth the risk to prevent further damage and death. The decisions were made in spite of the clear perception that the quality of life may be seriously impaired if the patients did survive.

Where there is some time available in dealing with the emergency as in the first case, the prognostic issues should be brought to the fore by discussing with the next of kin the consequences of a persistent vegetative state and the possibility of a ventilator dependent state. Although these issues may not be decisive in making the decision it sets the stage for reflection and to be better able to cope with the decisions that may have to be made subsequently.

- ***Should further therapy, surgery and artificial nutrition be offered?*** This question should only be raised when it is clear that the outcome is going to be poor and the quality of life will be unacceptable to the patient. Some professionals and laypersons may view ventilator dependency as an unacceptable way of living, whilst others may feel that as long as there is life that there is hope. Therefore, the question arises - what is an unacceptable quality of life and to whom? Is it unacceptable to the health care staff, the patient and their relatives or to the community?[212]

The ventilator-dependent patient who is not expected to regain consciousness may be viewed by the health care staff as unacceptable; they see futile and demanding work using scarce resources, which could be used to the benefit of someone else. Staff may also view the situation as one of working under a legal threat without the chance of a compensating reward of patient recovery. Many medical staff faced with life-threatening situations and current treatment options which appear futile, often opt to do something.[213] Doing something may involve the use of measures that the staff generally consider harmless like antibiotics and cardiovascular

[212] The Quality of Life: The New Medical Dilemma; J.J. Walter, T.A.Shannon. Paulist Press, 1990, ISBN 0-8091-3191-9

[213] Use of the Medical Futility Rationale in Do-Not-Attempt-Resuscitation Orders; J. R Curtis, D R. Park, M R. Krone, R A. Pearlman, JAMA. 1995; 273:124-128

support drugs; they seldom consider that such therapy may have hidden harms for the patient, other patients and to the institution. For example, the latest antibiotics are often used; and apart from any risks of toxicity to already damaged organ systems, such drugs may cause resistant organisms to emerge and be passed on to other patients.[214] Because such drugs are often expensive they may drain the budget to the point that even the simple and cheap drugs may become unavailable in some institutions. Intravenous alimentation is essential to the recovery of most seriously ill patients, it is however expensive and its appropriateness may be questioned in cases in which treatment is judged to be futile.

Unlike discussions about surgical procedures, such decisions can seldom be shifted onto the patient or their relatives, for it would be unfair if not unethical to ask for them to bear the burden of shifting resources from others, or to feel responsibility for harm that might come to others. Therefore, these decisions are best guided by institutional guidelines and protocols, along with mechanisms to discuss decisions in individual cases.

In the case reports the patients have been judged to be ventilator-dependent. The patient in the first case report is said to be unconscious but is described as having spontaneous eye opening, and the patient in the second report is described as awake; there is no statement on the consciousness of the patient in the third report. In the three cases the prospects for recovery are poor and discussion should be initiated about the possibility and consequences of stopping the ventilator, as was done in the third case report.

• ***Should supportive therapy be withdrawn when there is no hope of recovery?***
When the terms 'withdraw' or 'withhold' are used in relation to therapy it should be when treatment is considered futile, and such action is expected to hasten death. When this consideration is given in relation to a patient who is conscious, it has implications that transcend a similar decision in an unconscious patient. It is therefore vital when treatment is deemed futile, that who makes that determination is clear that the state of consciousness of the patient is clearly defined.[215] There are three states of being that have to be considered - brain death, a persistent vegetative state and those who are neither.

Brain death is a diagnosis that is made using objective confirmatory

---

[214] Management of Multidrug-Resistant Organisms In Healthcare Settings, 2006; J D. Siegel, E Rhinehart, M Jackson, L Chiarello, CDC; https://www.premierinc.com/informatics/tools-services/safety/topics/guidelines/downloads/mdro-guideline-2006.doc
[215] Medical Futility in End-of-Life Care; AMA Opinion; JAMA. 1999; 281: 937-41

tests.[216] There is the absence of neurological activity and spontaneous respiration is not possible in a patient with a diagnosis of irrecoverable injury and the absence of drugs suppressing brain activity. These patients usually die within 72 hours of the diagnosis being confirmed, and 'withdrawal' of supportive measures may be initiated if it has been agreed that the patient will be an organ donor, or if the supportive ventilation equipment is required for a patient whose life can be saved. Patients who are brain dead can look remarkably normal and therefore both staff and relatives must be made aware of the patient's condition and how the diagnosis was confirmed, if they are not to feel that some wrong is being suggested or perpetrated.

A persistent vegetative state is one where there is sufficient cortical brain damage that there is no expectation of regaining consciousness.[217] However, there is sufficient central neurological activity that there may be spontaneous movement that may support unaided respiration. There are no confirmatory tests for this state and the diagnosis is made by excluding recoverable causes of a coma and ensuring over a period of time that recovery will not occur. Although withdrawal of ventilation support may hasten death through the development of pneumonia, it may not. Discussions and court actions have centred on whether it is ethical to withhold water and nutrition in order to hasten death.[218]

Decisions in such cases should be done with the support of the health care staff and the written informed consent of the next of kin or the person with a legal power of attorney. There is a view that withdrawal of life support measures in such cases amount to euthanasia, and doctors, relatives, institutions and community groups have petitioned courts against instituting such measures. Petitions to permit such withdrawals usually come from relatives when doctors have refused their requests to do so.[219]

The conscious patient. Consideration of the withdrawal of life support measures in a conscious patient may be looked on in the context of euthanasia, which applies to patients who are not considered to be dying.[220] Dying is a state in which the patient will cease to be alive in spite of all known therapies. There are no objective criteria for the

---

[216] The Diagnosis of Brain Death E F.M. Wijdicks, N Eng. J Med 2001; 344:1215-1221

[217] Medical Aspects of the Persistent Vegetative State; N Eng. J Med 1994; 330:1499-1508; http://www.nejm.org/doi/full/10.1056/NEJM199405263302107

[218] From Quinlan to Schiavo: medical, ethical, and legal issues in severe brain injury R L. Fine; Proc (Bayl Univ Med Cent). 2005; 18(4): 303–310

[219] Cruzan v. Director, Missouri Department of Health, (88-1503), 497 U.S. 261; 1990

[220] The Definition of Euthanasia; Beauchamp, T L.; Davidson, A I. Journal of Medicine and Philosophy 1979; 4 (3): 294–312

dying patient although most people feel they know what it is. States of consciousness may vary from the perception of consciousness, such as spontaneous eye opening, to the explicit statement of being awake. Wherever a patient is conscious enough to be rational, they should properly initiate any discussion on the matter of withdrawal of treatment rather than have it come from the staff or relatives.

There are other life sustaining treatments, which are not as dramatic as ventilation and include antibiotics, cardiovascular support drugs, food and water. The withdrawal of antibiotics is intended to let sepsis take its course and is not obviously distressing to the patient. However, it should be discussed with the patient and / or relatives and the staff in case there is a challenge about the standard of treatment being given.

The withdrawal of cardiovascular support drugs can be more dramatic and the decision should be made openly if one is to avoid a possible legal challenge. The withdrawal of nutritional support remains controversial and the expected effect of starvation is repugnant to most health care staff. It is a consideration that has reached the courts via a petition from relatives of patients in persistent vegetative states.

Patients have tried to exercise autonomy over their bodies and the manner of their dying by the execution of 'Living wills' or issuing 'advanced directives'. These are imperfect tools and are seldom honoured in an emergency where health care staff opt for the preservation of life; and even when they are aware of the Living will tend to play it safe by doing what they consider to be right. In non-emergency situations 'Living wills' may be resisted when they conflict with the moral or religious values of the staff that are asked to implement them.

Relatives or staff can raise objections to the provisions of a Living will and take the matter to the court. A Living will to be effective must therefore be drawn up with the willing consent of the responsible relative[s] and the physicians who will deal with the situation. If a doctor is presented with a living will and feels unable to carry out its requests, that should be conveyed to the patient, their relatives and the authorities in the institution right away.[221]

In the first case report the patient is unable to communicate and her husband has not raised the issue of withdrawing life support. If consideration is given to stopping ventilation, discussion with her next of kin should be initiated in a sensitive manner.

In the second case, the decision not to ventilate after surgery may have contributed to the respiratory arrest and resuscitation with ventilation. A

---

[221] Twenty-five years after Quinlan (1976): A review of Jurisprudence of Death and Dying; N Cantor, J. Law Medicine and Ethics 2001, Vol 29:2; 182-96

decision to withdraw ventilation whilst awake can make dying frightening and uncomfortable.[222]

In the third case, the mother would need counselling and access to independent advice before consenting to the suggested course of action. If the mother is unwilling, consideration should be given to finding resources to do ventilation at home.

• ***Should the patient be resuscitated if cardiac arrest occurs?***
Resuscitation is now the normal standard of care for a cardiac arrest and therefore any decision not to resuscitate is a judgment that must be made by the doctor in charge of the patient's care. When resuscitation started, doctors were accused of playing God; a similar accusation may now be raised if one does not resuscitate. Therefore, a decision to not resuscitate, should be discussed beforehand in suitable cases with the patient or their relatives, and, if necessary, their consent obtained for this course.

The decision should be made in consultation with staff and communicated to them, for in the absence of support from the staff the order may not be honoured.

In the first case report the patient appears to have satisfied the criterion of a persistent vegetative state and the patient's husband appears to be receptive to a discussion aimed at having his consent to a 'do not resuscitate' order.

In the second case it appears that such a decision was made but was not honoured.

In the third case discussion on the withdrawal of ventilation should include the question of making a 'do not resuscitate order'.

---

[222] Withdrawal of Ventilatory Support From the Dying Adult Patient; L Marr, D E. Weissman, J Support Oncol 2004; 2:283–288

Managing the Last Period of a Life

Case report 1:

A 75 year-old man, diagnosed with advanced dementia and depression, was admitted to hospital with pneumonia. He was treated with intravenous antibiotics and discharged back to the nursing home when his temperature had settled and the acute respiratory distress was over. Two weeks later he was readmitted dehydrated and with an aspiration pneumonitis. He was again treated with intravenous antibiotics and rehydrated. Five days after admission, the nursing staff, out of concern for the lack of food intake, passed a nasogastric tube. The patient became more anxious and tried to pull out the tube, but was restrained from doing so by tying his hands to the bed.

When the patient's relatives visited they requested to meet with the doctor and expressed concern about the patient's anxiety, asked for him to be sedated, for the feeding tube to be removed, and requested that there should be no resuscitative treatment should he have a cardiac arrest. The doctor requested the nurses to remove the tube and prescribed a sedative to be given when necessary. The nursing staff refused to remove the tube stating that they would not be party to starving the patient to death. The doctor removed the tube, but the patient remained agitated and the doctor enquired whether the sedative prescribed had been given. A nurse responded that the agitation was due to hunger, and "a sedative can't cure that". In the background a nurse was also heard to say 'Kunta Kinte, there wouldn't be a special conversation for regular people like us'.

The doctor decided in consultation with the nursing home to discharge the patient and manage the treatment of the patient there until he died.

Case report 2:

A 98-year-old woman is admitted to hospital for treatment of pneumonia. She is frail, mildly demented and diabetic. She was active up to three years ago when she had bilateral amputations for gangrenous feet. The pneumonia is treated successfully and she is discharged back home. Shortly thereafter she suffers what appears to be a stroke and is readmitted to the ward where it is concluded that her condition is due to dehydration. After being rehydrated her mental condition improves and she is discharged home in the care of her nurses. After consultation with her physician the home nurse inserts a feeding tube. The tube causes discomfort and after she made several attempts to pull it out, the nurse restrained her arms. After a while she stops resisting and becomes unresponsive. Her physician is called to see her and makes a diagnosis that she has aspirated. Her nearest relative, a niece of her late husband, calls from abroad whilst the doctor is present and is told what is happening and that her condition is unlikely to improve even with further hospitalization. In the ensuing conversation the doctor states that the only way to relieve her suffering is to withdraw the feeding tube, sedate her if necessary and allow her to die.

Issues raised

- ### *Terminal illness.*

A terminal illness leads to death. However, not all illnesses that result in death are designated terminal for they may be recoverable in some patients. Therefore terminal remains a matter of judgment as to the underlying condition and the resilience of the patient. Elderly patients are not usually as resilient as others, particularly those with poor nutrition, heart disease, disseminated malignancies or major organ damage.

Dying is a diagnosis of a state where death will occur in hours, days or weeks but not in months or years, it includes the diagnosis of brain death.[223] The management of an illness as terminal depends on the assessment of the physician undertaking the care. The physician's decision will depend on the acuteness of the illness and the ease with which is it normally treated. Acute infections are often treated with antibiotics before the terminal nature of the illness is determined. Acute surgical illness in the elderly such as limb fractures, subdural haematomas and intra-abdominal infections are usually treated after the assessment of the risks through the informed consent process. Wherever possible treatment of a patient who appears unlikely to recover should only be undertaken after taking into account the wishes of the patient or their family and the laws and customs in the community. The role of physicians in these situations continues to evolve.[224]

In the cases reported, the patients are mentally impaired and although the acute illnesses are recoverable, they are likely to recur because of the underlying mental condition and dependency. In the first case report, when the patient's treatment makes him uncomfortable, it is the family that initiates a discussion on the issues of comfort care and no resuscitation efforts.

---

[223] Diagnosing dying in the acute hospital setting - are we too late? Gibbins, J.; McCoubrie, R.; Alexander, N.; Kinzel, C.; Forbes, K.: Clinical Medicine, Journal of the Royal College of Physicians, Vol 9, No 2, 2009, pp. 116-119(4)
[224] Physicians and Futile care: Using Ethics Committees to Slow the Momentum T.A.Brennan Law Medicine and Health Care 1992; Vol.20: 4 pgs. 336-339

In the second case report, the physician recognising the futility of on-going treatment institutes terminal care.

- ### When should restraints be used?

Restraints should only be used on patients who are a danger to themselves or others. When restraint is used on agitated patients, it usually makes the patient more agitated.[225] A diagnosis of the reason for the agitation should be made and where possible treated.[226] Common causes of agitation are hypoxia due to a respiratory cause or to hypovolemic shock; what appears to be a successful restraint in those patients who stop being agitated may actually be because the condition has worsened.

In both of the cases described the patients were restrained to prevent them removing an uncomfortable therapeutic device. The cessation of their struggling may either be due to exhaustion or hypoxia from aspiration.

- ### Family conferences

When a patient is not mentally competent, the admitting professionals should ensure that they speak to the responsible family members about the likely outcome of the illness. They should try and discern if they or the patient had any strongly held views about the treatment that may be required, and the consequences of using or not using such treatment. Such conferences should not be seen as the final word, for at times circumstances, views and the patient's condition might change unexpectedly. In such conferences, the various professionals involved in the patient's care should be involved. There are some institutions that engage professional liaison officers to keep in contact and provide counselling for the family.

When an impasse develops between the family and the health care professionals, or between the professionals, there should be a confidential, impartial committee of persons with ethics experience and expertise that can advise and seek to break the impasse. When such situations cannot be resolved one or the other party may resort to the courts for a resolution of the conflict. There have been landmark cases on disagreements over the withdrawal of ventilation, and of artificial

---

[225] Use of restraints for patients in nursing homes; Guttman R, Altman RD, Karlan MS. Arch Fam Med. 1999 (2): 101-5

[226] Agitation in the Medically ill elderly; A.O.Aloa et al WAJM, 2005; 24,2, p 171-4 http://www.ajol.info/index.php/wajm/article/viewFile/28191/21978

feeding.[227] [228] In one country, there has been a statute passed that takes away the rights of the family to make decisions about the treatment of their mentally incompetent relatives, but the directives of the patient made when they were mentally competent should be respected.[229]

In the first case reported the patient is mentally incompetent because of dementia and the family acting as his surrogate requested that measures that appear to be causing him discomfort be discontinued even if it led to his earlier demise. The physician agrees with the family and orders that the offending nasogastric tube be removed, but the nursing staff show their disapproval and refuse to obey the order or the use of sedation.

In the second case there is no immediate family and the nurses consult with the treating physician whenever a problem occurs, and carry out the orders given.

- *Advanced directives and surrogate decisions.*

Individuals will state that they do not wish to die 'before their time is up', yet the spectacle of being unconscious on a ventilator with tubes everywhere, for months or even years is not their idea of living. On the other hand, health care professionals are trained to save lives, and advances towards that goal constantly come on stream. Therefore, there may be a tension between the use of tools by health professionals and the patient's desire for comfort and dignity towards the end of life.

The tension between the technology of keeping people alive and the desire to end one's life in comfort and dignity has led to several court battles and to change in legislation in some countries.[230] Laws banning euthanasia have changed in some countries, and legislation has been passed in some jurisdictions to allow patients or their surrogates to use advance directives about the care they do not wish to receive if incapacitated.[231] [232]

- *Policies re dying - nutrition, sedation.*

There is no clear definition of dying; it is a process that can take a variable time, with a variety of levels of self-awareness and acceptance of the process.[233] It is a time of heightened religious or family awareness for

---

[227] In re Quinlan, 355 A. 2d 647 - NJ: Supreme Court 1976. In The Matter Of Karen Quinlan, An Alleged Incompetent

[228] Cruzan v. Director, Missouri Department of Health, (88-1503), 497 U.S. 261 (1990)

[229] Mental Capacity Act 2005 - Legislation.gov.uk; www.legislation.gov.uk/ukpga/2005/9/contents

[230] Where Is Euthanasia Legal? | New Health Guide; www.newhealthguide.org

[231] Advance Directives: Medline Plus; https://www.nlm.nih.gov/

[232] Medical Futility: Legal and Ethical Aspects E. R. Grant; Law Medicine and Health Care, 1992; 20:4 pgs330-335

[233] The Last Stages of Life | Kokua Mau; www.kokuamau.org/resources/last-stages-life

some, and a time of withdrawal for others. A consistent factor is the sense of physical debility and dependence on others for care and help with basic needs. Basic comfort care includes being free of pain and the anxiety when one is dependent on others for such relief. An agitated patient, who is hypoxic and is sedated without the use of other measures to relieve the hypoxia, may have their death hastened; and a patient who is in pain and is given an analgesic without consideration of the risk profile of the patient may also be put at risk.[234]

Dying patients usually lose their appetite and need assistance with feeding. When the process is prolonged care-givers may become concerned about the nutritional state of the patient and may try appetite stimulants and the use of a nasogastric feeding tube.

These tubes can be difficult to pass in the conscious patient, are uncomfortable and can be associated with an aspiration pneumonitis. The alternative to a nasogastric tube is a percutaneous gastrostomy; however, this involves doing an endoscopy under sedation or anaesthesia to achieve this aim.[235]

In the cases reported, the nurses took the decision to pass a nasogastric tube to enhance the nutrition of the patient, and had to restrain the patient from pulling it out. In the first case reported the decision is taken without the physician's consent and when the decision is countermanded, the nurses undertake to disobey the physician in more than one respect.

In the second case reported the tube is inserted with the consent of the physician and the physician makes all the critical decisions when the patient's condition deteriorates.

- *Applicable law.*

In most countries there are no laws that speak to the process of dying. There are a few countries where statutes permit mentally competent patients with an irrecoverable illness to request their physicians to end their lives with medication.[236] Where the patient is mentally incompetent the law allows a patient when they were mentally competent, their next of kin, or a legally appointed surrogate to direct what treatment measures should not be given when they are dying.

---

[234] The Double Effect of Pain Medication: Separating Myth from Reality; S A FOHR, Journal of Palliative Medicine 1998; 1: 315-28

[235] Percutaneous endoscopic gastrostomy: Indications, technique, complications and management; A A Rahnemai-Azar, A A Rahnemaiazar, R Naghshizadian, A Kurtz, and D T Farkas World J Gastroenterol. 2014; 20(24): 7739–7751

[236] "Reporting of euthanasia and physician-assisted suicide in the Netherlands". Buiting H, van Delden J, Onwuteaka-Philpsen B; et al. BMC Med Ethics (2009). 10: 18. doi:10.1186/1472-6939-10-18. PMC 2781018. PMID 19860873

In the report given, the patient's family are concerned when they observe that their relative is suffering and request a meeting with the physician in charge. They reach an agreement that their relative should be allowed to die in comfort. The nursing staff defy the decision on the basis that removing the feeding tube would starve the patient to death.

- ### *Professional interaction.*

When important and possibly controversial decisions are being made, there should be interaction between all of the parties involved. The common differences between health care professionals and the family relate to the need for ventilation, nasogastric tubes and adequate pain relief. A family conference should involve the various professionals involved and the decisions made recorded and disseminated among the staff. Where differences of opinion persist, there should be a confidential mechanism such as an ethical committee that could hear the contending parties, and suggest solutions for the parties to adopt.[237] Where an agreed decision cannot be arrived at, the parties have recourse to the courts, which may rely on reports from independent sources.[238]

When treatment orders are deliberately disobeyed in spite of adequate communication, there should be an institutional disciplinary process that is responsive enough to ensure that the patient does not suffer. Such a process should be thorough enough to discover and remedy any biases that exist, biases such as racial, ethnic, social, religious or cultural.

In the first report given the nurses have placed a nasogastric tube on their own initiative and after it causes distress refuse to carry out orders when asked to remove it. The nurses also refuse to participate in a family conference, with one of them implying that such a conference would not have been held for ordinary black folk.

In the second case the tube is placed after consultation with the physician and the nurses comply with the physician's orders when it causes distress to the patient.

---

[237] Health and Human Values–Society for Bioethics Consultation Task Force on Standards for Bioethics Consultation; M P. Aulisio; R M. Arnold; S J. Youngner, Ann of Internal Medicine 2000, Vol. 133. No. 1

[238] "Report of guardian ad litem," for "In re: the guardianship of Theresa Schiavo, an incapacitated person, Case No. 90-2908GD-003" (PDF). Hospice Patients Alliance. pp. 2, 8–11

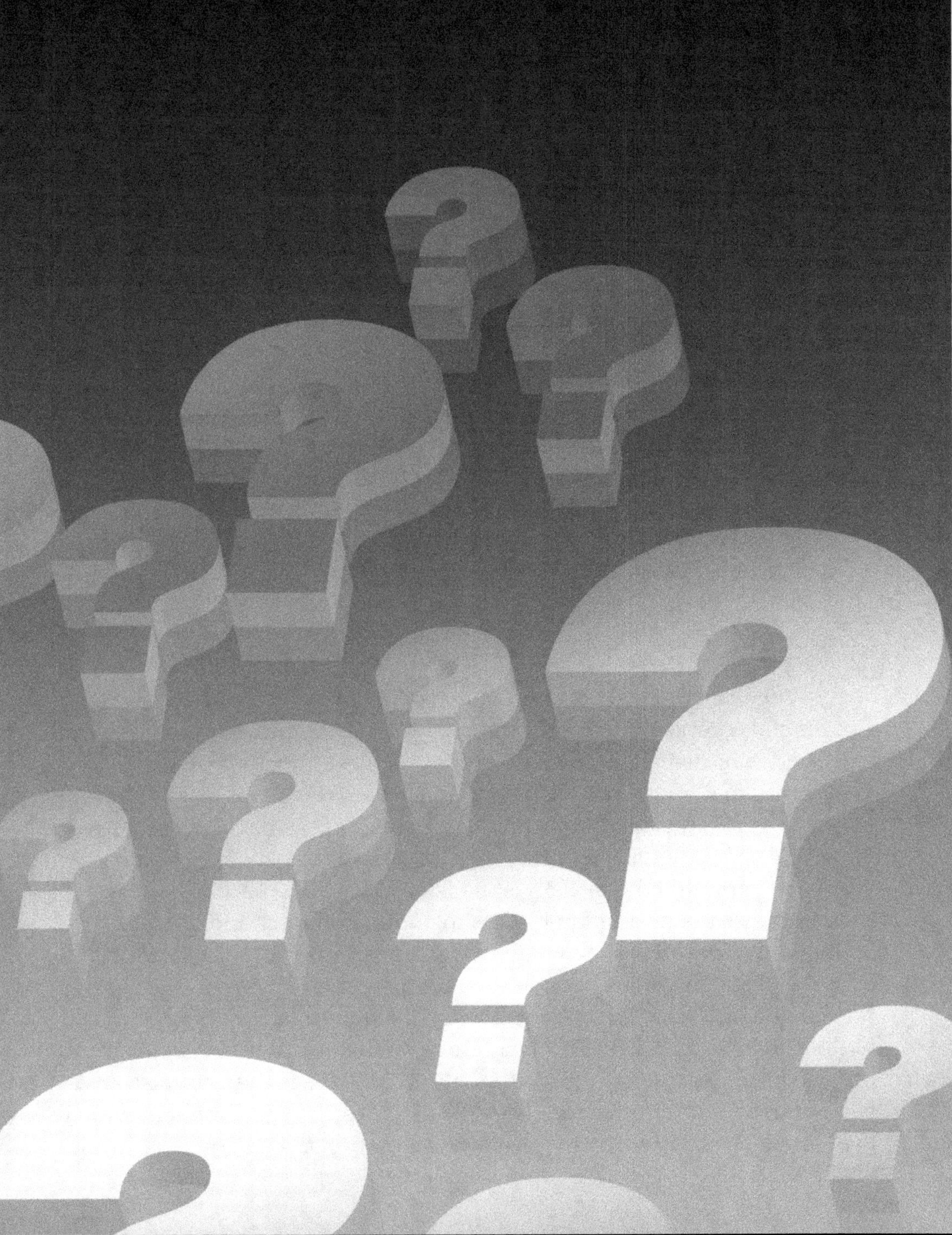

FUTILITY IN CARE

Futile Treatment

Case report:

An 85-year-old man was admitted complaining of abdominal pain, vomiting and distension of the abdomen. On examination he was fully conscious, vital signs were normal, but there was generalized abdominal tenderness with decreased bowel sounds. The full blood count, urea and electrolytes were normal. A differential diagnosis of acute diverticulitis or perforated appendicitis was made, and he was advised to have a laparotomy. His daughter was asked to sign the consent form and did so. At laparotomy, ischemia of the intra-abdominal organs was found - the intestines were dusky and there was a large quantity of altered blood in the peritoneum. The abdomen was closed without further intervention.

In the post-operative period the surgeon spoke to the patient's daughter and apprised her of her father's condition and prognosis. The patient was admitted to SICU and placed and maintained on a ventilator, total parenteral nutrition [TPN] and antibiotics. The biochemical parameters and haemodynamic status remained stable for one week after which his haemodynamic state deteriorated and required dopamine support. Ten days after surgery TPN, dopamine support and antibiotics were discontinued at the request of the relatives to 'let him die in peace'. Ventilator support continued and he had a cardiac arrest 14 days after surgery. Resuscitation efforts were instituted but were of no avail.

Issues raised

- ***Why was his daughter asked to sign the consent form?***
A mentally competent adult should sign their own consent form irrespective of their age. The patient may request the involvement of relatives in making their decision, in which case the relative could be used to witness the consent form of the patient. If the patient is confused or judged to be mentally incompetent the patient's next of kin or a previously appointed guardian is the legal consenting authority.

Sometimes the next of kin resides in another country and whilst the patient's condition may be discussed verbal consent should not be accepted over the phone but could be done by fax. Whatever consenting process is used, what is done for the patient should be clearly seen to be in the patient's best interest. Where there is no known or available next of kin, the legal guardian for institutionalised patients is the administrative head of the institution where the patient resides, or the hospital in which the patient is admitted. In an emergency situation the doctor responsible for the care of the patient can assume responsibility for the incompetent patient if other consent is not available.[239]

In the case described the man is said to be fully conscious, no other information is given about his mental state to justify asking his daughter to sign the consent form.

• ***Should the patient have been treated as an intensive care patient?***
A patient who undergoes surgery and the judgment is made that treatment is futile should be made comfortable and not seek to unduly prolong their life; measures such as parenteral nutrition, antibiotic therapy and circulatory support are not warranted. However, full supportive measures should be used if there is any uncertainty about the diagnosis or prognosis and a reassessment, including 'second look' surgery, made within 48 hours. The course of action decided upon should be noted and explained to all staff concerned in the care of the patient and to the patient's relatives.[240]

When a consensus is reached by the staff and the relatives, all supportive measures, including ventilation, could be removed to allow the patient to die. If no consensus can be reached and there are strong views on opposing courses of action, this can only be resolved by a court. However, recourse to the court is not desirable and disputes should be put before an ethical committee seeking reconciliation of viewpoints.

In the case report described, full supportive measures were employed in spite of an irrecoverable diagnosis being made. Why this is done is not stated and it is left to the relatives to plead for a stop to treatment. In spite of such pleas futile attempts at resuscitation were still carried out.

• ***Should the patient be taken off the ventilator in order to communicate?***
Any decision to take a patient off ventilation in circumstances judged to be futile must be made by treating physicians and conveyed to the patient's relatives. In situations of futility resources can be saved and it may allow a dying but conscious patient the opportunity to communicate with relatives. However, such decisions should only be made when the senior staff are involved and can take responsibility for the decision.[241]

In the situation described there appears to have been no consideration of taking the patient off the ventilator in spite of the observations made at operation.

---

[239] Assessment of Patients' Competence to Consent to Treatment; P S. Appelbaum, N Eng. J Med 2007; 357:1834-1840
[240] Medical Futility in End-of-Life Care; A Halevy, B A. Brody, R M. Tenery, JAMA. 1999; 281(10): 937-941
[241] Ethical Issues in End-of-Life Care; R M. Walker; http://moffittcancercenter.com/moffittapps/ccj/v6n2/article4.htm

- *Given the length of survival should the diagnosis have been
revised?*

A diagnosis of futility should be made on clear and irrefutable
observations. Health professionals may differ on their observations, and
on the length of time patients will survive.[242] Where there is doubt the
patient should be treated fully and further investigations or interventions
done to come to a clear conclusion.

*In the case reported the diagnosis of gangrenous bowel and hence the
diagnosis of futility should have been reviewed given the length of time of
survival. The senior person responsible for treating the patient should have
reviewed the diagnosis and taken such action as was considered necessary.*

- *Why was haemodynamic support started when the pressure
dropped?*

The use of haemodynamic support is part of the medication used when
one is trying to maintain life support. This is a decision that should be
made by the physicians in charge when the diagnosis is that there is no
prospect of recovery and the decision communicated to all staff. There
will be occasions when staff or relatives, particularly those with some
kind of health background, request such supportive measures. Such
requests should be granted while the futility of the patient's condition is
still being discussed. If necessary, the assistance of an ethical committee
should be obtained if discussions remain inconclusive. If the next of kin
adamantly objects to the withdrawal of support in an obviously futile
situation only the court can override their decision. When such situations
are not resolved early court action should only be entertained if the
ventilator is urgently needed for a patient with a chance of recovery.

*In the situation described in the case report there is no suggestion that the
diagnosis was revised and haemodynamic support should not be undertaken.
However, it appears that no clear decision of futility had been made or conveyed
to staff.*

- *What influenced the decision to withdraw supportive measures?*

Withdrawal of support measures is usually done when a consensus is
reached that further treatment is futile. Withdrawal of ventilator support
would be the final act in a dying patient; however, medical and nursing
staff are often reluctant to take this final step. In jurisdictions where there

---

[242] Medical futility: Predicting outcome of intensive care unit patients by nurses and
doctors — A prospective comparative study; S Frick; D E. Uehlinger; R M. Zuercher Zenklusen;
Crit Care Med 2003 Vol. 31, No. 2 http://med.stanford.edu/neuroethics/documents/
medicalfutilitypredictingoutcome.pdf

is a legal definition of brain death, staff are legally empowered to stop all treatment, and may make this decision more readily.[243] There are several instances that have gone to the courts where doctors and relatives have disagreed over the withdrawal of support in patients with persistent vegetative states; the tendency in the courts is to follow what is deemed to be the prior wishes of the patient. In the Quinlan case a suit was brought by the relatives to require doctors to withdraw ventilator support and allow the patient to die.[244] A similar request was made in relation to nutritional support in the Cruzan case in 1990.[245] In both instances the decisions were the subject of appeals and reverses with the eventual outcome of the relatives having prevailed.

It appears from the narrative given that the withdrawal of supportive measures was made at the request of the relatives. Ventilator support was continued probably due to the reluctance of staff, for resuscitation attempts were made when cardiac arrest did occur.

- ***Why were resuscitative measures employed?***

The institution of resuscitative measures is routine in modern medical practice. When a decision has been made and agreed upon, a 'do not resuscitate' [DNR] order may be given. Even when made, a DNR order may be ignored if all of the staff have not been informed or have been convinced that it is the right thing to do. When not fully consulted or convinced staff will ignore a 'do not resuscitate order' and do all they can to protect themselves from possible legal challenge and argue about the 'paper orders' after.

In the case presented there has been ambivalence by the staff on the outcome in the case and the issues had not been thought through and the staff given clear instructions.

---

[243] Medical and legal considerations of brain death, T. T. Randell, Acta Anaest Scand, Vol 48, 2, p139–144, 2004

[244] Quinlan 70 N.J. 10, 355 A.2d 647 ,NJ 1976

[245] Cruzan v. Director, Missouri Department of Health, (88-1503), 497 U.S. 261 (1990)

Discontinuing Life-support

Case report:

A 45-year-old woman travelling on a cruise ship in the Caribbean with her husband, his extended family, her daughter and the daughter's boyfriend, was admitted unconscious to hospital in an island when the ship docked. She had a history of treatment for depression, and the previous day her husband had died while snorkelling in the previous island visited. The patient and the family had decided to continue on the cruise, leaving the husband's body in the island where he died. Approximately one hour after the cruise ship left the port, the patient was found hanging in her cabin's bathroom.

The ship's medical personnel reported that she had been intubated and resuscitated for approximately 22 minutes, before spontaneous circulation returned. The patient was kept in the ship's infirmary and transferred as soon as the ship docked.

The patient was admitted to the Intensive Care Unit, where she required pressor support. No cervical spine injury was found on x-ray. The patient was noted to have fixed dilated pupils, but no other criteria for a diagnosis of brain death. During discussion with the patient's daughter, a registered nurse, she expressed the view of "not prolonging her mother's suffering". She said that she understood that her mother likely would have suffered anoxic brain injury, and in light of that she requested that the managing team discontinue the pressor support. She also requested that her mother get a CT scan of her brain prior to terminating support "just in case the CT showed any potentially treatable pathology". The patient's daughter was the only family member who remained in the island, the remainder of the family (the deceased husband's relatives) continued on the cruise. The patient was airlifted to her home state in the USA three days after admission still requiring minimal pressor support.

Issues raised

- *Was there information on why the family decided to continue the cruise?* This information is important in deciding the state of mind of the patient and of her daughter who has to make critical decisions in the situation. The factors that impinge on these decisions relate to previous relationships; the jurisdiction's regulations in regards to sudden deaths and moving bodies between countries; the cost to cancel the cruise and any health or travel insurance available.

These questions do not appear to have been asked but the circumstances of the husband's death almost certainly meant an inquest would have to be held and that would take time before the body could be released. The cruise ship will not delay its departure and the family probably had to make critical and emotional decisions in a short time-framework.

- ### Is there information as to events around the discovery of the hanging?

This is important in determining the patient's state of mind and whether any intervention by the family or the ship personnel could have stopped the incident.[246] The information is important from a medical prognostic viewpoint or any police investigation.

The patient was apparently very distressed and thought 'to be in need of constant support'. Relatives were with her when she went to the bathroom, and it was some time before suspicions were aroused and she was discovered hanging.

- ### Was information given on any assessment after resuscitation?

It is important to get information on the treatment given after resuscitation of a cardiac arrest in coming to a better assessment of the extent of the neurological damage and any deterioration or progress in the intervening period. This will help to determine the prognosis and decisions on treatment.[247]

There was no further information given as to the neurological state after resuscitation. The conclusion appears to be that there is severe anoxic brain damage, probably the result of hanging and the cardiac arrest.

- ### What other neurological criteria were looked at?

It is important to determine whether brain stem death has occurred, for it can be stated without equivocation that there will be no recovery and a number of decisions can be made by the family, particularly in relation to further medical treatment and possible organ donation. The criteria for brain death are quite specific to make an assessment.[248]

The statement was made that there were no other criteria of brain death. Accepting that assessment the best one can expect with the evidence of severe hypoxic damage is that the patient may go on to a persistent vegetative state.

---

[246] What physicians can do to prevent suicide D J. Muzina Cleveland Clinic Journal Of Medicine Vol 71; 3; 2004 http://ccjm.org/content/71/3/242.full.pdf

[247] Hypoxic-ischemic brain injury: Evaluation and prognosis G L Weinhouse, G B Young, http://www.uptodate.com/contents/hypoxic-ischemic-brain-injury-evaluation-and-prognosis

[248] The Diagnosis of Brain Death, E. F.M. Wijdicks, N Eng. J Med 2001; 344:1215-1221

- *What decision was made after cessation of life support was requested?*

Until a clear determination of the neurological status is reached, it is unwise to make any irrevocable decisions. The diagnosis of brain death should be made over a period of 48 hours, and a persistent vegetative state over a period of six weeks. This is particularly important where the neurological injury has occurred in circumstances where someone may be held liable for the injury; this includes the physicians at different points in the treatment given.

Decisions taken by surrogates can be challenged both in discussion and if necessary in court. They can be most successfully challenged when the decision cannot be shown to be in the best interest of the patient.[249] Institutions have also challenged decisions on withdrawing life support on the basis that they are not in the best interest of the institution itself and health care.[250]

It must also be recognised that in recent traumatic or catastrophic illness events, relatives of the patients may be overwrought and may not be in the best state to make irrevocable decisions; indeed they should be encouraged to take time and reflect before making their decision.[251] This has important considerations in the relationships between doctors and the patient's relatives if any legal actions were brought in the future.

It is clear from the report given that no cognisance was given to the daughter's request to discontinue pressor support. It seems clear that the daughter was in no fit state to make an irrevocable decision at that time.

- *Is another CT scan consistent with discontinuing pressor support?*

It is natural that in sudden tragic severe illness or injury, the patient's next of kin and other close relations would be confused and inconsistent in their thoughts and decisions. Doctors need to be conscious of inconsistencies that arise, but should not be dismissive of the legal rights of a patient's next of kin. Time spent to deal with inconsistencies should lead to more rational decision-making and avoid accusations of neglect of the patient.

In the narrative given there is no mention of the interactions that occurred, but events suggest that a state of consensus was reached between the daughter and the doctors.

---

[249] In the best interest of the patient. Applying this standard to healthcare decision-making must be done in a community context; Trau JM, McCartney JJ. Health Prog. 1993; 74(3): 50-6

[250] Cruzan v. Director, Missouri Department of Health, (88-1503), 497 U.S. 261 (1990)

[251] Surrogate Decision-making to End Life-sustaining Treatments for Incapacitated Adults; C. M. Hayes; Journal of Hospice and Palliative Nursing, 2003; Vol 5:2, 91 - 102

- *Was any interview of the other 'family' members done before they left?*
This has relevance in being able to assess the circumstances leading to the
patient's condition, and to the state of mind of the next of kin in making
crucial decisions. The sudden death of one relative, the near death of
his wife, and the relatives simply moving along on their cruise is not a
normal reaction, but cannot be assumed to be sinister.

*There were no enquiries made of the relatives by the doctors. The police may
have an interest in the events that occurred and keeping the patient alive should
remain a priority lest one be accused of facilitating the commission of a felony.*

- *What is the best prognosis for the patient?*
The prognosis is important in projecting the kind of advice that will be
given to the next of kin, as well as how far one is willing to comply with
any expressed wishes. In patients with severe brain injury the important
decision that has to be made is whether brainstem death has occurred
and what is the best treatment to preserve brain function.[252] If brain death
is excluded the questions are whether there will be some functional
recovery or will the patient go into a persistent vegetative state. The
latter diagnosis cannot be made until after a period of six weeks or more,
and is a state where the patient has progressed from a coma to a state of
wakefulness without detectable awareness.[253]

*From the limited information available it appears that a persistent vegetative
state is the best prognosis possible. Therefore, decisions about terminating
resuscitative measures would be premature without the kinds of enquiry into what
the patient's wishes might be if she were to be in a persistent vegetative state.*

- *Should an attempted suicide be indicative of wishes re resuscitation?*
Suicide is an illegal act which should not be facilitated by the profession,
just as euthanasia should not be performed where it is illegal.[254] The
profession tries to save the lives of persons who attempt suicide and
provide them with treatment; therefore an attempted suicide should not
be regarded as the prior wishes of a patient in relation to resuscitative
measures. A dilemma may occur if the patient obtains an enforceable
living will against resuscitation.[255]

---

[252] Treatment of comatose survivors of out-of-hospital cardiac arrest with induced hypothermia.
Bernard SA, Gray TW, Buist MD, Jones BM, Silvester W, Gutteridge G, Smith K; N Eng. J Med. 2002;
346(8): 557

[253] Medical aspects of the persistent vegetative state (1). The Multi-Society Task Force on PVS. N Eng.
J Med 1994; 330:1499

[254] Suicide attempts and resuscitation dilemmas. Karlinsky H, Taerk G, Schwartz K, Ennis J, Rodin G.
Gen Hosp Psychiatry. 1988; 10(6): 423-30

[255] Saving Life or Respecting Autonomy: The Ethical Dilemma of DNR Orders in Patients Who
Attempt Suicide Cynthia M. A. Geppert; The Internet Journal of Law, Healthcare and Ethics ISSN:
1528-8250

In the report cited the attempted suicide is as yet no more than hearsay and the health professionals should avoid making decisions that are properly those of the court. Therefore resuscitative and life support measures should be continued in spite of any expressed wishes of the next of kin.

Case report:
A 15-year-old boy presented to Accident and Emergency with a two-week history of discolouration of the toes following a trauma event. He had previous diagnoses of Rubenstein Taybi Syndrome, nephrotic syndrome, blindness from glaucoma, cognitive impairment and bilateral common iliac artery thrombosis. He had been seen twice by his GP prior to admission, and treatment with ice packs and $MgSO_4$ dressings was advised. On examination it was noted that the lower limb pulses were absent on the left and weak on the right. He was seen by the surgical service and taken directly to operating theatre. Bilateral femoral artery embolectomies were done with a fasciotomy on the left leg, and he was placed on a heparin infusion. Flow was not maintained on the left and with a mottled cold limb the decision was made to do an above knee amputation.

After amputation he was noted to have DIC, septic shock and hypoglycaemia. These were appropriately treated but investigations showed multi-organ failure. He had a seizure and deteriorated with episodes of apnoea and bradycardia; these were treated with adrenaline and he was intubated and ventilated.

The child's mother was updated about the events and advised of the child's poor clinical state and the plan for escalation of management including plasma, albumin, pressors, antibiotic changes, CVP placement and further resuscitation if required. She stated that she wanted to wait to discuss the case with the child's father. At a meeting with both parents and the treatment team, the parents decided that their son was suffering unduly and they wanted no further interventions. The consultant paediatrician counselled the parents and asked them to reconsider but they refused all forms of medical support for their child. The child became progressively unstable, eventually arrested and died.

Issues raised

- *Irrecoverable illness*

An irrecoverable illness is one where all known methods of treatment cannot prevent the death of the patient, permanent serious disability or ill health. In making such an assessment, one should know the natural history of the illness, the pre-morbid state of the patient, their previous illnesses, and their family and social history.

The issues in the irrecoverably ill include determining what the standard of care is and how this should vary with particular patients and existing circumstances. These include:
- the use or cessation of life support,
- the benefit vs. harm of narcotic analgesia,
- the quality of the life,
- whether a living will should be executed,
- handling thoughts of suicide and attempted suicide and
- within applicable law the possibility of euthanasia.

In the case as reported, there is information about the child's condition but nothing about the family and social history. It is clear that the child had a poor quality of life and with the possible loss of both limbs, the demands on his parents will increase substantially.

- ### *Who determines the quality of a life?*

Many persons including patients make a determination of the quality of a patient's life. The consequences of that determination and the decisions that follow will vary.

Physicians make decisions about the quality of life of a patient, and when the assessment is poor, thoughts may turn to 'do not resuscitate' orders. However, such decisions are seldom made where the illness presents as an emergency and physicians feel that one further measure will get the patient over the emergency. Patients and their guardians are least equipped emotionally to deal with difficult decisions in emergency situations.

Patients faced with making a decision about a poor quality of life usually cling to life and seek solace in their religion. However, there are those who despair and may think of suicide or seek help in terms of making a living will, and a few may make a request for euthanasia. Minors who are mentally competent are not usually allowed to make such decisions although they should be heard; even in a jurisdiction where minors can consent to their own treatment they are not allowed to refuse recommended treatment.[256]

When relatives, parents or guardians are required to make consent decisions where treatment may appear futile, they are faced with making a request to not resuscitate or stop treatment on their charge. Such decisions are not easily made, particularly in emergency situations. The patient who has executed a living will gives guidance to their surrogate, but in most instances a surrogate has to make the decision based on

---

[256] Family Law Reform Act 1969 UK; http://www.legislation.gov.uk/ukpga/1969/46

what they see as being in the best interest of their charge. This is a multi-faceted decision-making process and requires the best advice of health care professionals, the counselling of friends and religious leaders, and the provision of opportunities to discuss with ethicists who would not normally be available to them. When relatives have come to decisions not to treat, health care professionals have often resisted them and the cases may end up in court when both sides remain adamant in their positions. These kinds of court cases have resulted in landmark judgments in favour of the relatives' judgment as to what the patient would have wished, from removing the patient from the ventilator to stopping nutritional support.[257] These landmark judgments on patients in persistent vegetative states came from protracted court proceedings and could not be applied in acute situations. However, most jurisdictions have an emergency judicial process and it is likely that under such circumstances a judge would opt for the argument that offers the chance of life.

In the report presented, the doctors caught up in the treatment of an emergency were not prepared to give up on life, and disagree with the parents' decision to request no further measures, but are not prepared to challenge them. This may be because the quality of life was known to be very poor and the parents had been exemplary care-givers.

- *Responsibilities to the incapacitated patient*

An incapacitated patient has their family as the persons with prime responsibility for their welfare. The care that can be delivered by a family is determined by the resources, both human and material, available to them. When it comes to making crucial decisions about the care of the mentally incapacitated patient, a surrogate should respect the express prior wishes of their relative and always act in their relative's best interests, not their own.

A physician is expected to act in the best interest of the patient and any other patients who may be affected. In doing so they will see their first obligation as the preservation of life and the diminution of functional damage. All actions should be based on the best available evidence, taking into account the available resources.

The community's responsibility for those who are incapacitated is exercised through the laws protecting the rights, interests and beliefs of the individual and the community, and through specific laws to protect and assist persons with disabilities.[258]

---

[257] From Quinlan to Schiavo: medical, ethical, and legal issues in severe brain injury R L. Fine; Proc (Bayl Univ Med Cent). 2005; 18(4): 303–310
[258] Americans with Disabilities Act 1990; Title 42, chapter 126, Amend 2008 (P.L. 110-325), http://www.ada.gov/pubs/ada.htm

In the child whose illness was presented, the physicians have provided all the therapeutic care available and his survival would have needed additional resources for his care at home. There is nothing said about the support that the community can give a severely disabled child and should be factored into the decisions made.

- ### *Futility in medical care*

Futility in medical care is carrying out therapeutic measures that are useless in preserving life, useful function, relieving suffering or other symptoms.[259] Measures for the relief of symptoms should bring comfort to the patient and to their relatives. Physicians faced with life-threatening emergencies or apparently uncontrollable disease, may feel that something more can be achieved through intensifying treatment and applying additional measures. When such treatments fail, they are often thought of as being futile. When there is an unexpected favourable result, factors such as an unusual characteristic of the patient or the intervention of a deity are given the credit, unless the treating doctors can show that the result is a statistically valid result.

Today's futility is sometimes tomorrow's advance, and extending knowledge may have to be done against conventional wisdom, but in a calculated research manner. Therefore, an important tool in advocating measures thought by others to be futile is to be able to demonstrate any research data on the efficacy of the measures proposed. Alternatively, the doctor should show that what is being proposed is part of a research protocol, requiring the informed consent of the patient or their surrogate.[260]

In the report given there appears to have been no attempt to convince the parents that the measures being taken had any chance of success. This gave the distinct impression that the physicians themselves considered the measures futile.

- ### *The ethics of futility*

Therapeutic measures that may be futile should meet the ethical standards of beneficence, non-malfeasance, justice and autonomy. In difficult situations, beneficence and non-malfeasance are not simply two sides of a coin; for example, drugs used for the relief of pain may have serious side effects in the dosage required. The cost of the measures proposed might outstrip the resources the patient is able to raise, personally or through insurance mechanisms.

---

[259] When Is Medical Treatment Futile? D L Kasman; J Gen Intern Med. 2004; 19(10): 1053–1056
[260] 'Medico-legal aspects of Informed Consent' L.M. Nova, R.J. Rembert; Neurological clinics 1998; 16; No.1

When high costs are the path to life, it raises the spectre of whether justice is being done. In resource poor situations, the costs and complexity of the proposed treatment also raises issues of allocation of resources, both material and human. When allocation of resources becomes a major issue, the question of justice is an issue, not just for the patient directly involved but also for other patients. The standard of care by the professionals also comes under scrutiny when it fails to meet community expectations.

Community expectations are often expressed as values and these may be projected in both positive and negative ways. In meeting community expectations health professionals should reflect positive values to patients, their relatives, other staff and to the community as a whole. This is usually seen in emergency situations where health professionals will work long hours on difficult tasks to save lives.

Decision-making in emergencies has its drawbacks in that the immediate problem may be tackled but other problems remain unresolved. This becomes a reality when there is no opportunity to share decision-making among staff, relatives, religious counsel, ethicists and other advisors. Several factors affect decision-making, sometimes in sub-conscious ways; these include age, race, ethnicity, gender, social status and the pre-existing quality of life. Such factors are more apparent to some than others, particularly when there is an unsatisfactory outcome and a dispute arises.

In the report presented, there appears little doubt that the pre-existing quality of life would have a bearing on the parent's decision to discontinue treatment.

• *The legal parameters of futility decisions*
Some decisions that are made in situations of futility are in legal statutes or precedent. These include decisions arising out of brain death;[261] the withdrawal of ventilator support;[262] and the withdrawal of nutritional support.[263] These decisions were largely determined by the court establishing what the prior wishes of the incapacitated patient were, either through testimony or the execution of a living will.[264] In one jurisdiction, the law has taken away the decision rights of a next of kin for an incapacitated adult, unless the patient had previously executed a power of attorney to make such decisions on their behalf.[265]

[261] Diagnosis of Brain Death, Lancet 1976 ii 1069-70
[262] Quinlan 70 N.J. 10, 355 A.2d 647 ,NJ 1976
[263] Cruzan v. Director, Missouri Department of Health, (88-1503), 497 U.S. 261 (1990)
[264] Kutner, L. The Living Will: a proposal. Indiana Law Journal. 1969;44 (1):539-554
[265] Mental Capacity Act, UK 2005 http://www.legislation.gov.uk/ukpga/2005/9/schedule/3

Treating a patient without lawful consent could lead to a charge
of battery; on the other hand a decision not to treat or to withdraw
treatment can lead to an accusation of negligence or criminal neglect, if
such omission is carried out without communication with relations as
well as staff. Technical knowledge should not be exercised without taking
into account other intangibles in applying it to a particular person.[266]

- *Institutional guidelines and initiatives*

Institutions may have to bear legal responsibilities when difficult issues
arise and physicians and patients or surrogates have irreconcilable
differences. Administrators may be called upon to act as guardians when
none exist but must be wary of taking critical care decisions that conflict
with the professional staff.

Institutional guidelines and protocols provide legal protection
provided they are professionally derived, agreed upon and fit in with
the general professional standards of care in the jurisdiction.[267] Such
instruments should be subject to periodic peer review. A review process
should be open to all staff that may be involved and conducted in such a
manner that the proceedings of case reviews remain confidential.[268]

---

[266] The Concept of Medically Indicated Treatment F G. Miller J Med Philos (1993) 18 (1): 91-98. doi:
10.1093/jmp/18.1.91
[267] Reporting and preventing medical mishaps: lessons from non-medical near miss reporting systems
P Barach, S D Small, BMJ. 2000 March 18; 320(7237): 759–763
[268] Peer review committees--composition, purpose--immunity from civil liability, who, when-
-disclosure of records prohibited, exceptions--testimony before, discovery and admissibility,
limitations. Missouri Revised Statutes; Ch 537 Torts and Actions for Damages, Section 537.035, 2012
http://www.moga.mo.gov/statutes/C500-599/5370000035.HTM

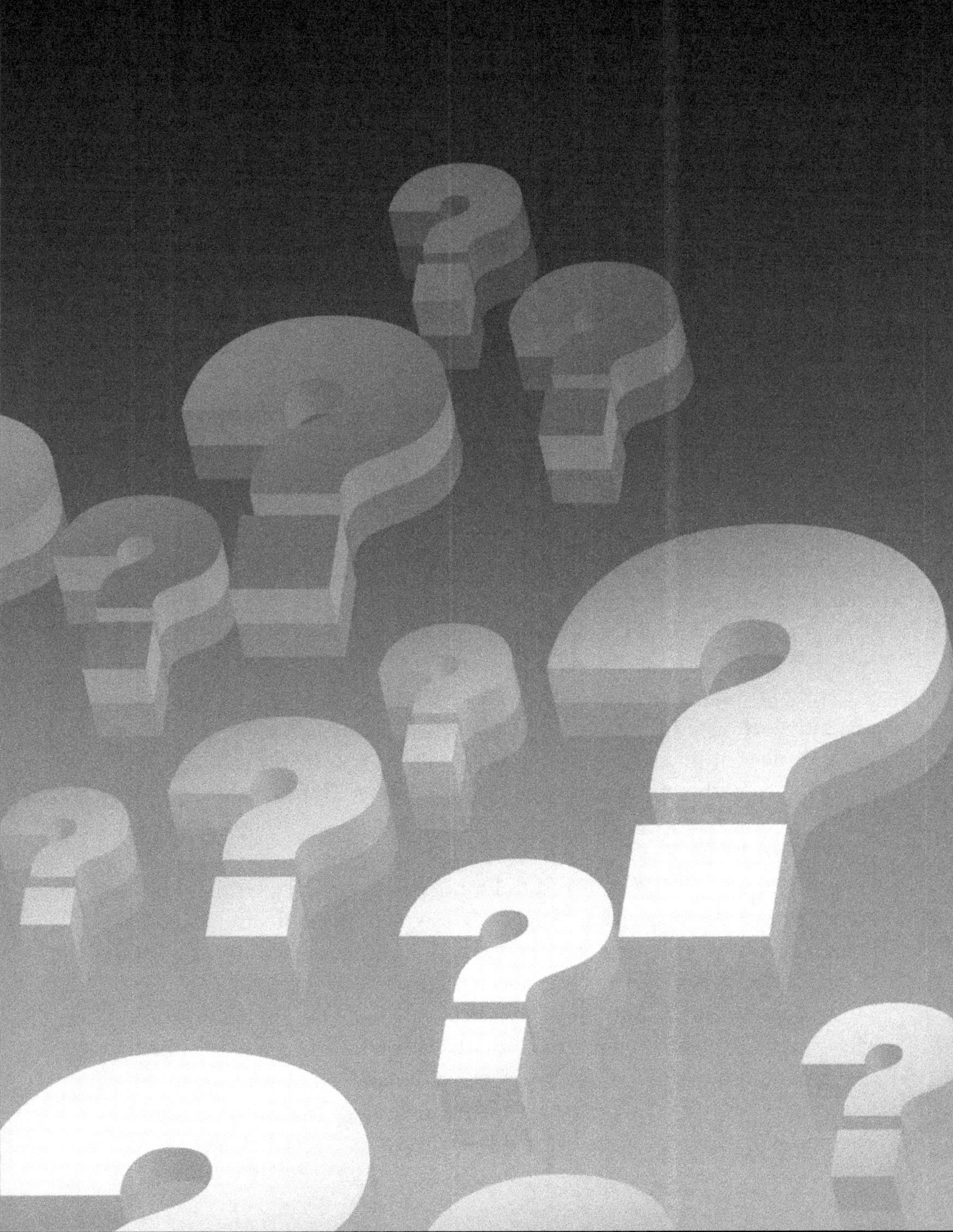

PROFESSIONAL CONDUCT
AND RISKS

Case report 1:

A patient is admitted two days before surgery to ensure that her diabetes and hypertension are well controlled. When seen by the surgeon she complained of an irritating dry cough that had not responded to the medicine recommended. On examination, her respiratory and cardiovascular systems were normal as were the chest x-ray and ECG. The surgeon tells the patient he will ask a consultant physician to see her.

The surgeon rings a physician [Dr Bentley] who agrees to see the patient later that day; the consultation request is written in the patient's notes. The following morning, the surgeon is told by the nurse that Dr Bentley called and said that she was unable to see the patient as arranged but would see her later that day. The surgeon apologized to the patient and remarked that he hoped that the physician sees her before the anaesthetist does. Some hours later Dr Bentley called the surgeon and said that she went to see the patient but was told by the nurse that another doctor had already seen the patient and prescribed medication. The surgeon expressed surprise that the anaesthetist had seen the patient so early, and thanked Dr Bentley for coming nevertheless. Shortly thereafter, the surgeon received a call from the nurse stating that she could not understand what the order for treatment was or who signed it. After a moment the nurse said that another nurse told her that the resident to Dr Grayson the physician wrote it.

The surgeon asked the nurse to have the resident call him. The resident called and said he was asked by his consultant to see the patient urgently and had done so. The surgeon then asked to speak to Dr Grayson urgently, who said that the patient's husband had called him and "out of the kindness of his heart he offered to help". Dr. Grayson said he would go and rectify the matter and ask Dr. Bentley to continue the patient's care.

Case report 2:

A family practitioner is referred to Dr Moses for surgery with a diagnosis of a benign gastrointestinal tumour. Dr Moses sees his colleague, suggests that the surgery is best done by laparoscopy and recommends that Dr Brody do it. Dr Brody agrees over the telephone to do the surgery and requests Dr Moses to prepare the patient to be admitted on the day of the operation. Dr Moses makes the arrangements and after admission, Dr Brody comes to see the patient, introduces himself and states that some of the equipment is not working properly so he proposes to do the surgery by the open method. The patient agrees to go ahead and the surgery is done that day.

On the second day post-op the patient has a high fever and complains of pain all over the abdomen. The nurse calls Dr Moses who advises that Dr Brody who did the surgery be called. Dr Brody is called and he states 'Get my resident to arrange a CT and I will come and see him when it is back'. The CT is arranged and the radiology consultant rings Dr Brody and states that the patient has air under both diaphragms, as well as a pocket of air and fluid in the left side of the abdomen. Dr Brody asks the radiologist to put in a percutaneous drain into the pocket on the left side. The radiologist remarks that this would not deal with all that he is seeing, but places the drain. Whilst writing the notes the radiologist notices that Dr Moses is the admitting doctor, rings him and expresses his concern that the patient needs an operation. Dr Moses states that he did not do the operation and will not interfere. The radiologist rings Dr Frank, another surgeon, and after discussing the case says the patient "called his name as someone he would like to do any further surgery". Dr Frank responds that he would be willing to help but he would have to get a consultation request from the patient through Dr Brody. The next day Dr Frank responds to another call stating that he has not heard from Dr Brody as yet.

Case report 3:
An 85-year-old woman presented with an incarcerated incisional hernia. She was counselled and advised to have surgery to relieve the obstruction. The risks of bowel strangulation, perforation and peritonitis were explained but the patient insisted that she did not want surgery under any circumstances even if this refusal led to her death. Her daughter was present and agreed that her mother's wishes should be respected, as this was the position she had held for quite some time. No questions were raised regarding the patient's competence to make her decision, and she was treated with analgesia, nasogastric tube decompression and intravenous fluid resuscitation.

During the time in hospital, other relatives voiced concern at her decision and requested a meeting to discuss it. During their visit she was briefly obtunded by a hypoglycaemic episode. A remark was made within the relatives' earshot by a surgeon from another team that 'since her clinical state had changed and she could no longer make decisions for herself, surgery should be offered with the relatives giving consent.' The hypoglycaemia was successfully treated and a CT scan showed that the bowel in the hernia sac enhanced normally, indicating its viability. When she returned to her baseline state she again refused surgery. Her relatives were updated on her state and told that the surgical team would honour her wishes. The hernia was reduced manually with resolution of her symptoms and she was discharged from hospital.

Issues raised

- ***Are the consultations professional?***

Consultation is an opinion obtained from a colleague with the consent of the patient. This is done routinely with the reporting of investigations and applies to other teamwork. Consultations carry no implication of taking over treatment unless explicitly stated but they do have medical-legal implications.[269] When patients are admitted to hospital it should be clear who is the physician in charge of the patient, and if there is to be joint care, that the roles are clearly distinguished for the health care staff.

Patients, relatives or friends who are not familiar with the code of conduct of the medical profession may try to initiate consultations without the knowledge of their principal physician. A recipient of such a request should explain the protocol and ask the patient or relative to inform their physician of their request or offer to do so.

When consultations are made to take over or undertake joint treatment, this should be made explicit to the patient and in the record. When joint treatment is being undertaken joint decisions should be made wherever possible.[270]

Practitioners should ensure that consultations sought are necessary and avoid the perception that consultations are being done in order to expand the business of partners. It is unprofessional, and in some jurisdictions illegal, to pay a fee to a physician or other health professional for sending a patient to you for consultation/treatment.[271]

Patients may be afraid of causing offence when they want a second opinion; however, second opinions are best done with the cooperation of the primary physician.[272] Direct communication between professionals leads to better outcomes for intangibles are better dealt with. Therefore, physicians should not offer a second opinion on a hospitalised patient without the knowledge and cooperation of the admitting physician.

---

[269] "Curbside" Consultation and Informal Communication in Medical Practice: A Medicolegal Perspective. B C. Fox, M L. Siegel, and R A. Weinstein 1996... www.jstor.org/stable/4459680
[270] Guide To Enhancing Referrals And Consultations Between Physicians; 2009; Coll. Fam. Phys. Can. and Roy. Coll. Phys. Surg. Can. http://www.cfpc.ca/uploadedFiles/Directories/_PDFs/Ref-Consult_Guide_new_title%20FINAL%20RCPSC%20(2). pdf
[271] Medical Professions Act 2011-1, sect 23(2)(g); Laws of Barbados
[272] AMA Code of Medical Ethics » Opinion 8.041 - Second Opinions http://www.ama-assn.org/ama/pub/physician-resources/medical-ethics/code-medical-ethics/opinion8041.page

It is natural to be concerned about a patient who is a friend or relative; however, this should not be allowed to cloud one's judgment or breach the appropriate lines of communication between colleagues.

In the first case reported the surgeon in charge of the patient has arranged for a consultation with a physician colleague. The consultation does not take place at the stated time and the patient's husband asked another physician to see his wife. That physician made arrangements for the patient to be seen and this is only discovered when the nurses could not decipher a prescription written. When confronted with the impropriety Dr Grayson states that he was only responding to the husband's appeal for help.

In the second case report, Dr Moses, who was asked to treat a colleague, recommended another surgeon, Dr Brody, to do the procedure by laparoscopy. Dr Brody, without seeing the patient, agrees to do the procedure; arrives on the morning of the operation and states that the laparoscopic equipment is not working but he would proceed with the operation. Two days later there is a complication, and when Dr Moses is called, as the admitting physician, he says that he is not responsible. Dr Brody, without seeing the patient, arranges for an investigation to be done and when called by the radiologist requests the radiologist to insert a drain, adding that he will see the patient later. The radiologist thinks the patient should be operated on and calls Dr Moses who again states that he will not get involved. The patient then asks the radiologist to get Dr Frank another surgeon to come and see him. Dr Frank responds that he will only do so if Dr Brody requests him to do so.

In the third case report an opinion is offered unsolicited by the physician the patient or the relatives whom it appears the opinion is addressed to. The approach is unprofessional and ethically flawed.

- **Investigation consultants**

Investigations are ordered to assist the primary physician in coming to a diagnosis and to guide management. Investigation consultants may have an opinion on how the patient should be managed, but that is not their role for they do not have the experience necessary to make a management decision that should usurp that of the primary physician. Where an investigative consultant is also involved in treatment they are entitled to an opinion on the intervention required, but cannot be seen as taking over the management unless they were given the primary responsibility.[273]

In the second case report the radiological consultant is asked to assess the patient when a complication occurs and properly rings the consultant who requested the investigation, when he thinks the findings warrant urgent surgical

---

[273] http://www.rcr.ac.uk/docs/radiology/pdf/Interventional_radiology_resp.pdf

intervention. In that conversation, the surgical consultant asks for a radiological intervention procedure to be done and the radiologist complies. The radiologist, on noticing that the admitting consultant is a different surgeon, seeks that consultant's intervention arguing that the patient requires an operation. The admitting consultant defers to the consultant who did the surgery.

In the third case report the radiological investigation gave the confidence to attempt treatment of the patient without surgery.

• ***Would the issues be any different if the patient were not hospitalized?***
Consultations should be no different if the patient is not hospitalized for there should be clear lines of communication and responsibilities between physicians. The reason for the consultation should be clear and patients should not be passed from one service to another for the purpose of expanding their earnings. Second opinions out of hospital can be more easily arranged by the patient but are best done with the cooperation of the practitioner who can supply all the previous findings and save time and expense.

When consulted, a practitioner should make an independent assessment even if it involves reviewing the records alone. It is unwise in agreeing to do an invasive procedure to not assess the patient oneself, even when one has confidence in other persons involved. Seeing a patient moments before doing a procedure and seeking to obtain informed consent can lead to misunderstandings particularly if the patient is anxious or sedated.

In the first case reported the patient would have been entitled to consult with whomever they wished if they were not hospitalized.

In the second case report it was unprofessional for Dr Brody to agree to operate on a patient without personally assessing them and to compound the matter further by behaving as if his colleague Dr Moses was not capable of doing the open operation, or to consider postponing the surgery until the equipment was available. It was equally unprofessional for Dr Moses to withdraw from the case he had admitted under his care. Dr Frank could have agreed to see the patient as an outpatient, and is right to insist that he would only see a hospitalised patient with the knowledge of the treating physician.

In the third report there is no basis for the unsolicited opinion given.

• ***Were there issues of consent?***
In obtaining informed consent a patient should be given all the information on the procedure, the alternatives and the risks involved.[274] This involves

---

[274] Gouse v. Cassell (615 A.2d 331) 1992

a full exchange of information between the doctor and the patient as regards previous illnesses, medications and any adverse effects. Changing the procedure should involve a further discussion and the patient given an opportunity to go over ground that may have been touched on before. Just before an operation, patients are anxious or may have been sedated and when faced with a change of plan may consent without thinking the matter through. If challenged in a suit of negligence, consent under such circumstances would be regarded as "not being fully informed".

A patient's autonomy gives them the right to determine what treatment they receive; this implies the right to refuse the treatment offered even if it is life-saving.[275] The refusal of life-saving treatment is a dilemma for the treating physician and usually raises the question as to the mental competence of the patient.

The mental competence of a patient may be brought into question by the effects of the illness itself, even though the patient may appear to be clear at the moment in time. The apparent competence of a patient may vary; e.g. in patients suffering from increased intracranial pressure due to an intracranial bleed, or those who are hypoxic. Such fluctuations can make objective assessment of mental competence difficult and the treating physician may decide that the condition should be treated irrespective of the patient's stated wishes, or ask a court to override the patient's refusal. The patient's competence may also change as a result of a medical intervention and this would hardly have been part of a patient's consideration.[276] A court may be asked to override the refusal of treatment when the public health is placed at risk.[277]

When the assessment is made that the patient is not mentally competent, the patient's next of kin or their legal guardian should be asked to make the decision. A decision to withhold treatment should be made in consultation with the next of kin, respecting any advance directives that may have been made, and any law or legal precedent in such situations, such as in the UK.[278] Advanced directives may turn out to be ineffective for they may not be known.[279]

---

[275] Taking No for an Answer: Refusal of Life-Sustaining Treatment ... AMA Journal of Ethics; S Cooper,
Virtual Mentor. 2010, Vol 12, No 6: 444-449.journalofethics.ama-assn.org/2010/06/ccas2-1006.html
[276] Overriding a Patient's Refusal of Treatment after an Iatrogenic Complication N Engl J Med 1997; 337:1477
[277] Refusal of Treatment - UCSF Missing Link
missinglink.ucsf.edu/lm/ethics/content%20pages/fast_fact_tx_refusal.htm
[278] Mental Capacity Act Code of Practice - Gov.uk
https://www.gov.uk/government/uploads/.../Mental-capacity-act-code-of-practice.pdf
[279] Hospital Do-Not-Resuscitate Orders: Why They Have Failed and How to Fix Them
J K. Yuen, M. Carrington Reid, and M D. Fetters, J Gen Intern Med. 2011; 26(7): 791–797. https://www.ncbi.nlm.nih.gov/pmc/articles/PMC3138592

In the first case reported, the surgeon in charge of the case is not aware of the assessment or medication prescribed and this could have compromised the patient's care.

In the second case, the process of informed consent was defective, for changing the procedure at the last moment gave no time for the patient to consider the alternative of postponement. When a complication arises, the surgeon directs the patient's investigation and treatment without seeing the patient who seeks other advice, for there is a loss of confidence in the surgeon's judgment.

In the third case, the issue of consenting to surgery is quite clear to the mentally competent patient of advanced age. The unsolicited opinion is given when the patient is temporarily incapacitated and would have been equally inappropriate if the patient was an outpatient and had made an advanced directive.

- ### *Role of relatives in decisions on treatment*

Parents and legal guardians of children or mentally incompetent adults have the right to make decisions on the treatment of their charges, but may be challenged before a court as to whether their decisions are in the best interest of the patient.[280] Where an adult patient is determined to be mentally incompetent by reason of dementia, the patient's next of kin assumes legal responsibility.[281] When there are other relatives seeking to determine the decisions on treatment, it should be made clear to them that whilst their opinions and support for the patient's welfare is valued, they have no legal right to determine the treatment that the patient can receive. When relatives seek to alter the decision of an elderly patient the physician should be wary of possible alternative motives and should seek the permission of the patient to involve the relatives in discussions regarding care.

In the first report, the patient's husband is concerned that a requested consultation has not been carried out, and seeks to arrange one himself. The inappropriate response to the husband's request comes to light when medication ordered cannot be understood.

In the second report, colleagues of the patient act as if they are anxious relatives and request opinions on the patient's management in an inappropriate manner.

---

[280] GMC | Consent guidance: Making decisions when a patient lacks ...
https://www.gmc-uk.org/.../consent_guidance_making_decisions_patient_lacks_capac...
[281] Making decisions in a person's best interests - Dementia - SCIE
https://www.scie.org.uk/dementia/supporting-people-with.../decisions/best-interest.asp

In the third report, the patient's decision to refuse surgical treatment has caused concern among relatives, in spite of the fact that her next of kin has accepted the decision. The surgeon agrees to meet the relatives and it is during that meeting that an unsolicited opinion is heard that the temporary incapacity of the patient should be used to override her decision.

• Is it appropriate to ask for a consultation on someone else's patient?

It is appropriate to seek the opinion and help of any other professional whom one feels can benefit a patient under your care. However, when patients are hospitalized one should follow a protocol for consultations and second opinions to avoid possible conflicts with colleagues or conflicting advice that may not benefit the patient.

A consultation is done amongst colleagues, and one should be sensitive enough to the patient's condition and their feelings to offer to have a consultation when things go wrong. When a patient initiates a second opinion, the treating physician should be sensitive enough to the patient's concern to offer to facilitate the second opinion with the doctor of the patient's choice. If the treating physician thinks that the patient's choice for a second opinion is inappropriate, they should explain why to the patient but still endeavour to cooperate if the patient wants to go ahead with their choice.

'Corridor consultations' are an important mode for the exchange of ideas and experiences, however, when they go beyond that to the day-to-day management of individual patients, they can lead to misinformation being circulated.

In the second case described, it is appropriate to try and get a second opinion; how it is done needs to be considered so that relationships do not break down. The admitting surgeon refused to accept any responsibility toward a patient who is officially under his care and the surgeon called in for a second opinion is sensitive to the fact that the principal surgeon may not have been told that a second opinion is being sought and requests that that be done.

In the third case it is totally inappropriate for the surgeon to give or attempt to give an unsolicited opinion to concerned relatives.

• When can a hospitalized patient call another doctor in consultation?

A patient always has a right to seek a consultation or a second opinion. However, when under active treatment in hospital, the principal physician should be aware of all that is going on for the safety of the patient. Since patients are not likely to know the protocol of seeking such opinions, doctors who are requested to give opinions should make it clear to the patient or their agents that the treating doctor should know of the request and preferably write the request for the opinion.

In the first case report, the patient and her husband are sufficiently anxious about a delay in the consultation promised that they initiated another consultation with a physician they know personally. That physician, seemingly unaware that this could cause a problem if the admitting surgeon did not know what was being prescribed for the patient, went ahead and arranged for the patient to be seen without informing the admitting surgeon.

In the second case, the patient is sufficiently anxious not having been seen by the surgeon when problems arose that a second opinion is warranted. The surgeon from whom the opinion is requested, having ascertained that it is not a life-threatening emergency, acts in a professional manner by outlining the proper mode of communication in answering the request.

In the third case, it would be entirely appropriate if the patient's relatives sought a second opinion. Nothing in the report given suggests that this has been done, and had it occurred, the approach of the surgeon who intervened would remain inappropriate.

- ### *Unsolicited opinions*

Unsolicited opinions are usually made with a partial factual basis and may miss the mark in complex situations. Persons who work in the health field often offer such opinions particularly when they work in countries they consider more advanced than in those in which they opine. When opinions are given in casual settings and are in conflict with those of the treating physician, it may damage the bond of trust between a treating physician and the patient or their relatives. Therefore, it is essential that when a physician feels that an incorrect thing is being done, they should approach the treating physician and express their concern.[282]

In the first report given, a consultation is carried out without the knowledge of the surgeon who is concerned about the control of the patient's diabetes. Medication is ordered, but the surgeon only becomes aware of this when the prescription cannot be deciphered.

In the second report the admitting surgeon is clearly aggrieved and refuses to deal with his colleague's patient when a complication arose. The surgeon is directing treatment without seeing the patient and this raises enough concerns for the radiologist and the patient to seek other opinions.

---

[282] Code of Conduct, Barbados Medical Council, 2015;2.6.Other Opinions and 3.1.1. Consultations and Second Opinions; www. arnottcato foundation.org/about. medical code of conduct

In the third report an unsolicited opinion is articulated in public in the hearing of concerned relatives and other patients. The opinion given is at odds with the position that has been made by the patient and accepted by the treating surgeon. The opinion is based on the deterioration of the patient's condition; however, the deterioration was due to poor medication control and was swiftly corrected.

- ### *Privacy in public settings*

Physicians may be called upon to make reference to patient care problems in public settings for the education of other physicians or members of the public, all patient identifiers should be removed in such communications. Permission should be obtained from the patient when being referred to outside of professional settings.[283] Offering opinions on patients should be avoided in any public setting and in carrying out care it is important to provide individual screening and lowering one's voice in the interaction.

In the first two reports the encounters occur in private settings, but the effects of the misconduct displayed ensured that the incidents would have wider discussion.

In the third case report the remarks of the physician involved are both unsolicited and loud enough to be heard by several persons who should not be involved. The remarks disturbed the physician in charge of the patient enough to ask whether the action required disciplinary measures.

- ### *Instituting a professional code of conduct*

A professional code of conduct is designed to guide practitioners as to how they should interact with their patients, colleagues and the public in general.[284] [285] [286] When guidance is sought or a complaint made, a code should be interpreted by a panel experienced in ethical conduct, and where necessary, recommendations made for rewriting of existing codes or the introduction of new ones.

In the three case reports there are practitioners who are aware and those who are not of existing guidance in giving second opinions. The lack of knowledge among some practitioners needed to be addressed.

---

[283] Ethics Conflicts in Rural Communities: Privacy and Confidentiality; T Townsend; 2009; https:// geiselmed.dartmouth.edu/cfm/resources/ethics/chapter-07.pdf

[284] Code of Conduct, Barbados Medical Council, 2015; www. arnottcato foundation.org/about. medical code of conduct

[285] GMC | Members' code of conduct; https://www.gmc-uk.org/about/council/register_code_of_ conduct.asp

[286] AMA Code of Medical Ethics; https://www.ama-assn.org/ delivering-care/ama-code-medical- ethics

Case report:

A patient with a colostomy was admitted for a bowel operation. The nurse told her that she had to drink a large amount to empty her bowel. She expressed concern about how this would be managed and was told that this was always done before this operation. The surgeon receives a call from the patient's husband, saying that his wife is weak and exhausted: 'She can't take the bowel cleaning; it is going into the bed and on the floor'. The surgeon shouts 'I didn't ask for any bowel washout! Let me speak to the sister!' The surgeon storms onto the ward, meets the sister and shouts: 'Sister what the hell are you all trying to do, who ordered a washout on Mrs Smith?'

Sister responds ' I am very sorry but I only just came on duty and heard that Mr Smith had called you and you wanted to speak to me. I went to see her with Mr Smith and I don't know why the nurses continued to push her in that state, the bowel washout was ordered by your registrar.' 'That only makes the whole damn thing worse, none of you use any commonsense; you all didn't care that she was messing all over herself – go and get that damn fool registrar to come and put up a drip!' With that the surgeon pushes his head around the door, and says 'Mrs Smith, I am so sorry, this should not have happened'. With that he storms off the ward and meets his registrar who had been called to meet him on the ward. The surgeon in an angry voice says 'What the hell are you thinking ordering a bowel washout on Mrs Smith!' 'I had noticed that you had not ordered any bowel prep, so I ordered it.'

Half an hour later, the surgeon rings the ward and sister answers, 'Sister, I wish to apologize for the language I used up on the ward; the last person that should have got that was you because you are one of the best nurses I know, please accept my apologies'.

Issues raised

- *Inappropriate professional interactions*

Inappropriate interactions take on many forms and are characterized by a lack of respect or consideration for others. They are most likely to occur when something goes wrong, professionals involved are under stress, are impaired from alcohol or drugs, or have poor relationships with the others involved.[287] It may be manifest by refusing to acknowledge a patient's

---

[287] WMA International Code of Medical Ethics; amended 2006; http://www.wma.net/en/30publications/10policies/c8/

problem by health care providers who view the patient as subservient, not knowledgeable about the care process or are seen as too demanding.

Another aspect of poor interpersonal relationships is characterized as sexual harassment, where women more so than men are subjected to unwanted advances, or are the object of crude sexual references or jokes.

The effect of poor interpersonal relationships is almost always detrimental. When key decision-making personnel are involved in a health care setting, patients are often affected by the dispute and harm may befall them if the situation is not resolved quickly.

In the scenario presented there has been an outburst of angry remarks by the surgeon to other professionals in response to something gone seriously wrong. The nursing staff had ignored the concerns of the patient resulting in great discomfort and humiliation for the patient. The mitigating factor is that an attempt was made by the surgeon to apologize.

- ***Perceptions of accountability to authority figures***

A perception that one must account to dominant figures such as doctors in charge of a service or heads of institutions, may lead health care providers to inappropriate actions, such as assuming orders or directions that will be given and not questioning orders that appear questionable. In some situations, there may also be a counter reaction of disobeying authority figures, which leads to conflict as well as poor care for patients.

In a field of diverse professionals and imperfect teamwork, there will be differences of opinion on what course should be taken. A sign of poor teamwork and relationships is when one professional decides that the decision is theirs alone and there is no need to entertain other views. Threats may be made in order to impose that person's point of view. Political influence may also be wielded inappropriately and is seen most often in small countries or within institutions that depend on government funding.

In the situation described, there is an apparent blind obedience to what the authority figure of the surgeon usually practises; however, the fact that there is no change of course or question asked when there is obvious harm being done may also be a rebellion against that authority figure.

The angry outburst of the surgeon could be symptomatic of an underlying problem.

- ***Reporting on unprofessional behaviour***

When unprofessional behaviour occurs, it places great strain on interpersonal relationships and is eventually reflected in poor patient care. There is a reluctance to report such behaviours for individuals do not like to be involved in disciplinary processes where their own behaviour will come under scrutiny. On the other hand, reporting unprofessional behaviour is one of the most important responsibilities if such behaviour is to be checked. The regulations of professional regulatory bodies do not normally speak to poor interpersonal relations per se, however, they do deal with a number of situations where poor relations may be a symptom of unprofessional conduct; e.g. substance abuse.

In the narrative given the surgeon in charge has reacted angrily to what is happening to his patient; the anger eventually abates and an apology is made. The nurses appear to have shown little regard for the patient's comfort or complaints, and this may result from a perception that what was ordered should be carried out without question.

- ***Unprofessional conduct and the health professions councils***
Professional councils or boards are set up to deal with complaints of unprofessional conduct such as - abandonment of a patient in danger without sufficient cause; the excessive ingestion of intoxicating liquor or drugs; knowingly practising medicine or treating a patient other than in a case of emergency while suffering from a mental or physical condition or while under the influence of alcohol or drugs to such an extent as to constitute a danger to the public or a patient; and the doing of or the failure to do any act or thing in connection with his professional practice, the doing of which or the failure to do which is in the opinion of the council unprofessional or discreditable.[288]

In the narrative given, a case can be made that the nurses' treatment of the patient has been unprofessional, as is the outburst of abusive language by the surgeon.

- ***How is poor conduct dealt with in institutions?***
In institutions poor conduct is usually dealt with at a departmental level, but is often not resolved when professionals who are accustomed to giving orders without question are involved. Furthermore, departments seldom diagnose underlying problems early, and often delay action until a crisis develops. Departments have no mechanism or authority to deal with problems that arise on an interdepartmental basis. Therefore, institutions should have an overarching mechanism that interdisciplinary/interdepartmental issues can be examined. A report to such a body should be open to anyone who has been a 'participant' or even an observer of such conduct.

---

[288] Laws of Barbados; Medical Professions Act 2011;CAP 1

Unfortunately, complainants often see themselves as either having to defend themselves, or as getting involved in an unpleasant and time-consuming process; the result is that many persons decide not to get involved. In some instances, a personal backlash is feared for getting involved; this is often the case with patients undergoing active treatment and with junior staff in departments.

In the case reported, no action is described to deal with the poor behaviour of the staff. This may be because of the apology tendered, and the acknowledgment that the patient has been badly served by the staff, who bore the brunt of the doctor's outburst. Nevertheless, the incident should be examined to ferret out the underlying causes so that faults can be corrected. The forum for such an examination could be an audit conference.

• ***What role should audit play in interpersonal relationships?***
Since poor interpersonal relationships adversely affect patient care, it is important to deal with it like other adverse events in patient care such as audit conferences or another confidential forum.[289] Although it is difficult not to continue discussion outside of the audit conference room, confidentiality should be kept in mind at all times. In any process where one searches for the truth, an atmosphere should be created where poor decisions or behaviours are brought up in a non-adversarial manner. This is a learnt behaviour and should be done in groups of professionals and trainees with the full expectation that there will be no adverse consequences for bringing the truth to light.[290] Nothing said in an audit meeting should be used as testimony at disciplinary or legal proceedings.[291]

In many societies poor behaviours are accepted or rejected depending on the position and social status of the persons involved. When one is dealing with poor behaviours or attitudes one often hears that a person's background is at fault, with the underlying assumption that little can be done to alter it. However, there are examples that show that behaviours and attitudes can be changed through training.

In the narrative given there is no mention of the matter coming up at an audit or any other forum, and the situation may remain until it surfaces again at a crisis level.

---

[289] GMC; UK; Confidentiality guidance: Disclosing information with consent; http://www.gmc-uk.org/guidance/ethical_guidance/confidentiality_24_35_ disclosing_information_with_consent.asp
[290] MPS; Raising concerns and whistleblowing
http://www.medicalprotection.org/uk/wales-factsheets/raising-concerns-and-whistleblowing
[291] O C R P R I V A C Y B R I E F; US Dept. Health & Human Services; http://www.hhs.gov/ocr/privacy/hipaa/understanding/summary/privacysummary.pdf

- *Professional reputation and behaviour.*

Damage to or enhancement of a professional's reputation is influenced by their personal behaviour to both patient's and colleagues. Sometimes having a scarce skill may lead a professional to think that poor behaviour does not matter. On the other hand, it is common to confuse acceptable behaviour with skill.

Poor personal behavioural patterns are seldom discussed openly with the family of the person involved, however, persons involved may disseminate stories of such behaviour widely and it may eventually reach home.

There is nothing in the report to suggest any factor other than professional hierarchy in determining the behaviour described. There may be other factors involved such as substance abuse or mental stress; however, none of this is obvious.

- *Legal consequences of poor behaviours*

Libel or slander. Outbursts, verbal or written, that are damaging to another person's reputation may attract a suit of libel or slander, particularly if shown to be factually untrue. The best way of avoiding slanderous utterances is to check the facts and let any feelings of anger cool before delivering an opinion.

Suits for negligence have been increasing against doctors and other health care providers; any poor behaviour over care will increase the risk of such suits. Poor behaviour by itself is not negligence, but if such behaviour can be shown to harm the patient, then a case may succeed.

Dismissal and non-renewal of contracts are possible consequences of poor behaviour. There should be a formal disciplinary process or contractual clause for such actions.

Censure or removal from the professional register by a regulatory body usually relates to criminal conduct within or outside of a professional's work; on occasion it may relate to particularly egregious conduct in the workplace.

In the report described the possibility of an accusation of slander is greatly diminished by the apology that was tendered. However, a suit of negligence remains a possibility if demonstrable harm has come to the patient.

- *Improving professional conduct*

Good professional conduct should be the aim of both individuals and organizations and can be accomplished in a number of ways.

Training in professional conduct at the basic, postgraduate and in-service levels is often neglected in favour of the quest for more technical training. In addition, there is a widely-held belief that attitudes are determined in the home and that training has little impact on them. As a consequence, little thought is given to the type of training needed to influence conduct and to measuring its effectiveness.

Socialization in the home is thought by many to be the main determinant of behaviour; however, there are other significant influences in schools, churches and the workplace. In high stress, multi-professional workplaces like hospitals, it is important that opportunities be sought for the staff to socialize so they may get to know one another at a personal level.

Accountability from top to bottom in an organization can improve both professional and social behaviour. Ethical codes of conduct provide a valuable guide to individual professionals, but do not usually cover all levels of staff. A code should contain clear guidelines related to making complaints and procedures for resolving them without feelings of victimization on anyone's part.

Sanctions should be the last resort for improving poor behaviour. Nevertheless, sanctions are important tools that must be applied after due and fair process, and must be proportionate to the offence committed.

In the narrative described there is a lot of room for improvement in the professional conduct of the persons involved and the incident could be used under the right circumstances as a teaching tool, apart from any other measure that may be taken.

Complaint 1:

A consultant physician writes a letter to the Director of Medical Services [DMS] in the institution where he works stating that a physician entered the hospital and sought to have a patient, whom he was treating, leave the hospital and transferred to his care in another clinic. The consultant physician goes on to state that he had heard from other physicians involved in the case that the DMS had called them to enquire on behalf of a government minister what was the reason the patient could not be transferred.

The letter goes on to question the bona fides of the physician who had sought the transfer and questions the policy of the hospital and of the ministry in relation to providing facilities for the treatment of the patient concerned. The letter is copied to all of the persons mentioned in the complaint, to colleagues in the department, heads of department in the hospital, the CEO and the governing board of the hospital, and to the Chairman of the Medical Council.

A press report appears quoting elements of the letter and states that the physician and the government minister are demanding an apology from the complaining doctor. Shortly thereafter, the board of the hospital demands that the complainant doctor withdraw the letter, and when he refuses to do so, suspends him from duty stating that he should not have written the letter using the hospital's stationery.

At the regular monthly ethics case conference the organisers decided to discuss the issues that can arise out of making a complaint. The hospital administration is invited to contribute to the discussion on the hospital's regulations related to complaints and how complaints are handled. The hospital administrator responds to the invitation by stating that no such discussion is to be held on the hospital's premises.

Complaint 2:

Letter to the Medical Council re Dr X. 'I would like to report Dr. X's appalling conduct and professional standards whilst I was hospitalized. What my wife and I experienced while I was in the resuscitation room is only what I can call as the most unprofessional, arrogant behaviour of a doctor we have ever experienced. Dr. X actually had the audacity to enter the resuscitation room and tried to shake my hand while I was in a critical condition. He then persistently lobbied my wife, and from my recollection maliciously, for at least ten minutes trying to persuade her to agree for me to be moved to his clinic. Initially we believed Dr X was a salesman or some kind of representative from a private hospital close to where I was being treated. He had telephoned my wife's mobile number several times unsolicited, and at no time did we initiate any contact with him. I believe our telephone invoices for that period will probably show his telephone number as an incoming call!

'During his intrusion Dr. X claimed he could do things better and that I would be safer in his clinic. How could he possibly know my condition without an examination or any details of my case? I for one would view this as gross medical negligence, actually highlighting the type of doctor he is, in actually being prepared to risk my life with no consideration. Thank God my wife Lorraine was strong, and guided by her instinct and also listened to professional nurses who were fighting to keep me alive only ever saying: "He has not stabilised; it is unsafe to move your husband at this stage". My wife then firmly insisted that he leave us alone, and requested that he leave the room and that he was to stop his pestering telephone calls. Eventually, the nurses protested to his presence and he left reluctantly. Lorraine and I have spoken and have agreed that if you required Lorraine to give evidence under oath she would fly back to the island as a witness.'

Issues raised

- *Why make a complaint?*

Personal 'injury' is the most common reason for a person to make a complaint. The complaint may be made to correct an on-going problem, prevent recurrence of an incident, or to punish the perpetrator of the injury. When setting out to punish, emotion may overcome good judgment and may result in false accusations being made.

Those with a strong sense of justice and those seeking leadership within the community often do the complaining on behalf of the vulnerable and powerless. Vulnerable persons may feel that they will be victimized if they complain, and therefore a more senior person or the doctor in charge of a patient may undertake the responsibility of complaining on their behalf.

Improving systems at work, or in a community, benefits both the individual and the community as a whole. Both patients and health professionals benefit from improvements in the quality of patient care; it may therefore be a focus for concerned complainants.

In the complaints reported, the target is a physician accused of soliciting patients; one is made by the physician treating a patient and the other by a patient. The physician complainant also complains about the complicity of officials in the institution and a government minister, as well as the facilities available for treatment.

- ### *Complaining about what?*

Breaches of law are the clearest of complaints for they relate to written statutes. Unlawfully practising as a professional may be practising without registration, or it may be that registration was obtained by false representation.

Professional misconduct is conduct that falls outside the acceptable behaviour as stated by the governing body of the profession. Misconduct is not uniform in all jurisdictions; e.g. advertising by the medical profession is not held in all countries to be misconduct, but the solicitation of patients would be widely held to be so.[292] Professional misconduct may rise to the level of a criminal complaint or a civil tort.[293] Criminal charges may include battery, sexual assault, manslaughter or murder. Civil torts are those related to negligence.

Ethical codes of conduct are the agreed conventions for the conduct of professionals in the communities they serve. Particulars in ethical codes do not always have the force of legal statute but can be persuasive in that regard. There may be national professional codes and agreed international codes such as the Hippocratic Oath and the Physicians Oath of the World Medical Association as the Declaration of Geneva.[294]

Institutional codes of conduct are usually contained in staff rules and cover credentialing of professionals, admitting and procedural privileges, lines of communication, disciplinary procedures, and in general rules that try to achieve an orderly conduct of the institution's business.

Solicitation of patients to provide them with services is generally forbidden to medical professionals. In one jurisdiction the law states that "any form of advertising, canvassing or promotion, either directly or indirectly, for the purpose of obtaining patients…" is professional misconduct.[295] It is considered bad for patients who may be misled by claims that may not be met, and also to be unfair competition for fellow professionals.[296] Solicitation or canvassing of patients is considered as distinct from advertising; the difference is that solicitation targets an individual patient whilst advertising is aimed at a wider audience.

---

[292] Laws of Barbados; Medical Registration Act CAP 171 Regulations Part V 21(2) (b)

[293] General Medical Council, UK; Guide to Professional Conduct; 2009 http://www.medicalcouncil. ie/Registration/Guide-to-Professional-Conduct-and-Behaviour-for-Registered-Medical-Practitioners. pdf

[294] Declaration of Geneva; World Medical Association 1948 amended 2006

[295] Laws of Barbados; Medical Profession Act; 2011-1; Sect 23 (2)(c)

[296] Advertising of Doctor's Services; D.H.Irvine; Journal of ethics, 1991, 17,35-40

Payment of a fee or splitting a fee for referrals of patients is a form of solicitation and is professional misconduct - "the division, with any person who is not a partner or assistant, of any fees or profits resulting from consultations or other medical or surgical procedures without the patient's knowledge or consent".[297]

In the first complaint a physician complains that another physician has solicited his patient to leave his care for another institution. He also complains that the Director of Medical Services, on behalf of a government minister, has made enquiries as to why the patient cannot leave the institution.

In the second complaint the patient states that his wife had been solicited persistently over the phone followed by an uninvited intrusion whilst the patient was being stabilized in emergency. The patient was clearly alarmed at the approach and felt his life was being endangered by such solicitation. The complaint could rise to the level of battery, for the physician in question had attempted to examine the patient without consent.

- ***When to complain***

A complaint should be made as soon as possible after the incident; this has the advantage of dealing with the matter when it is fresh in everyone's minds. However, there is the disadvantage of complaining too soon and not being able to gather all of the pertinent information related to the circumstances of the incident.

Unless available in writing, third party statements are a hazardous basis on which to base a complaint, for recollections vary with time, and may even have been transmitted in an incomplete manner. Complaints should be made within any statute of limitations for the particular infraction. Complaints related to negligence usually have a statute of limitation of some years, and relate to the time at which the 'injury' occurred or in some instances when it was discovered.

Third party statements form the basis for the complaint made by the physician. The complaint goes on to make accusations about the conduct of officials and questions the qualifications of the offending doctor.

The complaint from the patient is stated as the direct experience of the patient and his wife, and she has promised to fly back to the jurisdiction to give sworn testimony.

- ***Complaining - whom to?***

Anybody can be complained to. However, if the complainant is seeking a remedy rather than ventilating their feelings, they should choose the

---

most pertinent person or institution to complain to. Person to person complaints may be emotionally laden and lacking in form.

Institutions and government departments react poorly to complaints about them or their administrative staff, but when complaints are made about subordinate staff, there is often a lengthy process of enquiry as the institution or department seeks to protect itself.

Professions' regulatory councils / boards are made up predominantly of the professionals they are regulating and have a reputation of protecting the professionals who are complained about. There are regulations that define professional misconduct and categorize the offences that are subject to disciplinary action. These bodies have rules that govern enquiry into and adjudication of complaints. The sanctions are censure, reprimand, suspension or revocation of the professional's licence to practise.[298] A pattern of conduct may also be taken into account in coming to a decision by the disciplinary body. When the staff of an institution are found to be guilty of professional misconduct, the institution may become liable in civil proceedings for damages.

The police are the proper recipient of criminal complaints such as assaults, theft and fraud. When working within an institution such referrals are best made through institutional mechanisms, unless there is an immediate danger to life or serious injury.

The courts are the proper recipients of civil tort complaints, and should be approached through an attorney-at-law. In health care, the most likely related civil tort is that of negligence in the care delivered.

Public forums as a vehicle for communication of complaints are suitable for matters where the public's influence is sought in dealing with a matter. It may also be used in complaints of a general nature that affect the public welfare. Taking personal complaints into the public arena is likely to make a resolution of the problem more difficult.

The complaint in the first report is addressed to the head of the medical staff in the institution but is widely copied to those staff and to the Medical Council that may have a role to play in addressing the complaint. The press is not part of the distribution, but when matters are widely copied they do tend to reach the press. In the narrative given, the complaint has reached the public arena and a civil tort of libel is threatened against the complainant, presumably on the basis that what was in the complaint is not true. The institution also demands that the complaint be withdrawn and suspends the complainant on the ground that the complainant should not have used the institution's letterhead.

In the second complaint the patient has written to the regulatory body with

---

[298] Laws of Barbados; Medical Profession Act; 2011-1; Sect 39 (2)

a first hand account of his disturbing experience. There is nothing stated in the complaint as to how the physician complained about came to know about the patient.

- ***Where else should a complaint go?***

Complaints should be copied to all of the representative persons who should be involved at an administrative level within an institution, and to organizations that are intended to take action. They should also be brought to the attention of others involved or affected by the complaint under confidential cover. Wide distribution without confidential cover is likely to lead to wider dissemination than stated.

The first complaint has been appropriately copied to the administrative head of the institution and all of those departments that the complainant thinks should take action. It has also been copied to heads of clinical departments and the members of the physician's department.

The second complaint has not been copied to anyone; a copy to the patient's physician and to the head of the institution would have been entirely appropriate.

- ***Guidelines for writing the complaint***

An institution should have published staff regulations, which should state how complaints should be made. Regulations should have the disciplinary procedures for staff set out, and these may contain provision for the suspension of staff members, whilst an enquiry into a complaint is carried out against them. Institutional guidelines usually give some assurance of protection of complainants from retaliation in the workplace. This protection does not always operate if complaints are made against senior executives. This has prompted the passage of 'whistle-blower' protection laws in some jurisdictions. Whistle-blower protection is most often applied to financial infelicities, but can be applied to other types of administrative misconduct.[299]

It the narrative of the first complaint it would be quite unusual to have guidelines that call for the suspension of a staff member for writing a complaint to the institution on the institution's letterhead. The demand that no discussion of the institution's rules or regulations in relation to a matter that has occurred within the institution is repressive.

- ***Has a complaint been laid to the regulatory body?***

Council/board regulations should contain guidelines or statements

---

[299] Public Employee Free Speech: The Policy Reasons for Rejecting a Per Se Rule Precluding Speech Rights; M. M. Zack, Boston College Law Review, 2005, Vol 46; 4 /5

on how a complaint can be laid, and the matters that constitute professional misconduct.[300] Such regulations usually contain a requirement that the complaint be in writing, but may be accompanied by evidentiary attachments that may be visual or auditory recordings. Such a requirement not only allows the complaint to be distributed to the members of the regulatory body, it is the vehicle by which the professional complained about will have the chance to know what the accusation is and to be able to respond to it.

An unsolicited attempt to secure the transfer of a patient from one institution to another would constitute professional misconduct in most jurisdictions.[301]

When the *bona fides* of a physician to practise is challenged e.g. as a specialist[302] or as a result of fraud[303] the regulatory body has a duty to review the matter.

In the first report given, the complainant has brought his accusation of unprofessional conduct to the attention of the chairman of the regulatory body by a copy of a letter of complaint written to the institution. The letter contains two matters relevant to the regulatory body, solicitation and a challenge of the bona fides of the physician.

- ### Has defamation been committed?
Defamation is an unjustified injury to the reputation of another. It can be defended on the basis that what was said was true, had no malicious intent, and that it had not been distributed or published generally. Labelling a communication CONFIDENTIAL, demonstrates that it is not intended for distribution. Defamation and any consequential damages are determined in court, nevertheless, regulatory bodies may determine that damaging statements about others can constitute professional misconduct.

In the first complaint there is an accusation of administrative and political intervention on behalf of the physician being complained about. The latter if untrue could form the basis for a suit of defamation.

- ### Administrative misconduct
Misconduct may be committed at the institutional or governmental level. Misconduct committed at this level carries implications for future conduct. Threats of dismissal or other sanction may be used without due

---

[300] Laws of Barbados CAP 171 Medical Registration Act 1972 Regulations Part V sect 25
[301] Laws of Barbados CAP 171 Medical Registration Act 1972 Regulations Part V sect 21[2] b
[302] Laws of Barbados CAP 171 Medical Registration Act 1972 Regulations Part V sect 21[2] j
[303] Laws of Barbados CAP 171 Medical Registration Act 1972 Sect. 18

process and is often difficult to counter, unless the worker is prepared to bring a suit of wrongful dismissal.

In the instance described in the first complaint it is possible that the complainant may have been sanctioned out of hubris or embarrassment, for the reason given for the sanction, using the institution's letterhead appears to be a contrivance.

Conscientious Objection - or Patient Abuse?

Case report:

Two twenty-year-old women were admitted to hospital to have first trimester medical terminations of pregnancy. One woman requested her termination for socioeconomic reasons, as a single parent of a six-month-old baby whom she is struggling to support. The other was advised by her cardiologist to have a termination as she had severe peri-partum cardiomyopathy and a stroke in her last pregnancy.

Six hours after having medication inserted both women began experiencing severe cramping abdominal pain secondary to uterine contractions. A passing intern alarmed by cries of painful distress, stopped and inquired why the intravenous analgesia on the treatment order cards had not been given. The nurse, who was responsible for the care of the patients, informed the intern that she had not given the medication as it contributed to the abortion process, and abortion was against her religious beliefs. She added that the pain the women were suffering "served them right for the murder they were committing".

The intern said to the nurse that even though she was well within her rights to refuse to administer care based on her personal beliefs, she should have notified her senior or another nurse who could administer the medication. After discussion the nurse agreed she should have acted differently and one of her colleagues on duty administered the medication. No further action was taken.

Issues raised

- *Abortion as contraception*

Abortion has remained a lightning rod in many societies based on religious doctrine versus the right of a woman to control over her own body. Some religions extend their doctrine against abortion to contraception. Advocates against abortion and contraception see a woman as a receptacle for sperm, even when forced upon her during rape or incest.

Modern societies do not see women as simply vessels for reproduction and the rearing of children, and their wider roles have inevitably led to women gaining greater control over their reproductive ability. The voluntary termination of an unwanted pregnancy is now largely initiated by women who come to their decision based on societal pressures, their health and their assessment of their ability to raise the children.

Many societies, in acknowledgment of the worth of women, have changed laws from total bans on abortion to more nuanced laws which take into account the views of the woman, and protect the child being formed from being discarded capriciously. Such laws enacted against religious objections and threats to law makers have tried to accommodate religious sensibilities by looking at when a foetus can be viable without the support of its mother, and ensuring that no one with a conscientious objection should be compelled to take part in an abortion.[304] That accommodation is insufficient for some, who have resorted to terrorism and murder to impose their view.[305] Some have tried to redefine when life begins and may take part in medical services to frustrate or coerce women against seeking an abortion. It is also argued that where abortion is legal both men and women abuse the law by failing to prevent unwanted pregnancies. Unfortunately, available contraceptive measures have their problems and are not 100% effective. The effectiveness of any contraceptive method is determined by the education of the person using it, its availability and the judgments brought to bear by society, religion and medical attendants. Some health professionals who declare a conscientious objection to abortion have equated contraception with abortion and seek to block an unwilling woman from conceiving as well as from the abortion of the unwanted pregnancy.[306]

In the cases presented, there is no mention of using contraception to prevent clearly unwanted pregnancies. In one patient it was unusual to conceive so soon after birth, and in the other, the most effective contraceptive 'pill' would have been contraindicated.

* ***Conscientious objection - religious foundation and legal sanction***
Conscientious objectors to abortion state that their religious values are against the taking of an innocent life. Those professing the Christian faith quote the 6th commandment "Thou shall not kill' but state that this does not apply to their support for the death penalty or war. Not all believers are prepared to discount the views of women, who may be their mother, sister, aunt, grandmother, wife, girlfriend or fellow worker and face the possible tragic consequence of an unsafe abortion.[307] Debate on the morbidity and mortality of unsafe abortions has resulted in some societies enacting laws that take into account the circumstances and health of the mother and that of the unborn child, in deciding whether an abortion can

---

[304] Medical Termination of Pregnancy Act; Laws of Barbados, 1983 CAP 44A

[305] Abortion Clinic Violence as Terrorism; M Wilson; J Lynxwiler. J. Terrorism 1988 Vol.11 Iss: 4: 263-73

[306] The Limits of Conscientious Objection — May Pharmacists Refuse to Fill Prescriptions for Emergency Contraception? J Cantor, K Baum, N Eng. J Med 2004; 351

[307] Induced abortion: estimated rates and trends worldwide; G Sedgh, S Henshaw, S Singh et al The Lancet, 2007Vol 370, Iss 9595, Pg. 1338 - 45

be done legally. The debate included how one could respect the religious beliefs of health care workers and led to the conscientious objector clause, stating that a health care worker can object and not take part in a legal abortion.[308] These clauses do not state that one should participate and try to stop or sabotage it.[309]

In the report given the nurse is described as having a conscientious objection to abortion but has not declared this. She stays to 'take care' of the patients and deliberately denies them medication for their severe pain. When challenged she states that the pain medication aids in the process and she was entitled to not take part, furthermore the patients' suffering "served them right for the murder they were committing".

- ### *Conscientious objectors – defining not taking part*

Conscientious objectors are given a unique legal exception to escape a duty of care to patients who undergo abortion. There is no other conscientious objector clause in law; for example, a Jehovah's Witness health care worker is not accorded a legal right not to take part in the blood transfusion of a patient where it is the accepted standard of care. The statutes do not define taking part and some have sought to do so themselves. The decision by a secretary not to type a letter of referral for an abortion on the grounds of a conscientious objection, led to the judgment that taking part meant taking part in the actual procedure of an abortion.[310] Some pharmacists have refused to dispense drugs that they consider induce abortions on the grounds of being a conscientious objector.[311]

In the report given the nurse states that administering the analgesic is part of the process of the abortion. Her other remarks indicate that she decided to take part to punish the patients by withholding pain relief.

- ### *Patients' rights and professional abuse*

All patients have a right to be treated and to have relief of their suffering in a professional manner; this must be done irrespective of the race, ethnicity, social class, religion or culture. A health professional may have a view as to the origin of a patient's suffering, but that does not entitle them to a judgment that denies the patient treatment. The law denies or enforces medical treatment in few instances, and in general seeks to ensure that patients are not subjected to treatment against their will.

---

[308] Abortion Act 1967 United Kingdom c. 87; Sect. 4
[309] Abortion clinic violence as terrorism. M. Wilson, J. Lynxwiler, Studies in Conflict & Terrorism 1988, 11 (4): 263–273
[310] Janaway v. Salford Health Authority. UK. House of Lords. All Eng. Law Rep. 1988; 3:1079-84
[311] Conscientious Objection and the Pharmacist; H R. Manasse; Science 2005: 308; 5728 pp.1558-1559

In many countries the law still denies patients an abortion as a medical service; nevertheless, many women risk their lives and health seeking abortions outside of a regulated medical setting.[312] A number of countries in enacting laws to allow abortions have incorporated a conscientious objection clause to taking part in the procedure. However, such clauses do not throw out other professional obligations to patients, and a professional with a conscientious objection cannot forsake professional norms and seek to punish a patient or deny them care by another professional.[313]

In the report given, a nurse with a conscientious objection has forsaken her professional obligations and denied the patients pain relief. This comes to light when the patients' cries of anguish are overheard. The nurse has not taken part; she has deliberately denied care. When challenged, a remark was made that suggests that the patients were deliberately being tortured for availing themselves of a lawful abortion service.

- *Can a professional's conduct amount to torture?*

The United Nations Convention on Torture defines torture as "…any act by which severe pain or suffering, whether physical or mental, is intentionally inflicted on a person for such purposes as obtaining from him, or a third person, information or a confession, punishing him for an act he or a third person has committed or is suspected of having committed, or intimidating or coercing him or a third person, or for any reason based on discrimination of any kind, when such pain or suffering is inflicted by or at the instigation of or with the consent or acquiescence of a public official or other person acting in an official capacity. It does not include pain or suffering arising only from, inherent in, or incidental to, lawful sanctions."-1984.[314]

When applied to patients who seek an abortion one sees that deliberate obstructions, delays to make the pregnancy too late to terminate, and remarks intended to make patients feel guilty of 'murder' amount to imposing severe mental anguish.

In the narrative described the patients are deliberately left to suffer severe pain by withholding the medication that was prescribed.

- *Responsibility of employers, professional councils*

Employers, regulatory bodies, professional associations and insurance

[312] Abortion Around the World – Overview, M Abdullaeva, NOW Foundation, 2007
[313] Conscientious objection in medicine, J Savulescu, BMJ. 2006; 332(7536): 294–297
[314] Convention Against Torture and Other Cruel, Inhuman or Degrading Treatment or Punishment, 1984 United Nations, Treaty Series, vol. 1465, p. 85

agencies have responsibility for the proper conduct of health professionals. Such conduct must be monitored at all levels, and not wait upon challenges in the law courts or the court of public opinion. The confidential review of how cases are handled, both good and bad, is probably the best learning tool, as it is in other aspects of medical care.

In the narrative given there was no follow-up on the abusive conduct observed. This signals that such conduct will be tolerated until a patient challenges the conduct.

Case report:

A medical practitioner from overseas presented with progressive lower limb weakness and requested a particular investigation. The radiologist made a consultation request for management of delirium that hindered the investigation. The history was that the practitioner was last well five weeks ago when he was in the country for a minor surgical procedure. His post-operative course was complicated by delirium, and dissatisfied with the care he was getting, he had discharged himself and returned home. Within a few days of arriving home, he appeared fatigued and complained of lower abdominal and back pain. He prescribed himself NSAIDs, and later morphine, without relief. He then went to the local emergency room where he was treated with a narcotic and discharged. His condition deteriorated, becoming confused and dragging his legs. After a week, he was admitted to hospital where he had antibiotics for a "UTI", but frustrated with the lack of answers the family decided to return for better investigation.

The patient was alert but rambled and slurred his words. He gave a long history of depression – self-diagnosed, self-treated and well controlled. Examination showed bilateral lower limb paralysis. Imaging showed scattered oedema in and around the lumbar spinal cord and a loculated right pleural effusion. Blood tests, including HIV and HTLV1, were normal except for an elevated ESR >130mm.

The notes from the previous admission showed he had had a procedure followed on day 1 by delirium with chills and rigors. The surgeon was informed and directed the nurses to "discharge him to my office". The nurses asked the anaesthetist to see the patient, a diagnosis of bacteraemia was made and a cocktail of antibiotics given. He improved but did not see the surgeon and had signed his self-discharge on day 3 post-op.

Issues raised:

- *Physician self-treatment*

Medical practitioners who treat themselves or their close relatives are at risk of making a poor assessment of the condition being treated. A practitioner should not go beyond what would be expected of any other person in the application of self-treatment for minor ailments, unless they are in an isolated situation.[315] When a practitioner goes beyond the self-treatment of

---

[315] The AMA Code of Medical Ethics' journalofethics.ama-assn.org/2012/05/coet1-1205.html Opinion 8.19 - Self-Treatment or Treatment of Immediate Family Members

minor ailments, the practitioner may be more broadly impaired.[316]

In the history given, the practitioner has gone beyond the admonition to not treat oneself, by diagnosing and treating a psychiatric illness. The practitioner's self-diagnosis and treatment of back pain has failed, but when he seeks help, it proves to be inadequate.

• *The impaired physician*

An impaired practitioner has been defined as one unable to fulfill professional or personal responsibilities because of psychiatric illness, alcoholism, or drug dependency.[317] Impairment may be related to a physical or mental condition, or the adherence to cultural or religious viewpoints and/or practices that result in unethical or illegal conduct in relation to patients under their care. The mental states responsible may be spontaneous or induced, and include the various forms of dementia, persons with sociopathic and psychopathic personality disorders, as well as those secondary to substance abuse.

The impaired physician is often in denial about their condition and resort to self-treatment. They are usually a great success in their practice but may have a general disdain and lack of knowledge of psychiatric conditions. They may ignore the possibility of transmissible illness in themselves and tend to be intolerant in their religious views.

In the report given the practitioner patient appears to be impaired by virtue of his self-diagnosis and treatment of depression, as well as his self-treatment of back pain and weakness in his legs, and has to be persuaded by his family to seek further advice.

• *Reporting to authorities*

Reporting a practitioner to an authority is appropriate to correct malfeasance and dysfunctioning of a practitioner or for disciplinary action in relation to professional misconduct. Malfeasance includes poor clinical practice that endangers patients and poor conduct in relation to patients, colleagues and other workers.

Professional and illegal misconduct varies in different jurisdictions, but invariably includes improper relations with patients and abuse of alcohol or drugs to the point of affecting one's treatment of patients. It may involve a prohibition on advertising, the solicitation of patients and the splitting of fees among practitioners.[318]

---

[316] Identification of Physician Impairment; Pham JC1, Pronovost PJ, Skipper GE. JAMA. 2013; 22; 309(20): 2101-2

[317] The Sick Physician Impairment by Psychiatric Disorders, Including Alcoholism and Drug Dependence; JAMA. 1973; 223(6): 684-687

[318] Medical Professions Act 2011 sect 23(2); Laws of Barbados

In institutional settings poor clinical practice may be discovered through clinical audit or through a confidential complaints mechanism. These mechanisms give the opportunity to correct poor practice and conduct and may head off malpractice claims. Good medical records are the basis for defending any claim of negligent practice.[319]

As reported the patient practitioner is impaired by virtue of inappropriate self-treatment.

The reported responses of the surgeon amount to negligent conduct and ought to be addressed in an appropriate manner in the institution where the treatment occurred.

- ### *Referrals – opinion or management?*

When a referral is made it should be made clear to the patient and the physician to whom it is being made what the purpose is and any limitation of the referral. Thus there may be a referral that seeks a second opinion as to a diagnosis but does not request that the management of the patient be taken over.[320] If the management of the patient is being sought, it should be clear to all the parties involved if it is the total management of the patient, or if there is a limited service required. Patients, relatives or other health personnel should not refer without the knowledge and approval of the primary physician, particularly where the patient is hospitalised. Such referrals can result in conflicts of management, which could harm the patient. When a life-threatening emergency arises the most competent available physician or health professional should be engaged.

In the report the patient has made a self-referral to the radiological service; a physician is consulted by the service for control of delirium so that the investigation can be done. The investigation may well be misdirected without an independent assessment.

The notes of the previous admission describe the nurses asking the surgeon to see the patient who is very ill, but are told to discharge the patient. The nurses ask an anaesthetist to see the patient and emergency treatment for a bacteraemia was given.

The anaesthetist writes, but does not speak to the surgeon who in spite of requests from the patient does not see the patient and he discharges himself three days later.

- ### *Physician access to patient's notes*

A patient's record is a confidential document, recorded by the physician

---

[319] Medical records and issues in negligence; J Thomas; Indian J Urol. 2009 Jul-Sep; 25(3): 384-388. doi: 0.4103/0970-1591.56208

[320] Barbados Med. Council; Code of Conduct; 3.1.1. Consultations and Second Opinions; https:// arnottcatofoundation.org

and any other health care worker involved in the care of the patient. The patient can authorise access to their records for medical or legal purposes; however, the physician who wrote the notes might seek to embargo confidential information that refers to a third party.[321] It is therefore appropriate for individual practitioners and institutions to have some basic safeguards when a request comes for a patient's notes to be seen. The simplest authorization is to have a written request from the patient or their legal representative. However, in situations where the patient is under the care of a practitioner in an institution it can be assumed that the practitioner and those who work with them have that authority implied.

When records are being requested from another institution or practitioner, the patient should give written authorization, however, these may be forwarded to a 'trusted' practitioner in the form of copies. Trust facilitates use but may open the gate for abuse.

In the report given, the physician obtains the patient's notes from another institution without any written authorization from the patient. This is almost certainly on the basis of trust in the practitioner who also has privileges at that institution. The notes yield valuable information, but also reveal negligent management during the admission.

- *Physician to physician communication*

Clear, accurate, candid and courteous communication between physicians is important in the management of patients, or in dealing with infelicitous conduct of health staff.

Such communication is vital when referrals are made between physicians or when second opinions are being sought, either at the behest of the physician or the patient.[322] It is equally important to communicate effectively when another practitioner has made a significant mistake.

Communicating effectively with an impaired colleague is very difficult and consideration must be given to reporting the colleague to the appropriate institutional committee or regulatory body. Reporting to a regulatory body cannot be anonymous and should be done with the knowledge of a patient where one is involved.[323], [324]

---

[321] Medical records: Disclosing confidential clinical information; B Dolan; Psychiatric Bulletin, 2004; 28: 53-56

[322] Sharing information within the healthcare team or with others providing care; General Medical Council, UK; Good Medical Practice; http://www.gmc-uk.org/guidance/ethical_guidance/ confidentiality_24_35_disclosing_information_with_consent.asp

[323] Identifying and Assisting the Impaired Physician; Boisaubin, E V.; Levine, R E. American Journal of the Medical Sciences: 2001; Vol 322; 1; pp. 31-36

[324] How to investigate and analyse clinical incidents: Clinical Risk Unit and Association of Litigation and Risk Management protocol; BMJ Vol 320 Mar 2000 www.bmj.com C Vincent, S Taylor-Adams, E J Chapman, D Hewett, S Prior, P Strange, A Tizzard

*In the report given, the physician diagnosed as impaired is a patient, and
should be treated as a patient by giving him all of the facts and treatment
pertaining to his physical and psychological condition. Since there is no
evidence of harm to any other patient, it is appropriate to assess the response
of the physician patient before any report to a regulatory body. The situation is
compounded by the discovery of negligent conduct of another practitioner during
the previous admission and how this should be handled.*

- ## Consent for testing/reporting

Consent for any intervention with a patient was enshrined in the
Neuremberg Code formulated after the Nazi war criminal trials.[325] In
clinical practice consent may be oral, written or implied such as when
the patient presents for blood tests. Written consent should be obtained
for invasive procedures, which carry a risk of harm to the patient. Such
consent should be informed by making the patient aware of the risks of
the procedure and the available alternatives.[326] Where consent forms are
basic it is appropriate to write in the patient's notes about the consent
process that was undertaken.[327]

Blood tests are usually considered non-invasive and many like
blood counts are labelled routine tests and patients may not be aware
of what is being 'routinely' done. The societal explosion of stigma and
discrimination against those affected by AIDS required that those persons
being tested for HIV should be prepared by counselling.[328] This meant
that there should be explicit consent for testing for HIV from patients
who were able to do so. As treatment for HIV emerged the mortality of
AIDS diminished and the level of HIV could be reduced diminishing the
transmission of the virus.[329]

Treatment encouraged a drive for more persons to know their HIV
status and be offered treatment. This led to a call for 'routine' HIV testing
of persons attending health care institutions.[330] Routine testing was
interpreted as testing without the patient's knowledge or consent, and
referring those who were positive to treatment centres.[331]

In the report given, the physician patient is tested for HIV among a number of

[325] Fifty Years Later: The Significance of the Nuremberg Code; E Shuster, N Engl J Med 1997; 337:1436-1440
[326] Gouse v. Cassell (615 A.2d 331) 1992
[327] Informed Consent May Not Protect You in a Lawsuit. Medscape W J. Guglielmo, June 27, 2017
[328] Voluntary Counselling and Testing (VCT) for HIV Prevention; http://www.unfpa.org/hiv/prevention/hivprev5b.htm
[329] Effectiveness of Highly Active Antiretroviral Therapy in Reducing Heterosexual Transmission of HIV J Castilla, J del Romero, V Hernando, B Marincovich, S Garcia, and C Rodriguez, AIDS 2005, Vol 40 No 1, pg. 96-101
[330] WHO | HIV testing services; www.who.int/hiv/topics/vct/en/
[331] Guidance on provider-initiated HIV testing and counselling; www.unicef.org/aids/files/PITCGuidance2007

other tests without consent. The clinical picture required the exclusion of HIV as a possible cause.

- *Informing patients of defects in management*

Patients should know about the risks of treatment through an informed consent process.[332] When untoward events occur the patient becomes distressed even when they have been warned; it is made worse if the attending physician/surgeon appears indifferent. Becoming aware of problems is often made over the telephone, such calls usually contain the most alarming symptom/event to the person making the call, but there may not be enough information on which to make a critical decision. If such information is not available it is appropriate to arrange for the patient to be seen. Having ascertained the scope of the problem it is appropriate to express one's regret.[333] When the patient has been under the care of another practitioner, it is appropriate to give one's assessment of the problem to the patient. However, it is not appropriate to offer any opinion on any legal consequences as it relates to another practitioner. Offering of a legal opinion may be seen as bias if one were to be a witness in any subsequent legal proceeding.

In the report given perusal of the notes of a previous admission discovered what appears to be negligent conduct by the surgeon concerned. The patient is already aware of this conduct, having given the history of the previous admission and discharging himself.

- *Reporting malfeasance of colleagues*

Observation of the poor or unusual conduct of a physician may be the first indication that the individual is impaired. What to do is sensitive and most often little else is done than gossip about it with other colleagues. The observations made may be sensitive and colleagues will not want to be involved, particularly when taking action may lead to the loss of friendship. Observations on a concerning behaviour should be noted in an objective manner in personal notes or when appropriate in the patient's notes. Whilst it is tempting to approach a friend or colleague about their behaviour, it is almost certain to be met by denial, counter accusations and deterioration in one's working relationship. If a personal approach is decided upon, it is better to initiate it through a senior, respected and independent person - a colleague, a religious or other community leader.

---

[332] The duty to warn patients about risk. Chester v Afshar [2004] UKHL 41; [2005] 1 A.C. 134; [2004] 3 W.L.R. 927; [2004] 4 All E.R. 587

[333] 'Doing the right thing' after an adverse event; M Bismark, R Paterson NZMJ 29 July 2005, Vol 118 No 1219 Page 1 of 6; http://www.nzma.org.nz/journal/118-1219/1593/ © NZMA

If the impaired colleague is working in an institution, that mechanism should be defined in a code of conduct for the staff. If the physician is working independently, guidance should be sought from a professional association or the regulatory body.[334] Regulatory bodies should have a confidential system for enquiry into such complaints, and flexibility and confidence in the fairness of the system to the impaired colleague will give fellow practitioners the confidence to report issues with a colleague.[335]

The confidentiality of an ill practitioner is as important as that of any ill person. However, given their responsibility for the welfare of patients, the health and confidentiality of practising practitioners must be balanced against other interests. If the practitioner's health places patients' lives at risk confidentiality should be broken to the appropriate body that can prevent them from practising.[336] It would be for the regulatory body to take appropriate action to protect patients and to decide whether breaking the practitioner's confidentiality to individual patients or to the public is warranted.

In the report given, the patient physician was judged to be impaired by his admitted self-treatment of psychiatric illness and there was nothing to suggest patients have been harmed.

The consulting physician on perusal of the patient's notes of a previous admission noted what appears to have been malfeasance of the managing surgeon. The patient was aware of the surgeon's failure to see him and discharged himself in apparent frustration. The patient may not be aware of the relation of the neglect to his current condition.

- *Patient self-discharge*

When patients discharge themselves from care there is usually a breakdown in communication between themselves and the care-givers. Patients may discharge themselves to seek alternative care when the options offered are unpalatable. When a patient reaches this decision they should be seen by as senior a person as possible and the patient's fears and /or issues explored.[337] It should be reiterated why the treating team/ person thinks that the decision they are making is inappropriate, and

---

[334] Reporting Impaired, Incompetent, or Unethical Colleagues; AMA Code of Medical Ethics; http://www.ama-assn.org/ama/pub/physician-resources/medical-ethics/code-medical-ethics/opinion9031
[335] Identifying and Assisting the Impaired Physician; Boisaubin, E V.; Levine, R E. American Journal of the Medical Sciences: 2001; Vol 322; 1; pp. 31-36
[336] Tarasoff et al. V. The regents of the University of California et al. Supreme Court of California. 17 cal. 3d 425; 551 p .2d 334
[337] Assessing competence to refuse medical treatment. Biegler P, Stewart C. Med J Aust. 2001 21; 174(10): 522-5

failing the ability to change the patient's mind the process to be followed should be explained. Reassurance should also be given that they would be welcome to return for treatment.

Institutions should have a formal document for patient self-discharge that should state the reasons for their decision. A patient's self-discharge does not absolve the practitioner from responsibility for any defects in prior management.

In the notes of the previous admission the nurses record that the patient becomes delirious after surgery and that the surgeon is contacted. The nurses advised to 'discharge' the patient to the surgeon's office are dissatisfied with that advice and asks another doctor to see the patient. Emergency investigation and treatment is undertaken and the patient improves. The following day the physician patient asks to be seen by the surgeon who did his procedure, and when this does not occur, he discharges himself from the institution the next day.

- *Negligence*

Negligence is a civil tort in which a patient or their estate seeks damages for harm that has come to the patient as a direct consequence of a breach in the standard of care.[338] The breach in the standard of care may result from a failure of the consent process, the procedure or treatment regimen, or the failure to recognise or respond to complications in the treatment process.[339] When claims of negligence are contested, adjudication may rest on a determination of what was the standard of care at the time. Such a determination rests on expert witness testimony and the assessment of the bona fides and credibility of those experts.[340] Negligence may be claimed if the physician fails to treat when they have a duty of care to the patient, or when they treat without a duty of care to the patient.[341]

In the report given, there is evidence in the notes of a previous admission of negligence where the surgeon refuses to see the patient in an emergency situation post-op.

---

[338] Bolam v Friern Hospital Management Committee [1957] 1 WLR 582
[339] The Standard of Care in Medical Negligence – Moving on from Bolam? H Teff; Oxford J Legal Studies (1998) 18 (3): 473-484
[340] GRADE guidelines: 3. Rating the quality of evidence; H Balshem, M Helfand, H J Scheunemann, et al Journal of Clinical Epidemiology 64 (2011) 401-406
[341] Duty of care and medical negligence Contin Educ Anaesth Crit Care Pain (2011) 11 (4): 124-127. http://ceaccp.oxfordjournals.org/content/11/4/124.extract#

The Inconvenient Diagnosis

Case report:
A 55-year-old man was brought to the Accident and Emergency
Department complaining of generalised malaise, fever, pain and swelling
of the neck, difficulty in swallowing, wet cough, shortness of breath
and bloody green sputum for four days. He was alert in respiratory
distress, febrile 37.8°C, BP132/78 mmHg, pulse rate 149 b/min. There
was a diffuse tender neck swelling with subcutaneous emphysema with
no abnormality in the mouth or pharynx. Chest examination revealed
harsh breath sounds throughout with coarse crepitations bilaterally. No
abnormality was found in the heart or the abdomen. The arterial blood
gases showed a low pO2 66.1. The ECG showed fast atrial fibrillation.

The assessment made was supra-ventricular tachycardia, sepsis
secondary to lower respiratory tract infection or deep neck space infection
with gas forming organisms. The patient was started on antibiotics,
CT of the neck and chest ordered, and referral made to the ENT and
medicine services.

The ENT service did an examination of the upper airway and found no
abnormality; the x-rays showed multiple bullae in the upper lobe of the
right lung and bilateral pleural effusions and concluded that the 'free air
is likely tracking up from ruptured lung bullae'. The medical service was
informed of the CT report and advised referral to cardiothoracic surgery.
The cardiothoracic service on being informed of the CT findings advised
the patient should be managed by medicine. The medical service without
examining the patient stated THIS IS NOT A MEDICAL ISSUE.

The patient's condition deteriorated and he became unresponsive. The
A&E staff intubated him and placed a thoracostomy tube, which drained
brown, purulent, foul-smelling fluid. The patient died under the care of
the emergency staff some hours later.

Issues raised

- *What does a diagnosis determine?*

The history and examination of a patient should lead to a diagnosis with
a differential. The differential should determine the investigations to be
performed, appropriate referrals and the actions aimed at the treatment of
the patient. When diagnosis is substituted for by observations it can lead to
incorrect treatment, particularly in an undesirable patient. The denial of an
obvious diagnosis is an escape from responsibility for having to undertake
its treatment, which may include a difficult operation or a prolonged stay.

In the report given the referrals made are based more on observations rather than any specific diagnosis of the patient. On the basis of a rapid pulse rate a referral is made to the medical service, which rejects the referral. Referrals to ENT and Cardiothoracic Surgical Services on the grounds that there are signs in the neck and changes on the chest x-ray are also not accepted.

The diagnosis appears to be a mediastinitis, a lethal condition that should be treated by surgical drainage if caused by a ruptured oesophagus or pharyngeal infection.[342]

- ### *Responsibilities of a consulting service*

Any service consulted has a responsibility to undertake an independent assessment and diagnosis of a patient through taking the history, examination of the patient and doing the appropriate investigations. Having done so they should come to any alternate diagnosis and give advice on the basis of their opinion.[343] Giving an opinion entirely over the phone is fraught with error unless one can be satisfied that all of the relevant information has been obtained and that the source of the information is trustworthy.

In the report given the referral for an investigation of air in the mediastinum without a contrast study of the oesophagus was inappropriately ordered by the A&E staff, inappropriately accepted by the radiologist, and inappropriately ignored by both the ENT and Cardiothoracic Surgical Services. The medicine service stating that the referral was for a fast pulse rate has inappropriately addressed that only. The ENT service has responded to the referral of a possible ruptured airway, and without taking a history has examined the patient and the x-rays obtained and satisfied themselves that this is not an ENT problem. On being consulted the cardiothoracic service accepts the radiologist diagnosis given over the phone and gives advice. This seriously ill patient is left in the care of the emergency department staff, after three services have been consulted and each has said that the patient should not be treated by their service.

- ### *The undesired patient*

Patients may be rejected for a variety of reasons. Older patients with serious or terminal illness often go untreated, a poor prognosis is the usual excuse made and sometimes that the facilities are needed for younger persons. Ethnicity plays a role in many countries, as does social

---

[342] Descending necrotizing mediastinitis: An analysis of the effects of serial surgical debridement on patient mortality; R K. Freeman, E Vallières, E D. Verrier, et al, The Journal of Thoracic and Cardiovascular Surgery, 2000, Vol 119, 2, Pgs. 260–267

[343] GMC | Good Medical Practice Delegation and referral; http://www.gmcuk.org/guidance/good_medical_practice/working_with_colleagues_conduct_and_performance.asp

standing in how resources are marshalled to treat patients. The behaviour and/or appearance of a patient may determine how they are treated.[344]

An assessment as possibly having a contagious disease can be a powerful deterrent to some health care workers in dealing with a patient.

Institutional factors play an important role in a patient being undesired, for example, the time of day when most of the routine workers in the institution have left and the emergency staff feel under pressure by patients who are not seen as very urgent. Other schedules may affect the attitudes of staff, such as being in the operating theatre and on emergency duty at the same time, and without sufficient staff to separate both functions. The status of the wards in an institution can have a powerful bearing on the admission of patients from the emergency department and the attitudes of staff to patients where the workload is increased with inadequate facilities.[345]

Health professionals have inherent factors that determine their attitude to the 'undesired patient'; these include tiredness, poor health and substance abuse.[346] Reliance on telephone and other remote reports in making diagnoses is frequently used in dealing with an undesired patient. Another avenue of disaffection is poor relationships with colleagues resulting in turf wars amongst staff and departments.

In the report given all of the senior personnel have accepted the assessment of junior personnel without asking for critical information. All of the services made emphatic assertions as various times that the patient did not belong on their service, one of them without examining the patient. Institutional factors were on display, with personnel busy on other duties when asked for an opinion on an emergency.

- *Turf wars*

In any war there are likely to be winners and losers; in patient care the patient is almost certain to be one of the losers. Professionals lose in regard to their status among their peers and within the institutional framework. Such loss leads to a diminution in professional cooperation and a downward spiral effect on patient care.

Lawsuits as a result of poor patient care are a financial hazard and have a negative impact on the reputation of both the involved professional and the institution in which they work. Therefore, it is

---

[344] Dealing with the difficult patient. S. Smith; Postgrad Med J. 1995; 71(841): 653–657
[345] The Effect of Hospital Occupancy on Emergency Department Length of Stay and Patient Disposition; A J. Forster, I Stiell, G Wells, et al, Academic Emergency Medicine, 2003, Vol 10, Iss 2, pgs. 127–133
[346] Impaired healthcare professional. Baldisseri MR; Crit Care Med. 2007; 35(2 Suppl): S106-16

the responsibility of both the professional and the institution to foster
mechanisms to resolve disputes that arise over the care of patients.
These mechanisms usually involve a review mechanism, which may be
a departmental or institutional clinical audit, an ethics review board,
or a complaints/disciplinary mechanism to deal with poor patient care
outcomes.[347]

*In the report given there was a turf war denying responsibility for the care
of the patient. The most egregious was the medical staff who without examining
the patient or making a diagnosis asserted that it was not their responsibility.
Notably there is no appeal by any of the parties involved to an institutional
mechanism to intervene in the disputed responsibility for care of the patient.*

---

[347] Edwards MT, Benjamin EM. The process of peer review in US hospitals. Journal of Clinical
Outcomes Management. 2009(Oct); 16(10): 461-467

Case report:
A 30-year-old man, remanded in prison, was seen in surgical outpatients complaining of perianal pain for 4-6 weeks, accompanied by a swelling in the groin. There were firm lymph nodes in the left inguinal region and on a non-ulcerated mass on the left side of the anus. A diagnosis of rectal carcinoma was made and he was referred for colonoscopy and to be seen after that.

Three days later he was seen in emergency with the same complaints, as well as swelling in the leg, difficulty in passing stool and blood in stools. He was referred to the on-call surgical service, which made a diagnosis of anal carcinoma and discharged the patient with the following - analgesia; gastroenterology review; CT abdomen/pelvis; outpatients appointment [three months away]. Three days later the patient was back in emergency complaining that the symptoms were worse and accompanied by abdominal pain with defecation. Abdominal x-rays were ordered, and he was again referred to the surgery service on call. The x-rays were seen, no air-fluid levels were noted and minimal dilation of the bowel was noted. The on-call service made an assessment of partial obstruction and made the following plan - analgesia and discharge with follow-up by the primary managing team in outpatients once a colonoscopy was done.

A month later he was seen again in emergency with additional complaints of dry cough and chest pain. The prison doctor referred to the CT scan done on the first emergency attendance showing an 8x8 cm anal mass with enlarged inguinal and para-aortic nodes, as well as metastases to vertebral bodies and pelvic bones. He was admitted on this occasion, a biopsy was done but his course was complicated by thrombocytopenia and he died 10 days after admission.

Issues raised

- *Prejudice and discrimination*

Prejudice usually lies in the subconscious, but is expressed overtly in word and action. When expressed by actions alone, the prejudiced person may not realize that their action is prejudiced simply on the basis that they have not expressed it in words.[348] Prejudices are usually considered as being unfavourable, but they may also be expressed in

---

[348] What Is Prejudice? K Cherry http://psychology.about.com/od/pindex/g/prejudice.htm

favourable actions for a person or group. The most common form of prejudices are related to race, ethnicity, social and economic standing, and nationality. However, religion, age, cultural identity including criminal history, sexual preference and even health status are also the basis for discrimination.

In health care settings all of these factors may operate, and may result consciously or not in different or poor treatment of an individual patient.[349] Since the 1980s, the disease that was most overtly discriminated against was HIV.[350]

In the report described there are factors that may lead to conscious or unconscious discriminatory treatment; i.e. being a prisoner, and a clinical condition that may indicate a homosexual lifestyle and HIV disease.

- *Discrimination in medical practice*

Discrimination in medical practice is usually expressed through limitation of access, abandonment of care, and through the manipulation of 'research'. Each of these avenues has available excuses to avoid the appearance of overt discrimination.

Access to care particularly in emergency situations should be the right of everyone, even in those societies with a dominant private care system like the USA.[351] Access may be limited by a paucity of personnel and facilities, or the ability to pay. Most countries try to provide emergency services without the ability to pay at the point of delivery, but when services are crowded there is an opportunity to make discriminatory decisions on the basis that other persons required more urgent care.[352]

Access to care in non-emergency settings can also be deployed in a discriminatory way, by giving excessively long appointments for services; unusually long waiting times at appointments to be actually seen; and by invoking shortages of equipment or medications necessary to provide the required service.[353]

Abandonment of care by direct physical separation is rarely done except in situations where the care-givers feel that their life is in danger, even then the life of the patient should be considered the first priority for the

---

[349] Prejudice in medicine; Our role in creating health care disparities; J Guilfoyle; Can Fam. Physician. 2008; 54(11): 1511–1513

[350] Dealing with prejudice; A O'Rourke, J Med Ethics 2001; 27:123-125 doi: 10.1136/jme.27.2.123

[351] Emergency Medical Treatment and Active Labor Act (EMTALA) 42 U.S.C. § 1395dd

[352] National Transgender Discrimination Survey Report on health and health care; J M. Grant, L A. Mottet, and J Tanis, 2010; http://transequality.org/PDFs/NTDSReportonHealth_final.pdf

[353] GMC Good Medical Practice.2013 Treat patients and colleagues fairly and without discrimination; http://www.gmc-uk.org/guidance/good_medical_practice/treat_fairly.asp

care-giver.[354] Abandonment is done in less direct ways; e.g. by referrals to other services for problems that are not the priority problems while insisting that they are a pre-requisite for treatment. It can also be done by the withdrawal of empathetic communication in a variety of ways, often at the end of life.

Abandonment is a charge of professional misconduct in some jurisdictions, e.g. " Abandonment of a patient in danger without sufficient cause and without allowing the patient sufficient opportunity to retain the services of another medical practitioner or specialist."[355]

Research as a tool for discrimination was noted at the Nuremberg trials at the end of World War II.[356] Although ethical research protocols were formulated following those trials, discriminatory practices in research have persisted most notably on racial grounds.[357]

Avoidance of an obvious diagnosis can be done through ignoring or taking a bad history of the patient's complaint, misinterpreting or not eliciting examination findings, or making an uncommon diagnosis that would require treatment from another service.

Resource availability may be used as a way of discriminating in the provision of care. Beds not being available can be claimed in most hospitals that are running full; i.e. 80% occupancy. Appointments are full, including those for procedures, and therefore an unduly long period of waiting for a service must be endured. Medicines for the treatment of the diagnosed condition may be too expensive, or are in short supply.[358]

In the case described, access to care was used in a discriminatory manner by giving a routine outpatient appointment of over three months for an urgent matter. The patient was also referred to another service for an investigation that was said to be necessary before the assessment in outpatients could be made. However, there was no evidence that the appointment was made for the patient in any expeditious time.

The patient was abandoned by the responsible service on call by ignoring the urgency of the patient's condition and giving non-urgent referrals to services for further assessment. Investigations were ordered and the results not seen by the ordering service.

---

[354] Guidelines for Crisis Standards of Care during Disasters; 2013; Amy Kaji, American College of Emergency Physicians http://www.acep.org/uploadedFiles/ACEP/Practice_Resources/disaster_and_EMS/disaster_preparedness/Crisis%20Standards%20of%20Care%200613.pdf
[355] Laws of Barbados; Medical Profession Act 2011-1; 23.2(e)
[356] Fifty Years Later: The Significance of the Nuremberg Code; E Shuster; N Engl. J Med 1997; 337:1436-1440; http://www.nejm.org/doi/full/10.1056/NEJM199711133337200
[357] P A. Clark Vulnerability in biomedical research • spring 2009, Journal of law, medicine & ethics http://faculty.tcc.edu/CSeward/Journal%20Articles/Prejudice%20and%20the%20Medical%20Profession.pdf
[358] Health Care Refusals Harm Patients: The Threat to LGBT People and Individuals Living with HIV/AIDS http://www.nwlc.org/resource/health-care-refusals-harm-patients-threat-lgbt-people-and-individuals-living-hivaids

In the case described the diagnosis of a tumour arising outside of the intestinal tract, is set aside because of its location at the anus, and the patient is referred to a gastro-intestinal service for evaluation with no attempt to elicit urgent attention. Resource availability was not invoked in the narrative, but is the most likely reason for the long appointments given for the recommended services and follow-up.

• *Legal consequences*

There are legal consequences to delays in treatment depending on the outcomes. Without invoking discrimination or other motives for the delay, charges of negligent care as well as manslaughter have been brought against doctors involved in treatment delays.[359]

• *Poor end-of-life care*

Poor pain management is often a part of poor end-of-life care, and may be a consequence of poor knowledge compounded by poor surroundings and the embarrassment of care-givers who see being unable to cure as a defeat, or 'that's not my problem'. Such care-givers offer little or no psychological support to the dying person.[360]

In the narrative given an assessment of advanced disease could have been made six weeks before admission by looking at the CT scan ordered. What was offered was the repeated return to prison conditions with pain medication and no plan to monitor its effectiveness. When he was eventually admitted he died before a definitive diagnosis was obtained.

---

[359] Doctors and Manslaughter; P McDonald; Ann RCS Bull. 2014 No 4, V96, 112-3
[360] We need to talk about death: Complaints about end of life care; S Whitehouse; MPS Casebook / Vol. 21 no. 2 -2013; http://www.medicalprotection.org/uk/casebook-may-2013/complaints-about-end-of-life-care

Complaint 1. *Letter to the Head of Department from a Consultant Surgeon:*
I am writing about a situation that unfolded in the Operating Theatre
when I was assisting my resident in removing a breast lump in a 15-year-
old girl. I insisted that the comprehensive checklist be used and both the
nurses and doctors responded that there were no equipment concerns
identified. When we started, I asked for a small swab and was informed
by the scrub nurse that none were available. When I enquired why that
was not mentioned as an equipment concern, I was informed that the
situation had existed for two weeks and I should have known it. I was not
aware of this but started the operation using large swabs.

A cosmetic incision was made to reach the lump but on removing
the lump heavy bleeding came from deep in the wound. I instructed my
resident to enlarge the incision but still struggled to control the bleeder.
Recognizing that the large swab could not get down to the point of
bleeding, I asked for small wound dressing gauze to pack the wound. The
scrub nurse refused to take a packet of such gauze and said to the student
nurse that she is not to pass any unmarked gauze. I asked that the gauze
swabs be passed directly to me but all four nurses in the theatre and the
sister in charge refused to do so. I then asked the anaesthetist to pass me
the gauze and we were able to pack the wound, identify the bleeder and
secure it. Incidentally some small swabs appeared at the end of the ordeal.

I can no longer in good conscience continue to endanger patients
under "MY CARE AND RESPONSIBILITY" in this environment.
Until the situation is rectified I am not sure it is safe for my team to
operate. The Theatre Manager and the Director of Medical Services
were informed. The Theatre Manager did come and apologize to me.
However, this will happen again unless there are some consequences for
these actions.

Complaint 2. *Incident report to the Head of Department:*
I would like to report an incident where a nurse refused to carry out my
instruction to administer oral contrast to a patient. She said she refused
because she had not witnessed the contrast being removed from its
original vial.

I had gone to the radiology department to discuss an urgent CT scan
on a patient being treated conservatively for a diverticular abscess. The
radiographer drew up contrast from a vial into a 20cc syringe, labelled it,
filled out an instruction sheet and signed it. The contrast was sent to the
ward with the instruction sheet and the nurse refused to administer the

contrast stating that she had not seen the contrast drawn up herself. I told her that I had been present when the contrast was drawn from the vial but she did not relent. I spoke to the supervising nurse who responded that the nurse was correct to refuse to administer any unlabelled substance. I arranged for my intern to administer the contrast as per the instructions. I also spoke to the nursing office on the matter and the person on duty simply stated that the nurse was correct in her refusal.

Does a member of the patient care staff looking after a patient have a right to refuse to assist in the care of a patient? If so, should they not at least find some way that the care be administered rather than abandon the patient?

Signed

Surgery resident

Issues raised

- ***On being a professional.***

A professional is a person who has had special training and qualification in a particular discipline. Such training and qualifications may be set out in law and the functions and responsibilities of the professional outlined in law. The functioning of a professional may also be expressed in terms of how they should or should not conduct themselves.[361] When such conduct is defined it may be done in both technical and behavioural terms.

In medical practice there are several categories of professionals who more often than not work in teams in the care of the patient. Where there is teamwork the role of the team members is usually clearly delineated by the profession that they hold and the legal responsibilities outlined in law. However, there are some areas where responsibilities may not be clear or may overlap. When these situations arise in patient care it is prudent to have written guidelines or codes of conduct, and the clear delineation of legal responsibilities. The ultimate responsibility is usually that of the doctor whose care the patient has sought; however, clear communication is the responsibility of all.[362]

In the first complaint the nurses in the operating team clearly have a different view from the surgeon as to what their responsibilities are; this results in the use of inappropriate swabs in the procedure and resulted in conflict in an urgent situation. The surgeon salvages the situation in spite of the obstruction of the

---

[361] Professionalism in health care professionals - Health and Care ...www.hpc-uk.org/assets/.../10003771

[362] Teamwork skills: being an effective group member | Centre for ...https://uwaterloo.ca/.../teamwork-skills-being-effective-group-.

nurses and is making an appeal through the department to have some action to stop this impasse recurring.

In the second scenario a nurse is refusing to administer an 'unknown' substance, although the doctor contends that the substance is known and labelled. This contention can only be adjudicated with factual evidence.

- ### *Utilizing inappropriate equipment*

Utilizing inappropriate equipment in any procedure increases the chances that the procedure will be flawed. In medical practice should such flaws lead to compensable harm to the patient, the person responsible for using the flawed equipment would be considered negligent, particularly when they knew that the equipment was faulty.[363]

In a situation where the preparation of instruments for surgery is delegated to others, the person doing the operation retains the ultimate responsibility for the equipment.[364] For example, the person responsible for the procedure should be familiar with the procedures and labelling for the sterility of instruments, and through either formal or informal checks ensure that sterile instruments are being used. When deep or cavity procedures are being conducted instrument and swab counts must be conducted. Nevertheless, inaccuracies may occur.[365] In spite of a delegation of a duty to others, the person responsible for the procedure is indeed responsible for the instruments they use. Precautions should include instrument and swab counts, which if not done routinely should be done randomly, which would re-emphasize to the delegated person where the responsibility rests. Giving over total unsupervised responsibility to another person does not absolve the person responsible for the operation from legal liability.

The responsibility of administering medicines carries the legal responsibility to ensure that the medications administered are those prescribed, and that they are administered in the correct doses. If a prescription written is not clear, either as to the substance or the dose then the person administering the medicine must clarify it before doing so. Equally important, if the dose of a medication or its route of administration is considered dangerous, clarification or correction must be sought before it is administered.

---

[363] Working with medical equipment — Reducing the risks - Cmpa-acpm.ca
https://www.cmpa-acpm.ca/-/working-with-medical-equipment-reducing-the-risks
[364] Roles of Operating Room Personnel, http://work.chron.com/roles-operating-room-personnel-17867.html
[365] Risk factors for retained instruments and sponges after surgery. Gawande AA, Studdert DM, Orav EJ et al N Engl J Med 2003; 348: 229–235

In the first complaint it is said that both the nurse and the resident stated that the instrument check was correct, yet as soon as the surgery commenced a deficiency was detected. The nurse appears to justify the deficiency stating it had been so for the last two weeks. The surgeon accepted the deficiency and proceeded. However, the deficient swabs became a necessity and a substitute was requested, the nurses refused to cooperate. An unpleasant scene ensues and the crisis is overcome by bypassing the nurses. Although an apology from the theatre manager comes later, the surgeon is not satisfied that a similar situation will not recur.

In the second narrative there is a dispute about the fact as to whether a substance is labelled or not. The stated contention that the nurse does not trust a medication unless she has seen the original vial herself demonstrates a complete lack of trust between the doctor and nurse that is necessary for a properly functioning team.

- ***Assigning responsibility within teams***

Teamwork is an important part of modern medical practice. The team may consist of a variety of professionals and non-professionals and include individuals in training. Training should include a definition of individual roles, technical tasks, and an understanding of individual responsibilities and how these are carried out.[366] Carrying out responsibilities within a team requires an understanding of the responsibilities of other team members, and to understand who is responsible for decision-making should an emergency arise.

Good teamwork should result in few emergencies and it is important that the training of individuals within the team should be to recognize and handle emergencies. In some situations, simulation may be used in training, and it is important that written instructions should be available should there be any doubt about how the emergency should be handled. Such manuals may contain checklists that have been proven to reduce morbidity and mortality.[367]

In the first instance reported a surgical team comprising nurses and doctors purport to be employing a checklist prior to a surgical procedure. The checklist of the instruments and supplies is said to be OK by both the nurses and the doctor assigned to do the operation. However, at the very start of the surgery a deficiency is found and this is excused as a supply issue. The surgeon chose to ignore the deficiency but an emergency arose requiring the missing item. The

---

[366] Procedure for the checking of swabs, Instruments, sharps and needles; WAHT-THE-015, www.worcsacute.nhs.uk/EasysiteWeb/getresource.axd?AssetID=49632&type
[367] A Systematic Review of the Effectiveness, Compliance, and Critical Factors for Implementation of Safety Checklists in Surgery A Borchard et al; Ann Surg 2012; 256: 925–933

surgeon asked for an available substitute but the nurses refused to do so stating the substitute was unsafe. With the assistance of other doctors, the substitute was used and the emergency dealt with. An apology was subsequently tendered to the surgeon by the theatre management but none came from the nurses.

In the second complaint the nurse is absolutely correct to ascertain that what she is asked to administer is safe for the patient. However, there appears to be no trust between the doctor and the nurse and there is a contention as to whether a syringe is labelled or not and then whether the nurse saw the original vial from which the syringe was drawn. The supervisory nursing personnel, without checking the fact of labelling or not, simply asserts that the nurse is correct.

- ### *Resolving disputes*

Disputes arise when there are different interpretations of a given set of facts. In social and scientific discourse dispute resolution is done through a process of discussion and agreement on a way to proceed even when a given set of facts remains in dispute.[368] Such agreements are set out in documents that may be laws, agreed guidelines for procedures, or codes of conduct. None of these methods are eternal, for new discoveries, new skills or even different attitudes will influence how disputes are resolved.

In modern medical practice, there is constant striving to improve. However, because of the variability of the individual, the natural history of disease and the inevitability of death, some failure is inevitable. For many patients, surgical procedures are seen as the most hazardous of medical interventions, for there are issues of alterations of the body image going wrong and the fear of sudden death. Complex and risky procedures are best undertaken by teams of professionals who may enter their professions with different personal attributes, but are all looking for affirmation of their own self- worth. This affirmation of worth is expressed in terms of earnings, public approbation, and expressions of appreciation within the team. Team training and functioning requires both formal and informal ways of establishing relationships. Unfortunately, professionals who are viewed and feel themselves as subservient may be resistant to common training and may take an aggressive attitude towards those who they think consider them subservient. Such attitudes are dangerous when life or death issues arise. Therefore training should have multi-disciplinary components, which include behavioural modification. One important component of behaviour modification is the socialization of different disciplines by events where individuals are put on an equal social footing.

---

[368] Conflict resolution. Resolving conflict rationally and effectively ...www.campbell.edu/pdf/ student-services/.../conflict-resolution.pdf

When disputes are unresolved, and particularly if harm comes to a patient or any of the parties involved, the disputes should be enquired into and corrective or disciplinary action taken. Unresolved conflict leads to poor conduct embedded within institutions.[369]

In the complaints made there is a clear description of bad dispute resolution. Poor training is displayed when a checklist of instruments is said to be correct and almost immediately found to be incorrect, and in the other, whether a syringe is labelled or not is the contention. The aggressive response of the nurses in both instances on being asked for an explanation, may be a defiant response to what is seen as a challenge to their authority, or a response to the tone in which the complaints were made.

In the first instance the aggressive and defiant attitude persists in the face of an emergency. The fact that the missing swabs appeared after the emergency was handled bypassing the nurses, betrays a deeper dysfunction within the team and a lack of understanding of patient safety. In the second instance there is no trust between the parties for even the simple fact of a syringe being labelled or not is disputed. In both instances a complaint through the nursing hierarchy is adjudicated in favour of the nurse without any enquiry into the facts.

- *Patient safety*

With advances in medical care, there are more powerful drugs, complicated equipment and complex procedures that increase the risk of complications and mishaps. In spite of oversight agencies such as the FDA and scientific trials before new drugs or equipment is introduced, an absolute standard of drug, equipment and patient safety remains elusive. The weakest link is the human element, and this is expressed in the standard of care of a practitioner.[370] When a health professional acts outside the normal standard of care and the patient comes to harm, the law can consider them negligent. On the other hand, the professional is protected against the imperfections of medical practice by following the practices standard to the profession at the time. Invasive procedures test all of the sensitive points of patient safety and it is not surprising that checklists have become formalized to increase the safety of patients in the most hazardous areas of practice.[371]

In the administration of medication, it is vital that the correct medication, its dosage and the route of administration be specified and checked at every stage from its manufacture, its distribution, its

---

[369] Bad Blood: Doctor-Nurse Behavior Problems Impact Patient Care; C Johnson 2009 https://www. ache.org/policy/doctornursebehavior.pdf
[370] What is the Medical Standard of Care? - AllLaw.com www.alllaw.com
[371] WHO | Patient safety; www.who.int/patientsafety/

prescription and its dispensing. At every stage of this process correct and clear labelling is vital and checked by the persons/professionals involved in the process.[372]

In the first letter of complaint the safety of the patient is jeopardized by bleeding, fortunately not in a life-threatening way. The real hazard to the patient is that what was expected to be a minor operation with a cosmetic scar could have turned into a large scar due to the lack of standard small swabs being denied to the surgeon. On the other hand, the surgeon should not have started without the assurance that the swabs or a substitute would be available if necessary.

In the second complaint the nurse is properly going through the necessary checks before a medication is administered to a patient. However, the nurse's objection is variously stated as the syringe not being labelled to not having seen the medication drawn up herself. The fact that the doctor involved cannot assure the nurse of the authenticity of the process or the labelling on the syringe demonstrates a lack of trust between the doctors and the nurses involved.

- ***Role of a code of conduct/practice guidelines***

Professionals are trained and have to be qualified to formally enter their profession. It is acknowledged that at the point of entry the professional's knowledge will be further expanded, particularly in the practical applications of their discipline. Therefore, in situations with which they are not familiar it is good to be able to refer to more senior colleagues. However, it is preferable to have an authoritative source that can be referred to whether this is the law, professional or institutional codes of conduct.[373]

Laws describe professional behaviours in general terms of good or ethical conduct but are more specific in terms of misconduct. A code of conduct published by regulatory bodies or professional associations outlines acceptable and unacceptable behaviours to clients and between the professionals. [374], [375] Check lists are formulated for specific situations and are particularly important in surgery.[376] Such guidelines are only as good as those who use them and become a hazard if they are open to misinterpretation or are misused.

---

[372] Medication administration 3 - ATI Testing https://www.atitesting.com/ati_next_gen/.../medication-administration-3/.../safety.html

[373] WMA International Code of Medical Ethics; www.wma.net/en/30publications/10policies/c8/

[374] AMA Code of Medical Ethics - American Medical Association; www.amaassn.org/go/codeofmedicalethics

[375] Code of Ethics for Nurses - International Council of Nurses; www.icn.ch/who-we-are/code-of-ethics-for-nurses/

[376] A Surgical Safety Checklist to Reduce Morbidity and Mortality in a in a Global Population; AB Haynes et al- N Engl J Med 2009; 360:491-499; www.nejm.org/doi/full/10.../NEJMsa0810119

In the first complaint a checklist is used prior to the start of an operation, the listed item on instrumentation is said to be OK by the nurse responsible, but is found to be deficient at the start of the operation. The challenge as to why the checklist was said to be OK was met by an aggressive response suggesting that the deficiency was not important and that the situation had been known and accepted for some time. The surgeon signalled acceptance of the deficiency by starting the operation without any overt plan for a substitute if needed. When a contingency arose for which the deficient item is needed, the nurses become belligerent and obstructive disregarding the safety of the patient. This leads to an unpleasant scene in which the nurses are bypassed to deal with the situation.

In the second incident there is a total lack of trust between the nurses and the doctor involved. By the doctor's account even the fact of the substance in a syringe being labelled cannot be agreed on. When a complaint is made to the nursing supervisor, there is no check of the facts before deciding that the nurse is correct.

Case report:

A 40-year-old man experienced a sudden onset of sharp, sticking chest pain which radiated to the left side, was worse lying back and improved on leaning forward. A co-worker said he should have it looked at by the cardiac specialist she had seen on television. He went to the specialist's office, was told that he had "fluid around the heart" and needed an echocardiogram right away. He was told that it confirmed the diagnosis.

He was admitted and received a course of antibiotics as well as hydrocortisone injections three times a day for two weeks. Two further echocardiograms showed resolution of the fluid. He was discharged but the pain returned after two days and he was told that he needed further tests. A CAT scan, pulmonary angiogram, two exercise stress tests and cardiac catheterization were done and were reported normal. He was prescribed a course of steroids 60mg a day for four weeks. In the following weeks he noticed mood changes, weight gain, fatigue, blurred vision and easy bruising. After the medication was completed another echocardiogram was done and he was told that the fluid had resolved. A week later, he developed dizziness, nausea, "foggy-mindedness", headache, fatigue, and generalized muscle pain. He returned to the clinic and was told he should see a psychiatrist. He attended the psychiatrist who told him that his symptoms were in keeping with an organic disorder and recommended he get a second opinion. The physician concluded that the patient had adrenal insufficiency caused by prolonged high dose steroids. The physician added that the extensive workup had been unnecessary, as the patient had no risk factors to suggest coronary artery disease or pulmonary embolism. After getting this opinion, the patient thought he had been taken advantage of, and asked the physician whether he should pay the substantial bill he had received from the clinic.

Issues raised

- *Professional malfeasance/negligence*

Professional malfeasance is any conduct or practice that is contrary to law, medical ethics, professional regulations, or the existing standard of care.[377] Advertising one's medical service is against professional regulations in some jurisdictions, but not in others where it may

---

[377] Good Medical Practice; gmc.uk. section 53

still remain contrary to medical ethics.[378] In some jurisdictions it is unlawful to refer patients for services to a laboratory or other diagnostic service that the practitioner owns, particularly when there is no clear indication for such service.[379] The splitting of fees between practitioners either directly or indirectly is also against medical ethics.[380] It can be considered professional malfeasance to imply to a patient the improper behaviour of another professional, if one is not prepared to complain to a regulatory body.

Negligence is a form of malfeasance that carries legal liability to a patient who has been harmed as a result of care they received.[381] Medical practice is not perfect and both medications and procedures can have complications. However, negligence cannot be found in law unless the harm can be quantified and the practitioner acted outside of the standard of care existing at that time. The standard of care is that of the practitioner acting in the circumstances within which they are practising, and that which would have been carried out by their peers. Such standards are subject to change as advances are made; it therefore redounds on the court to be advised by experts in the field, based on the best available evidence.[382] In order to avoid such cases, clinical problems should be reviewed within institutions at departmental audits, mortality and morbidity reviews, or at an ethical board. When malfeasance comes to light outside of an institutional setting, a review may be conducted within a professional association such as an ethical committee. Such committees should be seen as advisory and do not replace regulatory bodies.

Regulatory bodies may receive complaints of professional malfeasance from the public or other professionals. These bodies usually have a quasi-judicial mechanism to enquire into complaints and to prosecute any charges that may emerge. Regulatory bodies do not have the power to compensate patients, but they have the power to suspend or revoke the licence of the professional charged.[383] Because of the consequences to a fellow practitioner, professionals are often loath to complain about other professionals to the regulatory body. This can end up making the situation worse as the malfeasance may become a pattern of behaviour.

---

[378] Medical Profession Act, 2011-1, Barbados; section23

[379] Insurance Fraud and Abuse: A Very Serious Problem; S Barrett, http://www.quackwatch.com/02ConsumerProtection/insfraud.html

[380] The Code of Medical Ethics of the American Medical Association; F A. Riddick, Ochsner J. 2003; 5(2): 6–10

[381] Bolam v Friern Hospital Management Committee [1957] 1 WLR 582

[382] GRADE guidelines: 3. Rating the quality of evidence; H Balshem, M Helfand, H J Scheunemann, et al Journal of Clinical Epidemiology 64 (2011) 401-406

[383] When Should a Doctor Lose His License? mdwhistleblower.blogspot.com/2015/11/when-should-doctor-lose-his-licence.html

The practitioner cannot escape responsibility by putting the onus on the patient to complain, for invariably an enquiry will unearth the practitioner who expressed concern to the patient about the alleged malfeasance.

In the case reported, the consulting physician, by virtue of the detailed commentary on the previous management to the patient, has clearly given the patient the impression that professional malfeasance had occurred in the patient's management.

- ### *Professionals handling professional malfeasance*

Professionals will encounter instances of professional malfeasance, either their own or that of colleagues. Malfeasance occurs when a practitioner incorrectly prescribes or performs a procedure, without a reasonable rationale to depart from the normal standard of care. When a practitioner becomes aware of their own malfeasance it is appropriate to review the record and enter date and time any necessary correction; and if there has been an adverse consequence to the patient to tell the patient what has happened and express one's regret. When working in an institution, the issue should also be brought up at the appropriate forum such as an audit meeting.[384] When working outside of an institution, the steps outlined in relation to the record and the patient should be observed. When compensable harm comes to the patient such conduct becomes negligence in law and the patient may wish to get legal advice on pursuing a claim. It is not appropriate for another professional to advise their patient to initiate a legal claim; the professional can supply a medical report and opinion to be used by the patient's lawyer.

When a professional discovers malfeasance in the work of another practitioner, one's opinion on such malfeasance should be recorded, and if responsible for giving a second opinion, the facts should be carefully recorded. Patients should be given the facts and one's opinion, without any conclusive opinion on the conduct of another practitioner. If a patient asks directly about the conduct of another practitioner, one's opinion on the treatment should be reiterated and an offer made to put the opinion in the form of a medical report. If a patient asks whether they should pursue a complaint against another practitioner, the patient should be informed of the avenues available to do so. Assurance can be given that as long as the complaint is made to the regulatory body and not publicised otherwise, they are protected from any threat of legal action by the doctor being complained about.[385]

---

[384] Guidelines for medical audit: seven principles. C. D. Shaw and D. W. Costain; BMJ. 1989; 299(6697): 498–499

[385] Making Complaints to Regulatory Bodies within the Protection of ...defamationlawblog.ahbl. ca/.../making-complaints-to-regulatory-bodies-within-the-pro. 2014

Professionals who know the offending practitioner in an institutional
or social setting will wish to consider informing the practitioner of their
opinion and any action that they intend to take, such as bringing the
matter to an audit conference. Where the practitioner does not know the
offending practitioner or does not have cordial relationships with them,
the practitioner has to decide whether the malfeasance should be brought
to the attention of the practitioner through a professional association
or by a complaint to the regulatory body. Professional associations will
vary in their effectiveness in dealing with such complaints depending
on the attitude to preserving the reputation of the profession or acting as
a sanctuary for its members. Providing good guidance for its members
and pointing out defects in conduct to individual members is the best
way by which a profession's reputation is held high. On the other hand
a professional association should not shrink from referring its members
for egregious offences or a pattern of misconduct after having issued a
warning about such misconduct.

Regulatory bodies are often made up of the professionals themselves;
such professionals should be persons of integrity and be prepared to
examine complaints they receive with a sense of fairness to both parties.
Regulatory bodies gain the confidence of the public when they include
lay representatives in their membership.[386] In making a complaint
to a regulatory body, the complainants should be advised that their
complaints will be sent to the party complained about for their response.
Patients should also be advised that compensation or the regulation/
retrieval of fees is not the province of regulatory bodies but that of a
court. When a disciplinary hearing is being conducted the complainant
may be subjected to cross-examination as in court proceedings. Whenever
professional malfeasance is complained about in relation to a specific
patient, it should be done with the explicit knowledge/consent of the
patient, for the regulatory body will not wish to deal with the matter
without hearing from the patient. Courts may also be called upon to
deal with fraud, such as unnecessary investigations or false billings done
without any medical rationale.[387] Such cases are usually brought after a
pattern of fraud has been established.

When a patient seeks advice, a professional should avoid giving direct
advice to sue or not pay a bill. The alternative is to offer to give a medical
report on which a legal opinion can be sought. Advice can be given to

---

[386] Whose interests do lay people represent? Towards an understanding ... C Hogg - 2001
onlinelibrary.wiley.com/doi/10.1046/j.1369-6513.2001.00106.x/pdf
[387] Insurance Fraud and Abuse: A Very Serious Problem; S Barrett, http://www.quackwatch.
com/02ConsumerProtection/insfraud.html

obtain a medical report of the questioned care with originals of X-rays etc., for obtaining an expert opinion through a lawyer.

A complainant doctor should not act as an expert opinion on their own complaint, but they may be called upon to provide references to back up their complaint.

A professional code of conduct can be helpful in providing guidance in dealing with malfeasance, as well as avoiding it.[388] They can also provide guidance as to how to make a complaint and what to expect when one is made. For example, a complaint to the regulatory body will be transmitted to the doctor complained about for a response, and the patient concerned will have to be identified so that the doctor involved can respond. If the complaints body finds that there is a case to answer, the disciplinary process is similar to a court process where evidence is given and is subject to cross-examination.[389]

In the case presented the opinion given by the physician has prompted the patient to question the conduct of the original physician as to whether they were taken advantage of and whether the bill should be paid. The best response would be that questions such as whether a bill should be paid are best done with legal advice.

- ***On being thorough vs. exploitation***

Concern is often expressed over 'unnecessary' and expensive investigations of patients. This is explained by some practitioners as being thorough and to avoid a possible accusation of negligence should the treatment outcome prove to be less than optimal. In addition, the training of the modern-day physician has placed clinical diagnosis as subservient to diagnostic imaging and laboratory results. Unfortunately, this trend has led to indiscriminate imaging and laboratory testing before assessing the patient, both before and during treatment.[390] Furthermore, the fear of malpractice claims drives some physicians to repeat investigations on the basis of being thorough.[391] The fact is that the increased costs of such practices may trigger the patient to seek to recover costs when results are unsatisfactory.

There is another dimension to over-investigation when physicians have an economic interest in the investigative facilities they use. This has resulted in overuse of such facilities to a level where some physicians

---

[388] GMC | Good medical practice; www.gmc-uk.org/guidance/
[389] Medical Profession Act, 2011-1, Barbados; Part V
[390] Overkill; A Gawande, Annals of Health Care May 11, 2015
[391] Defensive Medicine Among High-Risk Specialist Physicians in a Volatile Malpractice Environment D M. Studdert; M M. Mello; W M. Sage; et al. JAMA. 2005; 293(21): 2609-2617

have been accused of fraud.[392] The detection of such practices is seldom noticed in single incidents, and often waits until a third party payer has noticed a pattern of claims.

In the case report given, the assessing physician has made it clear that in their opinion a number of investigations have been carried out without any indication to do so. It is also implied that repeated investigative monitoring of the patient was unwarranted. This has resulted in a large bill and the patient asking 'were they taken advantage of?'

- ***Breach in the standard of care***

A breach in the standard of care may be brought about by the misdiagnosis of a patient; such mistakes may lead to delays in treatment or incorrect treatment. The standard of care may also be breached by applying the wrong treatment for the patient's condition, or by carrying out the treatment inappropriately.

A breach in the standard of care may be inconsequential, but if the patient is harmed the practitioner can be sued for negligence. In suits of negligence the standard of care is described as 'that standard which a responsible body of similar professionals would employ in similar circumstances.'[393] The determination of such standards is left to expert opinion, which may vary in any one circumstance. Because of such variability some jurisdictions require that contending parties in a suit of negligence agree on a single expert who can advise the court.

In the case presented the alleged breach in the standard of care is the high dose and prolonged use of steroid medication leading to adrenal insufficiency.

---

[392] 10 popular health care provider fraud schemes - ACFE.com; www.acfe.com/article.aspx?id=4294976280
[393] Bolam v Friern Hospital Management Committee [1957] 1 WLR 583

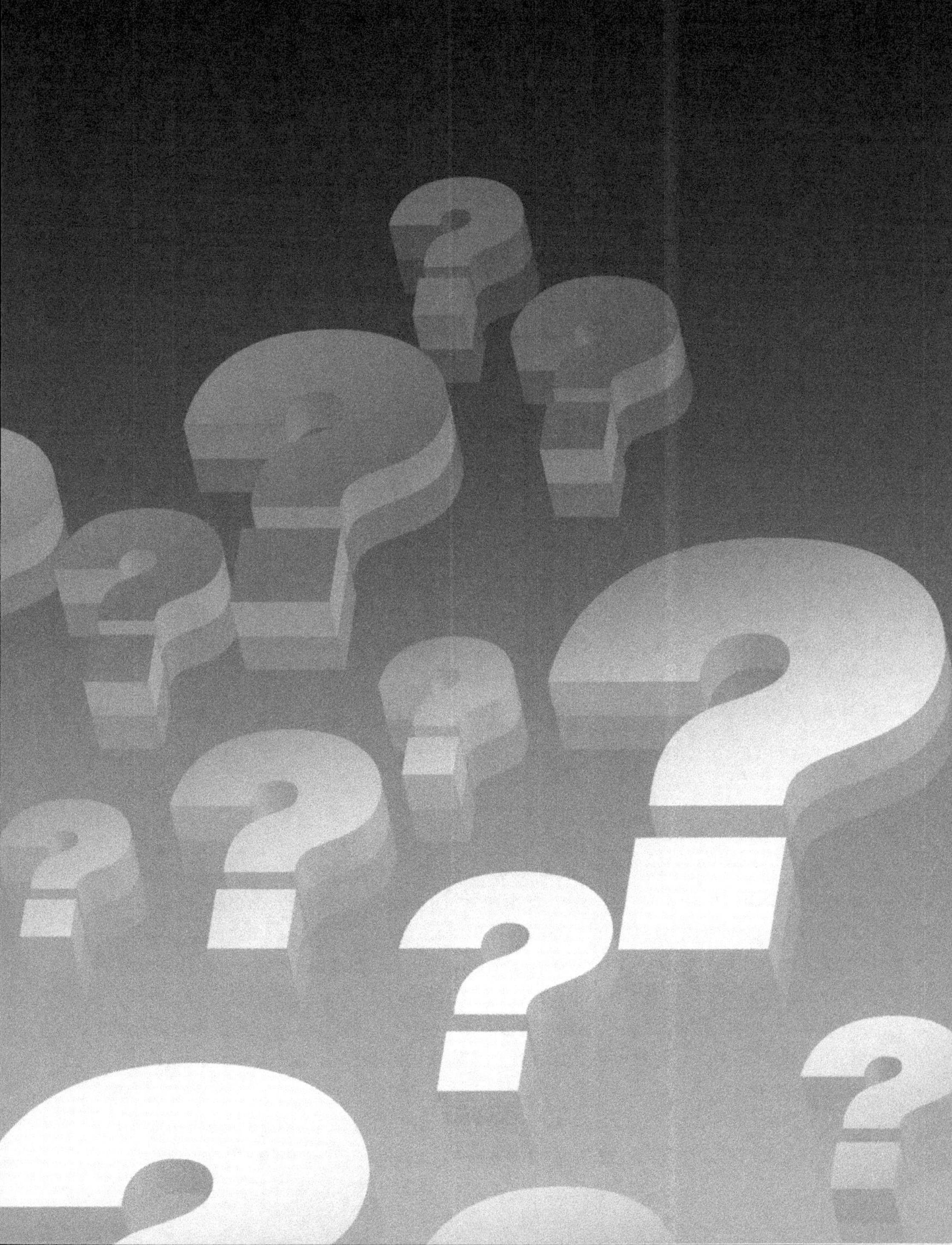
ALLOCATION OF
RESOURCES

Doing All That's Possible

Case report:
An 18-year-old man sustained an injury eight months ago and was
paralysed in all four limbs. He is now an outpatient with partial recovery
of his limbs on one side and a urinary catheter in situ. Prior to the injury
he had been in a training programme to be a draughtsman. He is from
a low-income family and is unable to attend for all the recommended
therapy because of the lack of suitable transport.

The physiatrist's assessment is that under the current circumstances
the prognosis is poor and is requesting that funds be made available
to send the patient abroad for rehabilitation for a minimum period of
12 weeks at a cost estimated at US$168,000. The patient has no medical
insurance and was not employed previous to the injury.

Physiatrist's presentation: With treatment in such a centre, the rate of
recovery of motor function declines after the first six months following
the injury. Expected functional outcomes were not being met; for
example, the patient has an indwelling urinary catheter, and this leads to
recurrent urinary tract infections and chronic renal failure.

The staff required for rehabilitation were available in the hospital or
in the private sector, and included an occupational therapist [OT] and
a psychologist. The deficiencies in the local setting were specialised
transport, wheelchair prescription and maintenance, and vocational
training facilities. An occupational therapy assessment obtained two
months after the injury stated that the patient required daily intensive
physiotherapy and occupational therapy, was developing contractures, but
it was noted that the household was partly adapted for the patient's use.

Issues raised

- ### *Exploration of the current status*
Determination of the effectiveness of public expenditures requires
an examination of the prospects for the patient under consideration
and other patients that may be in a similar situation. This requires
an examination of local resources inclusive of preventative actions,
emergency and rehabilitative treatment resources and plans for
improvement. Therefore, requests for resources to be spent abroad must
be justified for the individual patient requested, as well as a plan to boost
local resources.

*There was no current assessment of the patient's neurological status, the
course of the patient during hospitalisation was not clear and there was no*

existing protocol for handing such injuries. There was no assessment of how the patient was being managed at home and the national ambulance service used to bring the patient to the physiotherapy department was not available for all the sessions booked in the department, which would be inadequate even if they could be adhered to.

The data for recovery possibilities presented was for the immediate treatment of injuries and there was no data on likely progress with an injury after eight months. The one post of occupational therapist for the hospital was not enough and was not currently filled and the patient would have to go abroad to obtain a personalised wheel chair. There were no resources in the island for wheel-chair maintenance and there was no provision in the sum requested for training anyone in the household to assist the patient.

- ### *Why do all that is possible?*

A community depends for its well-being on its members being able to contribute to the society in a full and productive manner. Therefore, the provision of services designed to achieve full and productive lives is of paramount importance, as is the maximising of impaired lives.[394] A family and a community has to look after its members with an impairment, and a balance should be struck with regard to the resources used in maximising the life of an impaired person and the contribution such a person can make to the family and to the society. Discussion should occur as to when a life is no longer useful rather than simply symbolic or spiritual.

- ### *Avoid pursuing a futile course.*

The call to do all that is possible when no improvement can be expected is pursuing a course of futility; however, maintaining stability and avoiding deterioration is a crucial objective. In emergencies it is not always clear what the outcome will be, and advances in care have made what appeared futile in the past to be no longer so. In determining whether a course of action will prove useful the following should be considered: -

- Will the action save a life, preserve function or relieve a symptom, and without undue burden bring comfort to relatives, friends and the community?

- Can the action generate new knowledge that would benefit the community?

---

[394] Functional recovery measures for spinal cord injury: an evidence-based review for clinical practice and research. Anderson K, Aito S, Atkins M, Biering-Sørensen F, et al al J Spinal Cord Med. 2008;31(2):133-44.

*In the case presented the request is being made to try and maximise the
severely impaired life of a young man, who may be able to contribute to his
own upkeep within the community. However, the presentation does not make it
clear that the intended programme will be successful in producing a significant
improvement; that they are the only resources that will be needed; that any gains
will not be reversed on the patient returning to the local situation.*

*There are questions that remain to be answered, and additional information
such as an assessment of what follow-up visits would be needed abroad, what
facilities would be needed at a prospective workplace to make employment
possible. It is also necessary to determine the numbers of persons with similar
injuries, to assess their treatment and provide recommendations to correct any
deficiencies in their treatment.*

- ### *The implications of quality of life decisions*

Quality of life is measurable and will influence decisions.[395] The legal
implications of the quality of life are set out in law and decisions may
have to be made regarding withdrawal of life support in the brain-
dead patient, persistent vegetative states and patients on permanent life
support. These decisions can be based on the definition of brain death
and the prior wishes of incapacitated patients.

Advanced directives are for a patient to express their wishes about
treatment when they are no longer able to do so.[396] However, a directive
may be ignored if it is considered as an illegal request for euthanasia. A
decision not to treat opens a care-giver to an accusation of negligence or
criminal neglect; such charges can only be defended on the basis that the
caregiver had pursued what was considered the normal standard of care
in the treatment of the patient.

Standards may be presented in international terms but have to be
adapted to local circumstances, which cannot be reduced to nothing for
even severely deficient facilities can be utilized in an agreed institutional
protocol that sets out to achieve the best standard of care achievable
within the level of resources available. If it is not possible to achieve
a reasonable standard with the resources available then mechanisms
should be explored for transfer of the patient, or making the resources
and funds available in an emergency.[397]

In the case discussed there was insufficient information presented to determine

---

[395] Measuring health-related quality of life. Guyatt GH, Feeny DH, Patrick DL Annals of Internal
Medicine 1993, 118(8): 622-629
[396] Childress, J. Dying Patients. Who's in Control? Law, Medicine & Health Care. 1989;17(3):227-228.
[397] Defining standard of care in the developing world: the intersection of international research ethics
and health systems analysis. Hyder AA, Dawson L. Dev World Bioeth. 2005; 5(2): 142-52.

*whether a 'normal' standard of care had been met. With the clinical state
described it is highly probable that international standards had not been met.*

- ### *Making funds available*

Funds for unexpected or catastrophic medical treatment events are
often large and are usually required on an urgent basis. They may be
derived from a number of sources such as medical insurance, institutional
reserves, government, settlement of claims from insurance for personal
damages or medical negligence, personal savings or loans, and publicly
raised funds from NGOs, appeals, raffles etc.

Each of the sources has its own rules and limitations. The most
problematic is institutional reserves for publicly funded institutions can
expect a large flow of requests once such a resource is known to exist.
Any reserve funds should have clear mechanisms for how they will
be replenished.[398] Making institutional funds available must take into
account their most effective use and ensure that services and protocols
are put in place to try and reduce similar demands.

*In the case presented there was an explicit exclusion of medical insurance, a
claim for personal damages, no prospect of personal financing and no mention of
publicly raised funds.*

---

[398] http://www.ihs.gov/california/UploadedFiles/CATASTROPHIC-HEALTH-EMERGENCY-
FUND.pdf

Refusal to Dispense

Letter to the Hospital Director

Dear Sir, Mr P. Maddow aged 60 years [registr. no.123456] has recently been hospitalised for a deep vein thrombosis. I saw him on the 15th February in outpatients and ordered a pair of TED stockings. Mr Maddow's wife, a former staff nurse at this hospital, took the prescription to the Medical Supplies Department and returned stating that the department has refused to issue the stockings. I asked her if they had run out of them and she replied that one of the clerks in the department said that he was not giving them out because "this type of stocking is dangerous and should only be used on inpatients who are being monitored". Mrs Maddow said she told the supplies officer that she was a nurse and could supervise her husband at home, but was told that he didn't care who she was, he was not giving out these stockings to outpatients and the doctor should prescribe something else.

I wrote a note on the prescription pad stating that the stockings indicated were the type I wanted and asked Mrs Maddow to take it back to the Supplies Department. Shortly thereafter I received a call from the clerk who said, "I am not going to give out these stockings; they are dangerous and cut off the circulation." He then said, "I will not be dispensing the stockings unless I get an order from the Director."

I left my outpatients and came to your office, you agreed to see me and said that TED stockings were not routinely dispensed and that the hospital only dispensed them to outpatients who were indigent in order to save funds. When I pointed out that this was not the reason given for not dispensing the stockings you then phoned the Supplies Department and told them to issue the stockings to Mrs Maddow. I am writing this letter to ask what person or constituted body has the authority to challenge a hospital consultant's management of patients? I am also objecting to the manner in which Mrs Maddow was treated, and alarmed at the way my professional integrity was impugned in such an offensive manner. I await your appropriate intervention in this matter.

Yours sincerely, Dr H. Adam

The Hospital Director responds after two months:

Dear Dr Adam

Re. Issuing of TED stockings

I must apologise for any distress your patient and you would have suffered over this most unfortunate incident. There can be no dispute as to the authority and responsibility of the consultant in the management of patients in the hospital.

The Supplies Department is sincerely regretful that this incident had to occur. I have counselled the department of the danger of attempting to use medical reasons in the controlling of the supply of medical supplies. Following the discussions I have had, I am confident that a repeat of this incident is less likely to occur.

Yours sincerely, ...for HD

Issues raised

• ***Does anyone have the authority to question a consultant's management?***
A patient has the right to question their management, and health professionals have a duty to question the management of any doctor they think endangers a patient. Apart from questioning the doctor, a patient may refuse treatment and ask for other opinions. On the other hand, health professionals do not have the authority to refuse a treatment order of a practitioner in charge of a patient's care. A health professional who is concerned about the treatment ordered should contact the practitioner and express their concern; if after clarifying with the practitioner the health professional still considers that the treatment ordered dangerous, they should not administer or dispense it but refer the matter to the appropriate regulatory authority in an institution or the community.[399]

Lay staff including heads of institutions or government departments have no role in making medical judgment decisions, although they are called upon to make administrative decisions that impinge on medical decisions. However, ethical advice and court decisions do broaden decision-making beyond the medical practitioner.[400] A hospital director may be called upon to consent for the treatment of a mentally incompetent patient who has no available next of kin, but should have no role in challenging the medical judgment of the doctor unless judging it to be not in a patient's best interest. Similarly, an administration may be called upon to make judgments about obtaining medical supplies and should do so in conjunction with the medical staff.

In the instance described, the staff member is not a health professional and has made it clear that they do not respect the medical consultant's opinion. When

---

[399] Good Little Soldiers - NOT! Are you justified refusing an order or questioning a chart entry? G M. Clavreul, http://www.workingnurse.com/articles/Good-Little-Soldiers-NOT
[400] Lay Participation in Health Care Decision Making: A Conceptual Framework; C Charles and S DeMaio; http://reference.kfupm.edu.sa/content/l/a/lay_participation_in_health_care_decisio_65393.pdf

*challenged the clerk declared that only the Hospital Director can order them to do
so. The response clearly indicates a skewed line of command in which the medical
staff have no place. This will inevitably lead to conflict and build up frustration
and anger in the organisation.*

- ### *Should treatment be characterised as dangerous to a patient or relative?*

A health professional who thinks there is a serious error should not
characterise the treatment as dangerous to a patient or their relative.[401]
The correct course is to discuss one's view with the doctor involved and,
if necessary, through the heads of departments. Nevertheless, there is a
duty of health professionals to act on matters they consider dangerous.
For example, a pharmacist may say to the patient "I do not understand
the prescription as written, I am going to ring the doctor to clarify
what is required". A pharmacist also has a role in informing patients
about complications of a drug but must be prudent about how such
complications are characterised, for conflicting information from health
providers will lead to non-compliance in many cases.[402]

*In the instance described the clerk involved is not a health professional but
has been assigned a role in 'dispensing' medical supplies. Any person assigned
a responsibility must be trained to perform the task, which would be to ascertain
that the correct size of stockings has been ordered and the administrative lines for
handling problems that arise.*

- ### *Did the consultant handle this matter in a proper manner?*

Disputes can be provoking and may induce anger and inappropriate
responses. Submitting a patient or relative to abuse is never warranted.
When problems cannot be solved by a simple corrective, they should be
addressed through management.[403]

*In the situation described it was not appropriate for the consultant to
have sent the patient's wife back before trying to solve the problem with the
department. Direct communication is tried only after the patient and his wife
were subjected to further trauma, and then the line of management is ignored
and the top administrative official approached. The consultant was in fact pointed
to the Hospital Director as the only person who could resolve the problem and
proceeded directly to the director's office.*

------

[401] GMC; Good Medical Practice: Respect for colleagues; 2012; http://www.gmc-uk.org/guidance/
good_medical_practice/working_with_colleagues_respect_for_colleagues.asp
[402] The Pharmacist as Patient Educator; L Raman-Wilms Can J Hosp Pharm. 2009 Mar-Apr; 62(2):
93–94.
[403] Dealing with the difficult patient. S. Smith Postgrad Med J. 1995; 71(841): 653–657.

*The practitioner's response was made in anger and there is no indication
that thought was given to the other patients who were left unseen in the
clinic. Fortunately, the problem was promptly resolved and the consultant
probably derived some satisfaction in finding a quick solution for the problem.
Nevertheless, the consultant subsequently writes a letter stating that they are
unresolved issues related to the challenge to his authority.*

• *Did the Hospital Director deal with the matter in an effective manner?*

Senior administrative officials have a responsibility to act in a fair manner
and to ensure that all staff act within an established code of conduct. In
a hospital where some responsibilities are clearly drawn, administrators
should know what the boundaries are for all staff. Without such
knowledge administrators may issue directions that lead to conflict
between staff, and may be unable to resolve issues when they arise.

There is no doubt that a hospital administration has the responsibility
to regulate supplies, however, it is fraught with danger to do so without
an input from the medical staff who have responsibility for treatment.
Any policy made should be disseminated to those affected and should
contain mechanisms to determine conditions within the policy.

*The Hospital Director must be commended for resolving the immediate
issue by seeing the consultant who has arrived at his office unannounced, and
in spite of the explanation of the hospital's policy, ordered the supplies to be
dispensed in apparent contradiction of that policy. However, the resolution of the
problem should involve corrective action in relation to the staff of the Supplies
Department, and clarification of the 'policy' related to providing medical supplies.
The staff member has not been called upon to apologize to the consultant, and this
is the minimum of disciplinary action that should be expected.*

*The Director's response to the consultant's letter apologizes for the distress
caused to the patient, and expresses a qualified regret for the department but
there is no apology to the consultant. The regret that the incident 'had to occur'
suggests that the department was acting within the directives given. This is
supported by the contention of the clerk that the item would only be dispensed on
the order of the Director, and the counselling not to give medical reasons for their
actions. The letter also appears to give the department carte blanche to use 'other
than medical reasons' to deny or refuse a consultant's order, and states that he is
'confident that a repeat of this incident is less likely to occur'.*

• *Should outpatients be treated differently from inpatients?*

There are no clear guidelines on how rationing should be done in health
care settings and this matter is under debate in all health care systems.

Distinctions can be rationalised on various grounds, such as the urgency of the matter, expected outcomes, scarcity of the resource, costs and the ability to pay.[404] As technology has evolved fewer and fewer treatments are being restricted to inpatients only.

While it is acknowledged that social services departments should have the expertise to determine who is unable to pay, is it a prudent use of resources to make such determinations for dispensing an inexpensive item that may be required immediately? Policies should be based on evidence, consultation with relevant staff and widely disseminated.[405] When this is done there should be a high degree of confidence that policy can be carried out with the interest of the institution as a whole.

There is no evidence that relevant consultations have been done in deriving policy in this matter and as such disputes 'had to occur'. What is of greater concern is that no lessons seem to have been learnt by the administration and policy appears to have been altered to rationalise the immediate problem without further consultation.

- ### *Is the supplies clerk practising medicine?*
The practice of medicine is defined in law as carried out by qualified medical practitioners. There are medical practices that are carried out by other qualified health professionals, and there is nothing that prevents someone giving home remedies or medical advice. What is illegal is when one purports to be qualified as a health professional and gives medical advice or carry out procedures that are considered medical and as a result cause harm to another person.[406]

With the widespread availability of medical information sources, many persons feel that they have the information with which to challenge a doctor's opinion. However, it should be realized that articles even in the most prestigious medical journals are subject to critical analysis and the conclusions of the authors may not stand up to the scrutiny of other experts in the field. Furthermore, with the spread of direct and comparative advertising, and the prohibition of advertising by doctors in some jurisdictions, it is likely that challenges to medical opinion are likely to increase rather than decrease. [407]

---

[404] What Is Healthcare Rationing? From Denial of Care to Healthcare Reform, Rationing Is a Consideration; T Torrey, About.com Guide, 2012, http://patients.about.com/od/patientempowermentissues/a/rationing.htm

[405] Decision making in health and medicine; MGM Hunink, et al Cambridge University Press; 2003; http://faculty.ksu.edu.sa/AlBarrak/Documents/Decision%20Making%20in%20Health%20and%20Medicine.pdf

[406] Laws of Barbados 1972; Medical Registration Act CAP171. Sec 18

[407] Use and abuse of advertising in medicine. Advertising and the pattern of prescribing. G. Teeling-Smith, Proc R Soc Med. 1968; 61(8): 748–750.

The supplies clerk has clearly purported to give a medical judgment without being qualified to do so. However, the clerk is working within a hospital and any such person purporting to give a medical judgment in the course of their work should be subject to disciplinary action. There is no indication that disciplinary action is contemplated in spite of the senior administrator recognising that an inappropriate medical opinion has been given. This has left the consultant involved dissatisfied, particularly in relation to characterising, to the patient's relative, that the consultant's treatment is dangerous. The consultant could justifiably feel that they have been slandered, the question would then arise as to what responsibility the institution will take for the acts of its employees?

- ### Has the issue been resolved?

Issues are resolved when all parties feel the problems have been satisfactorily addressed. In matters involving health care, mechanisms are required to ensure that the medical staff are involved in decisions about the acquisition and prioritising of medical supplies and other matters involving the care of patients.[408]

It does not appear that the underlying issue in the situation described has been resolved, although the hospital administrator considers the incident has been dealt with. The supplies department appears to have been cautioned not to give medical reasons when refusing to release medical supplies.

---

[408] Principles of Justice in Health Care Rationing' R. Cookson, P. Dolan, J. Med. Ethics 2000; 26; 323-9

Pay First or No Treatment

Case report 1:
A three-month-old infant suspected of having biliary atresia, is referred for treatment in a public hospital in a neighbouring country. The parent is told that treatment would have to be carried out urgently to have a reasonable chance of success. The parent and the referring doctor are informed that the child would not be accepted unless the estimated cost is paid in advance. The parent makes urgent attempts to obtain the sum quoted and travels with the child to the hospital and offers 10 per cent of the estimated cost that was raised. The accounts office refuses admission for the infant and when told about the urgency of the situation informs the surgeon that at least 50 per cent of the cost would be required as a deposit. The parent confesses that they had said that they could raise the money but was unable to do so and given the urgency of the situation had lied about it. The surgeon approached charitable organizations about donating the money but was unsuccessful. Meanwhile, the money raised was being exhausted on accommodation expenses, but after further efforts 40% of the estimated cost was realized. After further pleading the 40% was accepted as a down payment and the infant admitted.

The surgery was carried out without recourse to some of the elements in the estimated cost, however, no revision of the estimated cost was done. The infant was discharged from hospital, but was refused a follow-up appointment in the outpatients department until the rest of the money was paid.

Case report 2:
A 75-year-old man was referred from the publicly funded geriatric hospital to the public general hospital with a complaint of bleeding per rectum. On examination a rectal mass was found and biopsied. Because of the workload and the anticipated time for the biopsy result to be obtained, the patient was discharged back to the geriatric hospital with an appointment to attend surgical outpatients in one month's time. When the biopsy result is obtained, the surgical service asks for the patient to be readmitted for further biopsy and were told that the patient cannot be readmitted until the bill is paid for his previous admission. On enquiring why the patient was billed, the service was told that he was not a national.

Two years later the patient was again referred back and admitted to the ward, where an advanced carcinoma of the rectum was diagnosed. When an enquiry was made as to why he had not been referred back earlier, it was said that the billing for the indigent patient domiciled in the geriatric hospital was referred to the Ministry of Health and the decision made that he should not be billed was not conveyed or noticed until the patient had further alarming symptoms. The patient was demented, had no relatives living in the country, but had resided in the country for over 30 years.

The patient was treated by neo-adjuvant therapy followed by a radical resection of the rectum and succumbed to complications one month after surgery.

Issues raised

- ### Public vs. private financing of health care

In every country there exists a mixture of public and private provision of health care. Public care is provided for by government through the collection of taxes and generally seeks to provide all levels of care. Private care funded through personal payment, either directly or through third party payment, is often valued by the individual for having direct and quicker access to the physician of their choice and is said to have better outcomes.

The assertion of better outcomes in privately funded care is challenged by studies of health care in industrialised countries with government funded universal access to health care, as in the UK, as against the USA where universal access is not assured. In a study of outcomes such as life expectancy, infant mortality, quality of care and access to care, the USA was found to spend twice as much per capita than 10 other countries, yet was rated last in the assessment of outcomes.[409]

In the first case the hospital concerned is a publicly funded entity in which paid treatment is available for persons who are not citizens.

In the second case the patient is indigent and has been in a public institution for the elderly indigent for many years, from which he was referred. The outcome in this case illustrates the oft-times insensitivity of public services to individual needs.

- ### The ethics of withholding access to care

The ethics of the medical profession commands beneficence and justice for patients; neither can be realized without access to health care facilities. It is particularly egregious to withhold access to care in emergencies

---

[409] Mirror, Mirror on the Wall, 2014 Update: How the U.S. Health …ww.commonwealthfund.org/…/ mirror-mirror

for lack of the ability to pay; yet it is done where services are provided privately. In most countries there is a public emergency service, but laws have been enacted to ensure that emergencies presenting at private institutions are not sent away without essential life-saving care.[410]

Children and the indigent are particularly vulnerable where medical care is accessed through payment at the point of delivery. Furthermore, neonatal and congenital disorders may require very expensive care beyond the ability of most individuals or families to afford. In addition, third party payments through health insurance imposes limits on the amount of money they pay, or the coverage they will give to 'pre-existing' conditions such as a congenital disorder. It is therefore imperative that in systems where health care is accessed through payment at the point of delivery, that consideration be given to children's disorders through charitable and other financial arrangements.

In the first case report an infant with an urgent condition is being denied access to care on the basis that the parent is unable to pay in advance for the estimated cost of services.

In the second case an indigent patient is billed on the grounds that he is not a citizen, this in spite of his being resident in another public institution for indigent persons.

- *Billing of indigent patients*

An indigent person is one who is penniless and unable to pay for the services required for daily living. Such persons may be homeless on the streets, seek shelter in facilities run by charities, or accommodated in government-run institutions. Governments undertake such care for persons who have exhausted all of their resources and turn over their pension to the institution. Billing of such patients becomes an exercise in futility.

In privately-funded health care institutions patients are not accepted unless they can show an ability to pay, or when there is a source of charitable funding. The use of charity funding for the treatment of indigent patients usually relates to teaching and/or financing research. Such arrangements are difficult to make in emergencies and patients may be left unattended or sent to other facilities.

Where private and publicly funded services are undertaken in the same institution confusion may arise over the entitlement of those who are not to pay. Assessments should be made with explicit guidelines, based on humanitarian policies and undertaken in consultation with medical staff that can assess the urgency of the patient's problem.

---

[410] EMTALA statute - 42 USC 1395dd, part of the U.S. Code

In the second case report, a resident of the country, recognized to be indigent and domiciled in a public geriatric home is sent a bill for services as a non-citizen. Although a cancer is diagnosed and was being confirmed, there was no one in either institution that advocated for the patient until his cancer reached an advanced stage.

- ### *The rights of residents to public services*

In most countries citizens and legal residents have a right to the services that authorities provide. However, access to services may be limited by legal or bureaucratic means and may be particularly difficult for the poorest and indigent in societies. These difficulties become almost impossible to surmount when the individuals are weakened by illness. In many countries, the right to public services may be denied by the authorities on the basis of racial, cultural and religious identities.[411] Prejudicial treatment is often based on the minority status of the person and may be for or against a minority group depending on long-standing historical, cultural and economic factors. There are even some countries where residents may by deprived of their status for lack of papers or for minor infractions of law, and rendered stateless and devoid of all rights including humane treatment when they are ill.[412]

In the second case report, the patient is recognized as being resident and indigent by being admitted in a public institution for such individuals. The staff responsible for billing patients takes no notice of such residency and sends out a bill that cannot be collected. The professional staff in the institutions showed little interest in the problem until the patient has reached an advanced stage in his illness two years later. As a result more was spent on the treatment of the patient than was necessary.

- ### *Governmental responsibility for provision of health care*

Governments should exercise responsibility for the populations they serve. The responsibilities include the ability to have food, shelter, health and education. Governments vary in the level of responsibility they exercise in providing these essentials and the provision of comprehensive health care shows the greatest variation in governmental provision worldwide. The variation is evident in both rich and poor countries, and is the subject of much policy discussion given the high cost of medical care. Costs driven

---

[411] Unequal treatment; B. Smedley, A. Stith, A. Nelson; 2003, National Academy Press http://www.nap.edu/catalog/10260.htm

[412] Limitations on universality: the "right to health" and the necessity of legal nationality; L N Kingston, E F Cohen and C P Morley; http://bmcinthealthhumrights.biomedcentral.com/articles/10.1186/1472-698X-10-11

by the pharmaceutical and medical equipment industries makes it very difficult for non-industrialised countries to provide the 'modern' care that their populations come to expect from the global communications network. Many governments provide what they can afford, and the well-to-do in the community uses 'private' services within the country or abroad. This dual system gives an impression of inadequacy of government provided services, even when government has superior professional and technological services compared to privately-owned services.

In the first case presented the hospital is a government-funded facility, providing the professional resources that would do the procedure at no cost to its citizens. The infant is from a nearby territory and there is no agreement for sharing medical resources.

In the second case the patient is recognisable as a long-standing resident, but is not a citizen. The ministry recognises that there is a responsibility to provide this resident with care, nevertheless there is a two-year delay for their authorization to be realized.

- ### *Estimating the cost of care*

Costing of health care can be a complex undertaking particularly when it comes to hospital services. The estimate of costs given to patients varies widely as health care organizations attempt to estimate the patient's ability to pay, as well as trying to recover losses made from unrecovered bills. Patients hearing of such variation in charges may be less than truthful about their ability to pay, even when they have health insurance. Health insurance agencies may be equally opaque about what they will pay and may leave patients to meet large out of pocket payments. Even when patients get an estimate of costs, the actual bill sent is often much larger.[413]

In the first circumstance described the parent is clearly unable to pay out of pocket for her infant in need of an urgent procedure. She pretends to be able to do so and there is some negotiation that goes on between the finance department, the parent and the doctor carrying out the treatment. In the end a down payment is accepted and the treatment carried out on the promise of further payment later.

In the second case report it is clear that the patient is unable to pay, being in an institution for the indigent and having no known relatives to call upon.

- ### *Should there be humanitarian policies for patients who cannot pay?*

A key principle in medical ethics is beneficence towards patients including the indigent. Administrators in health care do not have the

---

[413] Negotiating Medical Bills http://healthcaresavvy.wbur.org/resources/negotiate-medical-bill/

same ethical obligations and may remain inured to the plight of the indigent or others for whom they have no obligation. This attitude does not enhance the reputation of institutions or the professionals employed within them. Professional reputations depend on both knowledge and experience, and the latter may depend on the number of patients who come for service but cannot pay. It is also in an institution's interest to attract the rare and uncommon disorders so that their professionals can have increased experience and enhance the institution's reputation.[414]

In the cases presented, the hospital has no humanitarian policy towards those in need who are not citizens of the country.

- **Is an ethical code of conduct applicable to administrative staff?**
Ethical codes should exist for all staff that provides services for the public.[415] Health professionals abide by a written professional code but there is seldom a written code for the non-professionals with whom they work. Nevertheless, the public expects that those staff should abide by similar rules as the professionals to whom they come for service. As organizations get larger, administration becomes more remote from professionals and the personal transmission of modes of conduct may be lost. When this occurs it is likely that staff will insist that they have a different set of rules that are distinct from those of the professionals in the organization. In health care the important core values that should apply to all staff, are confidentiality, equitable access and compassion.

There is nothing in the case reports to suggest that the administrative staff have an ethical code and take little or no account of the urgency of the patients' problems.

- **Is access to care a professional's responsibility?**
Access to health care is a right of all persons, and is a core responsibility of the health professional. Exercising that responsibility equitably is challenging given the financial, nationality or cultural barriers the patient may face. These barriers are set up in the practical governance of an institution. The philosophy varies from governments that provide services for all its citizens, to those who leave it mostly to market forces. The systems leave professionals to make or influence decisions on access of patients to care.

---

[414] Surgeon volume compared to hospital volume as a predictor of outcome following primary colon cancer resection. Schrag D1, Panageas KS, Riedel E, Hsieh L, Bach PB, Guillem JG, Begg CB; J Surg Oncol. 2003; 83(2): 68-7.
[415] Code of Ethics and Standards of Practice - NAHQ.org; www.nahq.org/uploads/files/about/codestandards.pdf

In the first case, the doctor shows a high degree of interest in getting access for the child.

In the second case there is little attention by the professionals to the effects of administrative action on the patient until the patient's condition progresses.

- ### Is delay in access to care negligence?

Negligence arises when a breach in the standard of care is directly linked to the harm that comes to a patient. For a delay to be negligent, the delay would have to be outside the current practice and shown to have a direct relationship to the harm of the patient. A misdiagnosis causing a delay is not by itself negligent except if it is established that the misdiagnosis was itself due to a breach in the standard of care.[416]

In the cases reported the delay is occasioned by institutional rules on payment that would have to be challenged in court to establish whether they were outside of the legal standard. There is no doubt that the delay in access caused considerable harm to the patient in the second report through progression of the disease.

---

[416] How the wrong diagnosis or late diagnosis from your doctor can lead to a medical malpractice lawsuit. K Michon, https://www.nolo.com/legal-encyclopedia/medical-malpractice-misdiagnosis-delayed-diagnosis-32288.html

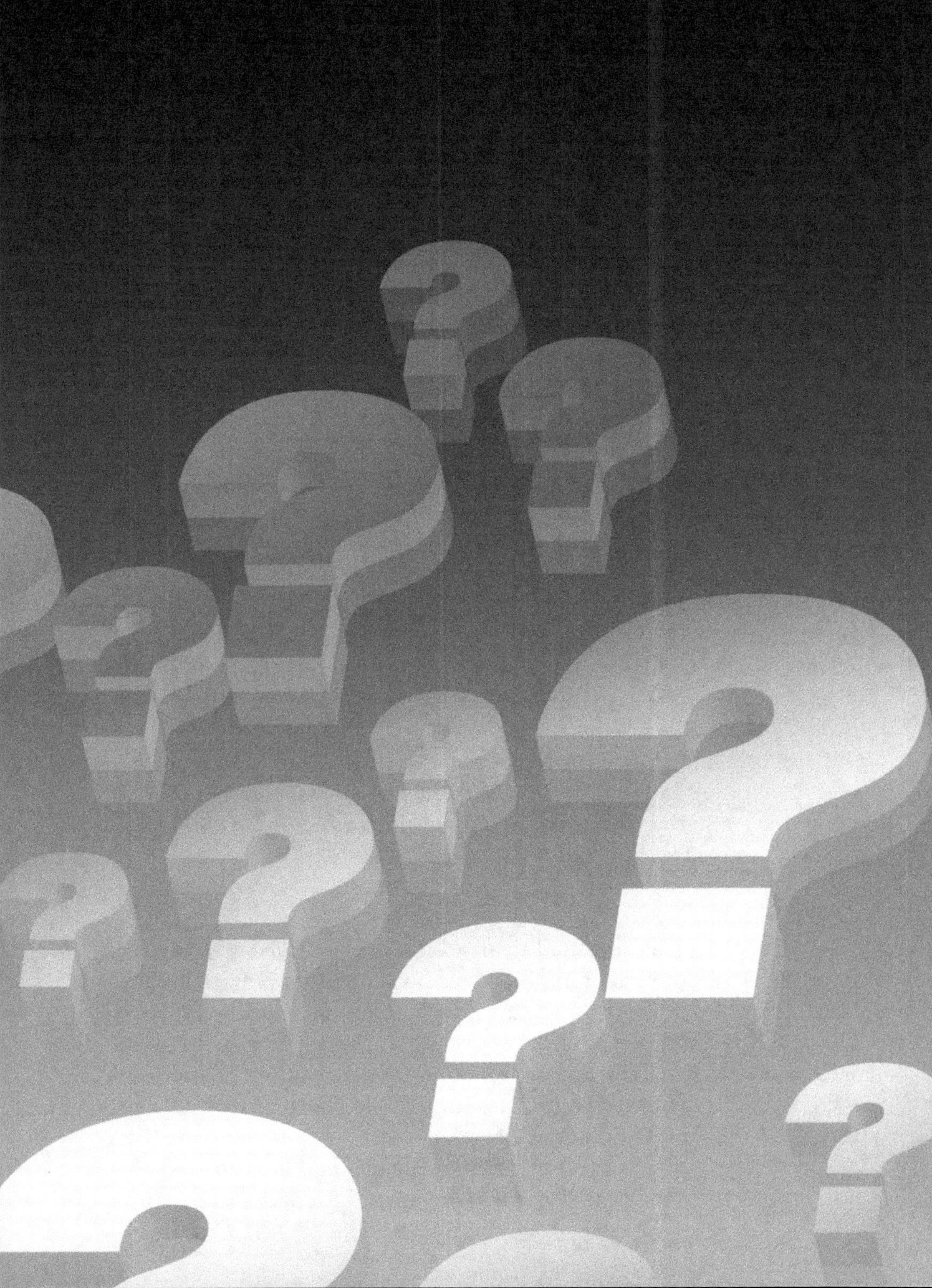
CHILD ABUSE

Case report 1:

A girl aged 11 years was admitted with a painful swelling on her right buttock associated with fever and headache. She had not yet started her menses. There was a tender swelling on the right buttock and a lax anal sphincter on rectal examination. A diagnosis of an ischiorectal abscess was made and anal sexual activity suspected. On drainage of the abscess both the anus and the vagina were noted to be gaping. There was an offensive greenish black vaginal discharge and plaques on the vagina and cervix.

The child denied any sexual activity and referral was advised to the psychiatric and social services. When asked by the psychiatrist why she looked sad she replied that she was always a quiet person and asked to go home to avoid missing school. The nurses arranged for the parents to see the psychiatrist separately on the next day. The notes state that the surgical findings were read to the mother and she was asked if she had considered that the child had been sexually abused. A similar interview was conducted with the father and the parents told that the child 'will remain hospitalized because these issues took precedence over her returning to school'. The child was transferred to a psychiatric ward and a gynaecologist of the parents' choosing confirmed the vaginal findings.

The parents wrote a letter to the hospital director complaining that the psychiatrist had 'insinuated that the mother had prior knowledge of this alleged abuse, that the child 'would not be allowed home unless it could be ensured that the home was safe, and that, if necessary, the child would be forcibly taken from their care'.

The social services investigated the matter and reported that there were two older daughters living in the home who stated that they did everything together and there was no opportunity for the child to be sexually abused.

Case report 2:

A 14-yr-old girl was admitted to an adult ward with a complaint of generalised abdominal pain; there was no vomiting or alteration in bowel habit. She had the build of an adult, but spoke as if she was 10 years old. She was tender all over the abdomen, the adjacent chest wall as well as her thighs; there was no rebound tenderness and bowel sounds were normal. The blood count, abdominal and chest x-rays and a pelvic ultrasound examination were normal.

On review of her notes it was noted that she had had several admissions from the time she was six years old for abdominal pain,

with no abnormal pathology being found. It was decided that a review
of her history was necessary, and in spite of her adult build, she should
be transferred to the children's ward. She was asked if anyone had
'interfered' with her and her response was that her father had been
having sex with her up to two years ago when her mother found out and
stopped it. Her mother was contacted and when told what her daughter
had said, she confirmed it, and said that when she found out she went
to her priest and they decided that the father should be prevented from
seeing the child and that there should be no report to the police, since she
did not want to drag her child through the courts.

A consultation was arranged with a psychiatrist, and the Social
Services Department was asked to look into the family circumstances
with a view to reporting the matter to the child protection service. The
psychiatrist thought that the matter should be reported to the police
immediately, rather than going through the child protection agency.

Case report 3:
A 14-year-old girl presented with severe abdominal pain of several
days duration. She was noted to be febrile with abdominal tenderness,
guarding and rebound. Pelvic examination revealed cervical excitation
and adnexal tenderness and a diagnosis of pelvic inflammatory disease
was made. She was admitted and commenced on antibiotics and
improved over the next three days.

She had a history of sexual activity, which at first she said was with a
14-year-old boy, but she subsequently said that it was with a man in his
twenties, who lived in the same house. Further enquiry revealed that she
was involved sexually with several adults in the neighbourhood. The
child, her mother and two siblings resided in the home of her mother's
same-sex partner, her two children and her brother - the alleged assailant.

The matter was referred to Social Services as well as the Child
Care Board.

The child's mother confronted the man who apologized and admitted
that he had betrayed her trust. The mother's partner reminded her that she
had warned her that her brother liked little girls, and she had responded
at the time that he was nice to them, and that the children needed a father
figure. The partner persuaded her brother to stay away from the house
when they were around and not asleep, while the family looked for
alternate accommodation. The girl's mother was unable to provide for
alternate housing for the family, and the decision of the Child Care Board
was to place the girl in a state-run children's home. The mother expressed
great distress that her daughter was removed from her home to be in

care, rather than the police removing the assailant from the home. The mother reached the point of attempting suicide and during her psychiatric consultation she revealed that she had also been sexually abused as a child.

Several calls to the police from the paediatrician went unheeded.

Issues raised

- ### The diagnosis of childhood sexual abuse

An acute illness or injury is the most common presentation of childhood abuse. Suspicion is usually raised because of additional findings that do not fit in with the history of the acute illness. Signs of an old injury or of repeated abuse are also common. The presence or absence of a hymen does not exclude vaginal penetration.

Sexually transmitted disease in a child is indicative of sexual abuse. Evidence of penetration of the vagina or the anus is usually chronic rather than acute. The skin manifestations of other diseases may be mistaken for STDs or trauma.[417]

Gynaecological examination of a child must be conducted in a forensic manner where an accusation is made of a sexual assault, irrespective of when the assault occurred. Photographs and swabs for infections and sperm should be taken. An intact or absent hymen is no guarantee that sexual abuse has or has not occurred. False accusations or denials may be made for other reasons including issues of child custody or the protection of a person or family's image in the community.

Behaviour change particularly becoming unruly or withdrawn is a sign of childhood abuse. Children may become violent acting out their abuse on others, and in the case of sexual abuse may themselves become sexually promiscuous. They may become withdrawn, appear depressed and may suppress the episodes of abuse, which may emerge many years later in adult life.

Direct observation of abuse or the circumstances highly suggestive of abuse. Usually these are reports made to the police or to a child care authority. Affected children may be brought to the practitioner for a forensic examination similar to that applied to rape victims. Forensic evidence should be gathered as soon as the child is referred with a diagnosis or suspicion of abuse. Pathological specimens and photographs should be obtained and opinions sought from specialists that a court is likely to rely on. A gynaecologist should examine a female and a sexually transmitted

---

[417] Skin signs of sexual abuse; W Lambert, Univ. of Miami School of Medicine, CME Medscape; June 2002

disease specialist may be consulted appropriately. Appropriate professionals should do the social and psychological examinations.

Obtaining a history should be done without mention of the clinician's suspicion. Detail about life-style can be obtained in a non-threatening atmosphere, particularly from a child whose abuser is an authority figure, as the child may feel that they will be rebuffed or punished for saying what has happened. A child may also feel that the abuse is their fault since they did not raise an alarm. Where possible a child psychologist or a social worker who deals with children should do the questioning. In spite of any possibility of parental involvement, questioning of a child should not be undertaken without the consent of the parent or legal guardian. It is an area where there are strong value judgments, and the professional can come to the wrong conclusion or even suggest to the child what it might say. Caseworkers have been the subject of lawsuits by the persons accused on the basis of how the evidence given was obtained.[418], [419]

Questioning the parents when suspicion falls on them must be done on the background that they remain in authority over the child and have the right to determine how the child is treated, including approval of referrals.

In the first case reported the observation of a lax anal sphincter in the presence of a painful tender abscess, and a gaping vagina with a discharge, is highly suspicious of sexual abuse. In the third report the child presents with pelvic inflammatory infection from her admitted sexual activity.

In the second report there is no sexually induced disease but the child presents with considerable psychological symptoms and readily admits to the sexual activity.

In the first report with the most compelling physical evidence of the child's sexual activity there is a denial of sexual activity. On being questioned by a psychiatrist sadness is observed but the child responds that she is normally a quiet child and just wishes to return to school. The psychiatrist also interviews the parents who, apart from denying abuse, write a letter complaining about the insinuations made by the psychiatrist about them abusing or knowing of the abuse of their child, and the threats made to remove the child from home. The family circumstances were not investigated until several days after the parents felt that they were being accused, and the siblings denied that there was any possibility of abuse occurring at home.

In the second and third case reports the children present with mental

---

[418] Interviewing Methods and Hearsay Testimony in suspected child sexual abuse. JK Adams, Oklahoma Family Law Journal, 1995; 10(4), 105-111. www.ipt-forensics.com/journal/volume9/j9_1_4.htm
[419] Child eyewitness testimony in sexual abuse investigations. Bruce Mapes. Wiley, Chichester, 1995

problems, which were not diagnosed in spite of a long history. In both instances it was known that the abuse was going on; in one instance the child's mother knew it, and in the other known to the mother's same-sex partner.

- ***Abuser's profile***

In 90 per cent of child sexual abuse cases, the offenders are male and are often described as being unassertive, withdrawn, and emotionless. Other common characteristics include a history of abuse (either physical or sexual), alcohol or drug abuse, little satisfaction with sexual relationships with adults, lack of control over their emotions, and occasionally, mental illness.[420] Abuse is most likely to occur in the home with a family member or close friend; the possibility that it could occur at school or at church with an authority figure must also be entertained. Sexual intercourse among 'consenting' minors of similar age is difficult to characterise as abuse and may have to be treated through counselling and behaviour change.[421]

When parents are accused of abuse they may be from a troubled family known in the neighbourhood, or the family may appear to be entirely respectable in the community and the entire family denies its occurrence to avoid public exposure. There are also reports where abuse in the home has occurred with all the children, who form a protective bond of denial both against the abuser as well as the disapproval of the community. Incest raises strong feelings about the character of both abuser and victim, particularly when the family appears to be devoutly religious. In either case an accusation produces problems within the family, and accused parents or relatives are put in a position of having to fight to avoid criminal conviction. It is therefore vital to obtain as much information as possible before accusations are made, and to be prepared to remove the child from the care of the parents.

In the first report there is no profile of the parent who feels they are being accused. The child was seen by a psychiatrist without the parent's knowledge. The parents when interviewed by the psychiatrist are asked to interpret the medical findings and feel they are accused of the abuse to the point of writing a letter of complaint.

In the second report the character of the accused father is not explored, neither is why the mother does not wish him prosecuted.

In the third report there is no mention of the child's father at any point, and no authority has sought to profile the alleged abuser.

---

[420] Synopsis of Psychiatry Behavioral Sciences in Clinical Psychiatry, 7th Ed. A Kaplan, B Sadock, J Grebb, Williams&Wilkins 1999
[421] Child Sexual Abuse; F W. Putnam, J. Am. Acad. Child Adolesc. Psychiatry, 2003, 42(3): 269–278.

- *What enquiries were made about other sexual encounters/ partner/s?*

It is important to have on record any other sexual encounters than that offered by the patient. It allows a correlation between the examination findings and the history, which is very important before this kind of serious accusation is made to the police. Children who are abused may become sexually seductive and promiscuous, and this may complicate matters in any intended prosecution.[422]

In the first report no enquiry was made as to other possible abusers in the family, at school or at church. It is noted that the parents appear to be more outraged at being accused than they are about the diagnosis that the child has been sexually abused.

In the second narrative, there does not appear to have been any enquiry into any other sexual history before a decision is made to report the matter to the authorities.

In the third report the girl's story changes to that of a promiscuous life-style. However, all of the enquiries appear to relate to only one of the men claimed by the girl to be having sex with her.

- *What is expected from a psychiatric referral?*

A psychiatrist is expected to treat patients with mental disorders and try to get them better; this depends on the information obtained during the examination of the patient. Psychiatric referrals may be necessary for all of the actors involved, parents, guardians, siblings and suspected perpetrators of abuse. In dealing with criminal matters the issues of confidentiality become important, and in the absence of law compelling reporting of a suspected felony, poses a dilemma for the professional in a doctor-patient relationship. Corroboration of a child's story must be considered before referring issues raised in consultation to the police.

In the first case report the approach of the psychiatrist to the child's parents results in a letter of complaint from them, and has elicited no useful information.

In the second case described there is a call by the psychiatrist to immediately report the matter to the police. However, this action appears to be against the wishes of the child's parent who is responsible for her care, and who has stated that she did not wish the matter to go to court.

In the third case there is no referral of the girl to the psychiatrist although she is said to be mentally underdeveloped. On the other hand, the mother, after learning of the abuse, becomes suicidal and has to be treated. It is of interest that the police remained unresponsive to the reports that the child had been abused.

---

[422] Long-term Effects of Child Sexual Abuse, P E Mullen, J Fleming; Issues in Child Abuse Prevention, 1998, no 9

- *Social worker/services enquiries*

Social services personnel should have the training to enquire into the social circumstances of a patient who may not have been elicited in a doctor's consultation. In accusations of abuse it is important to check the domestic arrangements, including income and apparent expenditures. Social services will not have the powers that the police have to investigate a crime, but should have the ability to gather information that could guide how a patient's case should be handled. The information obtained should be used by the medical practitioner or in determining what route of reporting should be done by the service responsible for the patient's care, as well as assist in the therapy.

In the first case reported, the Social Services Department's findings elicit denials of abuse from the rest of the family, but there is no report on the child's activities outside the home or any report on visitors to the home that should be investigated.

In the second case, a referral is made with the suggestion that the department is expected to make the decision about reporting the matter to the child protection agency. However, the psychiatrist involved wishes a report to be made to the police; these are not mutually exclusive.

In the third case, the social services report complicated domestic arrangements in economic, socio-sexual arrangements, and relationships in the neighbourhood. These may have an effect on the attitudes of the police in dealing with the reported issue.

- **Is the child's behaviour / history consistent with the diagnosis of abuse?**

Some of the behaviours of children who have been abused are:
- the child appears withdrawn or engaged in fantasy or infantile behaviour;
- begins wetting or soiling the bed;
- has poor peer relationships;
- is unwilling to participate in physical activities;
- engages in delinquent acts;
- reports sexual abuse;
- engages in inappropriate sexualized behaviour; devalues sexual acts and acts sexually permissive;
- fears a certain person or certain places;
- exhibits depression, anxiety, guilt, fear, sexual dysfunction, eating disorders, substance abuse, prostitution; aggressive, disruptive, and sometimes illegal behaviour;
- experiences feelings of sadness;

- difficulty with bowel movements, urinating, or swallowing;
- recurring complaints of stomach-aches and/or headaches;
- displays an unusual or unexpected response when asked if he or she was touched by someone;
- has an unreasonable fear of a physical exam;
- creates drawings that show sexual acts or that seem overly focused on sexual body parts; more knowledge about sex than is normal for the child's age; seems preoccupied with or overly concerned about sexual acts and words;
- runs away.

An abused child's caretaker may be extremely protective or jealous of the abused child; encourages the child to engage in prostitution or sexual acts; may have been sexually abused as a child; experiences marital difficulties; misuses alcohol or other drugs; and is frequently absent from home; has difficulty in interacting with other adults.[423]

Child abuse is more likely to occur when any of the following exist in families: an adult in the family was abused as a child; a child is viewed as being different from the parent's preconceived expectations, or is seen as having special needs with extreme overprotection but with poor adherence to medical recommendations; there are crises in the family such as job loss, financial burdens, illness, death, separation, or divorce with parental depression or mental illness; parental chronic physical illness; physical abuse of the mother by the father or father figure; marked aggression among siblings and other violence in the home; alcohol or other drug abuse by parents or caretakers.

This list contains a number of the features described in the case reports, the sadness and withdrawal of the first child, the ready admission of the second child with psychosomatic abdominal symptoms and the infantile and promiscuous behaviour in the third report. The family's response to the situation included stigmatization in the three reports; the denial and aggression that occurred in the first report; the determination to keep the matter out of the public eye in the second, and the dysfunctional family arrangements in the third with the mother expressing suicidal intent on discovering the abuse, which she has also suffered as a child.

In the cases reported the profile of the abusers is not extensive, but there is difficulty in all the cases of relating to adults emotionally.

---

[423] Childhood sexual abuse, K L. Kinnear; ABC-CLIO; 2007

- *What is the health worker's role in pursuing a situation of childhood abuse?*

The role of health workers is to act in the best interest of the patient and to alleviate their condition. Part of the aims of treatment would be to stop the abuse and this may involve the prosecution of the abuser. To be successful in a prosecution the health workers should collect any forensic evidence of the abuse as soon as possible.

In some instances it is the parents who are the agents of such abuse and given the opportunity they may try to prevent enquiries into the matter. Therefore, enough information should be sought in emergency situations before having to involve the suspected parents in any situation requiring their consent, and to be prepared to have the child placed under protection from their parents if necessary.

In the absence of a mandatory requirement of reporting, the health care worker, a priest or any other responsible person should act in the best interest of the child, and not that of the parents or even themselves in not wanting to be part of a court proceeding. The effects of childhood abuse last long after the abuse has stopped and the best interest of the child is usually served by bringing the abuser to justice, and the child shielded before, during and after any court proceedings.

In the reports given there are few statements on the collection of forensic evidence; this could hinder a prosecution if one were brought. In each of the cases the health professionals wish the matter reported to the police, however the alternative of putting the children in care takes precedence. In the third case, putting the child in care creates a household crisis, including a suicide attempt by the mother.

There is no information on the long-term outcome.

- *The role of priests and other community leaders*

Priests and community leaders have an acknowledged role as spiritual advisors, confidential counsellors and confessors. These roles become somewhat ambiguous where crimes have been committed and are hidden. When priests are complicit in hiding crimes they could be viewed as facilitators of such crimes but are seldom treated as such. The trust placed by communities in priests and others such as teachers is not always reciprocated, for some have become opportunistic perpetrators of sexual abuse of children.

In the second case reported the priest has acted as facilitator for the mother's wish to hide the abuse that the child's father has committed. The child has not been counselled or helped in any way, and the child's mental trauma has continued unabated.

- *Child protection*

Many jurisdictions have a child protection agency that is responsible
for protecting children from harm. Such agencies have the power to
remove children to a place of safety, and to protect them, including from
their parents. These agencies should be equipped with professional staff
capable of investigating abusive situations, and in the best interests of
the child and of the community report crimes to the police. Removal of
a child from the parents' control can be done with the help of the police,
must be approved by an application to the court within a four-week
period.[424]

*In each of the reports as given the staff think of the child protection agency
and the police. In the first case the child is retained in hospital presumably under
a child protection order, while that decision is explicitly made in the third report.*

*In the second case report removal of the child is not being considered probably
on the thinking that the abuse has stopped.*

- *The police*

The police have the responsibility to apprehend suspected criminals
and gather enough credible evidence that persons suspected of criminal
activity can be successfully prosecuted in a court of law. In accusations
of sexual crimes, forensic evidence collected medically may be of
critical importance, and should be collected as soon as possible. Witness
statements are likely to be conflicting and are best collected by trained
personnel before accusations are made.

In jurisdictions where there is mandatory reporting to the police or a
related agency, there are specially trained police officers to investigate
abusive situations.

*In the case reports as given there is dispute among the care-givers as to which
agency should be given the lead responsibility for dealing with the accusation
of child abuse. In the third case report both the Child Protection Agency and
the police have been contacted, but there is no report of any police action in
the matter.*

- *Legal issues*

The Age of Consent to sexual intercourse varies with jurisdictions and with
the type of sex and gender. In most countries the age of consent to sexual
intercourse is 16 years but varies from as young as 12 years old for girls
to when they reach the legal majority of 18 years.[425]. An adult found to

---

[424] Laws of Barbados LRO 1985; Prevention of Cruelty to Children Act; CAP 145
[425] Age of Consent; www.ageofconsent.com

be having sex with a minor below the age of consent could be charged with the felony of statutory rape; however, there are circumstances where the charge may only be a misdemeanour. For example, in a jurisdiction where the age of consent is 16 years, sex with a girl of 14 years old can be considered a misdemeanour, if the man is 24 or younger[426].

Child neglect and abuse. Any child who is neglected is at risk of being abused. The abuse most often occurs by the parents, members of the family or household. Sexual abuse, in particular, occurs mostly at home. Older persons who abuse children or condone such abuse have often been abused themselves as children, and may see the abuse as a right in return for the economic support of the child. When monetary benefits play a definitive role in the sexual abuse of girls, the mother of the child may be in a competing relationship with her daughter, expressed in jealousy or even fights. This is frequently not prosecuted because it is difficult to obtain the appropriate witness statements. In other instances, there has been a period of grooming by the abusers, the parents and others in institutional care.[427]

Childhood marriage is practised in some cultures. In some religious cultures legal statutes may back it, and children [particularly girls] may be forced into premature sexual intercourse on the grounds of being married. (In some countries there are separate marriage laws for different religions.)[428], [429] Such children may be married as young as nine years old. There have been situations reported where sexual abuse has been reported to the police, and the parents have allowed a marriage to take place to avoid a prosecution. Tampering with or blocking the legal process for financial gain, is suspected as being the main reason why childhood sexual abuse appears to continue unabated in many countries.

Reporting felonies to the police. All citizens should report felonies to the police; the same duty applies to health care workers, taking into account the confidentiality of the patient and their wishes. Many felonies go unreported for fear of getting involved in the judicial system as a witness and sometimes the threat or feeling of a threat from the party reported. In many jurisdictions, the system is very wasteful of the participant's time, and persons who get involved as witnesses may feel that their livelihood is threatened in one way or the other. Court appearances for health care workers as witnesses is complicated by the fact that they will be called

---

[426] Barbados: The Sexual Offences Act CAP 154 L.R.O.; 1993
[427] Setting 'Dem UP'; Personal, Familial and Institutional Grooming; A-M McAlinden; Social Legal Studies, 2006 vol. 15 no. 3; 339-362
[428] Trinidad and Tobago: Muslim Marriage and Divorce Act Chapter 45:02
[429] Trinidad and Tobago Hindu Marriage Act Chapter 45:03

upon to interpret the testimony they have given.

Reporting of sexual abuse cases has been further complicated for health workers by some of the accused persons having brought civil suits, claiming that the evidence with which they were accused has been wrongfully obtained, maliciously given or interpreted.[430] Nevertheless, health care workers should not choose to ignore instances of abuse and abrogate their duty of care to the patient. Health care workers also have a duty of confidentiality to their patients, and must take that into account in proceeding along the path of prosecution. To determine what is in the best interest of the patient, the physical, history and psychological evidence must be obtained in the most thorough manner. Such evidence may not be obtained when premature reports are made to the police against the patient's wishes. The timing of a report to the police must therefore be carefully considered. The fact that not all cases of abuse are reported to the police has called for mandatory reporting where it does not exist.[431] Mandatory reporting may lead those who are reluctant to do so to 'hear and see no evil'; particularly if there is nothing to alleviate the fears of reporting that already exist.[432]

Consent for a minor. In general, a minor has no legal capacity to consent to medical treatment unless specific provisions have been made in law or judicial precedent. In general the age of consent to sexual intercourse is before the age of majority, as is the age at which one can legally work and obtain a driver's license. Therefore, in most jurisdictions [the UK is an exception[433]] minors are legally entitled to consent to sexual intercourse, but are not entitled to consent to the medical treatment that may be required as a result of their legal activities.

Parents have the legal power to consent to the treatment of their minor child, including their further investigation and referral. In situations related to sexual matters, parents are often conflicted about how their children should be treated. Such disagreements are likely to occur where there is child abuse and the parents or siblings are thought to be involved. With active obstruction by parents it may be difficult to obtain evidence that can be successfully used in a prosecution. When a dispute with parents cannot be resolved, the child can be taken into care and can be treated

---

[430] Ridicule or recourse: parents falsely accused of past sexual abuse fight back, J.M Whitesell, J Law & Health, 1996; 303

[431] Perceptions of, Attitudes to, and Opinions on Child Sexual Abuse in the Eastern Caribbean. Research Team A D. Jones E Trotman Jemmott et al UNICEF/Governments of the Eastern Caribbean 2008-2011; http://www.actionforchildren.org.uk/media/143143/child_sexual_abuse_in_the_eastern_caribbean.pdf

[432] Child Abuse: A Guide for Mandatory Reporters; 2011; http://www.dhs.state.ia.us/policyanalysis/policymanualpages/Manual_Documents/Master/comm164.pdf

[433] UK: The Family Law Reform Act; 1969

without the parent's consent. There are other legal provisions that vary in jurisdictions that can allow physicians to treat minors without the consent of their parents and even without their knowledge. One such provision is the Gillick precedent[434] where it was ruled that a child who understood the situation could be prescribed contraceptives over the objections of the parents, if the physicians thought it was in the best interests of the child.

Confidentiality of a minor. The right to confidentiality of a minor is like that of any other person, and it is considered more precious than that of adults by protecting the child's identity in legal actions. This is done through a prohibition on the publication of the minor's name or any other identifiers. However, the legal capacity of a minor to maintain their confidentiality in medical matters is curtailed by the limitations on their capacity to make medical decisions for themselves. From time to time health care workers come to the conclusion that the best interest, of the child would not be served by full disclosure to the parents, and they will either have to rely on judicial precedents such as the Gillick precedent, or lose the cooperation of the minor in resolving the problem.

In the first case reported the way in which the parents were handled led to a complaint from them and complicated the investigation of the suspected abuse.

In the second report the child is 14 years old and looks like an adult, but the sexual abuse is reported to have occurred between the ages of six and 12 years old, and could not be pleaded as a misdemeanour on the basis of her adult looks. However, the mother has been avoiding police action, and forcing such action may fail for lack of cooperation.

In the third report the sexual activity is allegedly with young men who may be able to plead a misdemeanour with a 14-year old who looks like an adult. Reports have been made to the police by both the mother and the practitioners but with no response from them.

- ### When children appear in court

Children may have to appear in court to give evidence against the person who is accused of abusing them and this can further traumatize the child. Judges will try to shield the child as much as possible and in some jurisdictions the child's testimony is given on videotape. The child's testimony may be challenged on the grounds that it is fabricated along with the person(s) who examined the child. Such challenges are particularly traumatic for the child and they frequently change their testimony.[435]

---

[434] Gillick vs. West Norfolk Health Authority- 3 A.E.R. 402; 1985
[435] Easing access to the courts for incest victims; J Lamm, The Yale Law Journal Vol. 100, No. 7, May, 1991

- ***Counter suits by the accused***

There have been cases where during trial the persons who have interviewed children or adults who are alleged to have been abused as children, have been accused of suggesting the abuse to the victim. There have been suits brought against such professionals and in one instance the suit succeeded; in this instance it was held that suppressed memories were elicited and then the 'victim' was pressed to bring charges on the basis of the recovered memories.[436]

In the first case the parents wrote complaining of their treatment by and allegations made by the psychiatrist.

- ***What happens on reaching the age of majority?***

When a child reaches the age of consent to sexual intercourse, their sexual contacts other than with the immediate family, or by force are not illegal. However, the child may still be in need of protection particularly if their mental age is low. In the absence of adoption, child protection agencies relinquish responsibility on reaching the age of majority. Nevertheless, individuals who are mentally subnormal remain vulnerable and are protected in law from sexual abuse.[437] Such acts are defensible if the 'abuser' did not know that the person was mentally subnormal.

In the third case report the child is reported as behaving well below her age but no formal assessment has been made.

- ***Accusations years after***

There are several instances where an adult only brings charges of sexual abuse as a child when they have reached adulthood. They usually state that they have had psychological difficulties and bringing the case at this stage is seen as a catharsis. These allegations are particularly difficult to prove and there are often duelling psychological or psychiatric experts who give testimony.[438] It is therefore important that when an examination is made in childhood that the records of such examination are kept. The circumstances and setting under which such examinations are done must be appropriate and videotaped if within the law.

---

[436] Hungerford vs. Jones 97-657 US district Court 1998
[437] Barbados: The Sexual Offences Act CAP 154 L.R.O.; 1993
[438] Recovered Memories of Sexual Abuse; J Hopper 2011

Case report 1:

A 14- year- old boy was admitted to the adult psychiatric ward after attempting to jump off the roof at school. He did this because the cell phone, which he had without his mother's permission, was stolen. He believed that attempting to end his life would shift attention from disobeying his mother. He was diagnosed as displaying "conduct disorder". The Social Services department was asked to investigate and found considerable psychosocial stressors related to his mother who was unemployed, had 3 children at home, and also cared for the 3 children of her brother who was in prison.

Five days after admission he was extremely tearful and on being prompted said he believed he had made another patient pregnant. He confided that he and the 11-year-old girl had had sex 2 days previously during the nursing staff's evening handover shift. The girl corroborated what had happened. The nursing staff informed the managing team and nursing office about the incident. Nursing office informed the clinical risk officer who in turn informed the hospital lawyer and the police were called. Guardians of both children were informed about the incident and were very angry about the lack of supervision of the children. The 11-year-old girl had been admitted for a behavioural disorder, and had a history of many years of sexual abuse.

A meeting was held with the consultant psychiatrist, the clinical risk officer, the hospital's lawyer, a social worker, a childcare officer, a police officer and the CEO. Plans were made to separate the minors, as they both required on-going admission. The police officer said that in cases like this the boy could be charged with assault. The police interviewed the girl but not the boy. The staff expressed concern about understaffing and their legal liability.

Case report 2:

A 15-year-old girl was referred complaining of daily thoughts of death and killing herself by hanging. Her appointed guardian was her 26-year-old half sister. She showed the behaviour of a 10-year-old child, and a speech impediment was noted. Intelligence testing using the Wechsler Intelligence Scale showed an I.Q. of 51, equivalent to an eight-year-old. A hearing impairment was ruled out.

Her mood was of sadness and anger and she stated that while living with her father "he feel me up and put his penis in my vagina." She had been living with her father from four years old after her mother's house burnt down. She was fearful of her father and thought daily about what he did to her. After an investigation the Child Care Board placed the girl with her sister Mary, who lived with her boyfriend and their two children.

She improved and was discharged but reported after three months that her suicidal thoughts had returned, after she saw her father walking past her school. She said that she had had sex with her sister's boyfriend on one occasion, and had run away after her sister threatened to beat her. She was readmitted, her suicidal ideation increased whenever she saw her father, such as on an occasion while she was walking with a nurse in the hospital. While in hospital she reported that her mother repeatedly said that her father was the person whom she "should like". Because of this she did not want to live with her mother again.

She was placed in a foster home but ran away after two months. She then said she had lied when she said she had sex with her sister's boyfriend, and her sister accepted her back into her home. Nine months later she regressed, admitted that she was in fact having sex with her sister's boyfriend and that she had gotten pregnant on two occasions for him. She was eventually placed in a children's home.

Issues raised

- *Unlawful sexual conduct or just 'rudeness'*

When sexual intercourse occurs with children and adults, the sexual acts are unlawful in most but not all instances depending on the law. When it occurs between minors, it is most often not unlawful, but may be unlawful depending on the nature of the contact and the ages of the children. Depending on the law in the jurisdiction, an accusation of unlawful sexual intercourse with a minor, may be charged as a misdemeanour, rather than statutory rape depending on the age difference of the child and the adult.

The age of consent for a minor to have sexual intercourse varies in jurisdictions, and may vary for girls and boys. Most jurisdictions have an age of consent at 16 years but this may be a low as 12 years for girls in some jurisdictions, and as low as nine or 10 years in some marriage laws. For example, in a jurisdiction where the law related to unlawful sexual conduct states that the age of consent to sexual intercourse for males and females is 16 years, exceptions are made for children under the age of 14, if the child is a spouse. Adults up to the age of 24 years having sex with a 14-16-year-old could be charged with a misdemeanour, rather than statutory rape, if it was successfully argued that the adult was unaware of the age of the minor; and children under the age of 14 years are 'deemed incapable of rape'.[439] Nothing in the law speaks to 'consensual sex' between children under the age of 14 years.

In the first case report both children were under the age of consent and in spite of the consensual nature of the sex, members of staff still felt some crime had been committed and summoned the police.

In the second case report, the history suggests that incest and statutory rape have been committed by the father, and statutory rape by the sister's boyfriend.

- *Liability of the staff and institution*

Institutions have a duty to protect all patients who come under their care. This duty is especially apt for the incapacitated physically or mentally and for children. Civil liability resides in showing that the actions and procedures of the institution and its staff were negligent and harm resulted, either physical or psychological. Criminal liability would rest where the negligence has been so gross as to cause the death of a patient, or a serious criminal act such as the rape of a patient. Negligence could be argued on the grounds of acts of commission or omission; e.g. the patient may be placed in a known unsafe situation, a failure to provide adequate supervision, or failure to heed warnings of impending harmful acts.

Criminal liability would require it to be shown that a crime had been committed or that the institution and /or its staff had shown a reckless disregard for obvious dangers, or had not provided the minimum protections in law.

In the absence of coercion, a big disparity in ages, or a specific law, it is difficult to state that a crime has been committed when sexual acts occur between minors. That does not mean that the behaviour should not be corrected or be tolerated. Corrective behaviour would normally be left to the parents or guardians, and if the parents are unable to control the children, or are not fit to do so, making them a ward of the state and moving them to a place of safety should protect the child.

The institution and its staff could be liable for child endangerment; for admission of children to an adult ward, with patients with mental disorders and mixed genders, is compounded when it is known that the child admitted is known to have been sexually abused for a long period and has been admitted for related behaviour which could not be controlled by her guardian. Under such circumstances how would one justify the routine sequestration of all staff for an indeterminate period of time, without any means of observation of patients admitted for behavioural and mental disorders?

---

[439] Laws of Barbados; Sexual Offences Act CAP 154 LRO; 1993

In the first case report, the mother of the boy has threatened some kind of legal action against the hospital and its staff, presumably for a lack of supervision in preventing the boy from having sex with another child on the ward, and is now under threat of prosecution by the police. The children had been admitted to a ward with adults, who are being treated for mental illness, and had the incident occurred between an adult and the children a serious criminal offence would have been perpetrated, facilitated by the unsafe situation in which the children were placed. The nursing staff appear to have a system of 'handover' that is in need of review. When the incident shows up the faults there appears to be an overreaction to label the incident a crime and the police are called. This seems to be trying to deflect responsibility away from the staff and with little thought for the consequences there might be for the children or their families.

Damages could be pursued by the families for any of the physical or psychological consequences of the incident.

Negligent placement of the girls could be argued, for both girls had a history of longstanding childhood sexual abuse, and it is known that such children may engage in inappropriate even seductive sexual behaviour.

- ***What action could the police take?***

The police, faced with situations of child abuse, may apprehend and prosecute the offender, or they may take the child to a place of safety, such as a hospital. When the abuse is alleged the police should investigate the matter with a view to the prosecution of the offender. Adults can be prosecuted for statutory rape of a child, and in the case of a minor for a sexual assault. In cases of childhood abuse the police should be specially trained to investigate such cases and in particular in the interviewing of children. They should also have facilities for videotaping the interviews with children in particular.

In the first case report the police were called when two children admitted to having sexual intercourse on a hospital ward. A hospital would normally be considered a place of safety for children and why the children were no longer safe there should be answered. The police opined that the boy in the incident could be charged with an offence but does not state what offence.

In the second case report the 15-year old girl is admitted and in an equally hazardous situation. In addition, the narrative shows up problems in the placement of such children in the services outside of the hospital, for this child has been moved from one abusive situation to another. There has been no call for police action in this case, the reasons for which were not articulated.

Battered Child

Case report:

A toddler presented with a story that he had fallen off the bed and injured his shoulder. A fracture of the clavicle was diagnosed and a referral made to the emergency department where the fracture was confirmed and treated with a collar and cuff. Three days later the child presented again with a story of having fallen when getting out of a chair, his complaints were abdominal and lower back pain. The doctor arranged an ambulance to the hospital, where it was noted that he had a haematoma on the forehead, the clavicular injury, and swellings over the sacrum, both buttocks and thighs. He was investigated with a CT scan of the brain, facial bones, abdomen and pelvis, and referred to Paediatric Medicine for assessment of 'non-accidental' injuries.

Referrals were made to the social services department, the Child Care Board, the orthopaedic and surgery departments. Further investigations including a skeletal survey showed him to be anaemic. The social history was that the mother and her boyfriend lived with the child's twin sister and an older child, and that her grandmother looked after the children when they were out at work. After two weeks the social worker reported that having interviewed the mother and her boyfriend, and the child alone, she concluded that the injuries were accidental and the child could be discharged home if he was well. The child was discharged that day. Two days later, the child was brought back to the emergency department in cardiac arrest and could not be resuscitated. The mother and her boyfriend said he was well until the day of his death, when he began to feel unwell, complained of abdominal pain and vomiting which did not respond to medication. The post-mortem examination found cerebral oedema and gangrenous small bowel due to a mesenteric injury from a blunt abdominal injury.

Issues raised

- *The battered child syndrome*

Battered children pose a diagnostic dilemma, because a history of accidental injuries is usually given by the parents or other care-givers and may be corroborated by the children out of fear for the consequences of contradicting those who have injured them. Medical professionals may not look beyond fractured bones at other soft tissue injuries to see that they may not fit in with the 'accident' said to be responsible for the injury. The penny often drops only after repeated bony injuries or the death of the child. The classic paper on the Battered Child Syndrome published in 1962, was largely based on multiple sequential bony injuries in children, aged three years and under.[440] The parents or foster parents were the usual perpetrators, and seldom owned up to beating the child. The parents may have emotional and psychological problems, drug abuse or criminal histories, may have been subjected to similar beatings as children and will consider beating as the normal way to discipline children. Unfortunately, the diagnosis of abuse is reluctantly made, and in many instances, only on the death of the child. The reluctance comes from not wishing to believe that a parent or care-giver would be so brutal to a child, the child's inability or unwillingness to relate what has happened to them, and the reluctance to use authorities to separate children from their parents.

In the case reported, the medical findings did not fit in with the accidental falls described and the primary care doctor and the emergency department promptly recognized this. The child is admitted for investigation; however, reliance was placed on the limited investigation by a social worker who reports that the parents and the child corroborate the story of a fall. The social worker did not talk to the other care-giver or visit the home and advises that the injuries occurred as related by the parents. The child is discharged as soon as this report is received and there is no account given of what examination of the child was done before it was sent home. The post-mortem report does not state whether the abdominal injury was fresh or from the previous admission.

- ***Suspicious injuries***

Healthy toddlers are very resilient and their bones are not broken except with great force. Multiple broken bones simultaneously or sequentially must raise suspicions of non-accidental injuries. Multiple bruises do not result from a simple fall from household furniture, and bruises around the head and abdomen are not normally associated with an accidental fracture in the limbs. In a study of suspicious bony injuries in battered children, fractures of the lateral clavicle, the ribs and the scapula were flagged as requiring further attention as being non-accidental.[441] Abdominal injuries are unlikely to be the consequence of a fall from domestic furniture.

There appeared to be no suspicion raised when the child first presented with a bony injury, and a limited examination was done. However, on the second presentation within two days, the child's ill state and multiple soft tissue

---

[440] The Battered- Child Syndrome, CH Kempe, et al - 1962 JAMA Jama.Jamanetwork.Com/ Article. Aspx? Articled=327895milaama

[441] Patterns Of Injury And Significance Of Uncommon Fractures In The Battered Child Syndrome M S. Kogutt, L E. Swischuk, And C J. Fagan, American Journal of Roentgenology 1974

injuries raised an alarm. The suspicion/diagnosis of non-accidental injuries was investigated but was unfortunately set aside on an inadequate investigation by a social worker.

- ### *Reporting and investigating childhood abuse*

The protection of children is a universally held aim in communities. However, there are cultural issues in some families and in communities that may value some children differently from others. These differences may be expressed in terms of gender, order of birth, ethnicity, and state of health or abilities, both physical and mental. These cultural differences may result in children being treated differently within families and within communities whether it is in terms of inheritance, disposition of resources, education opportunities, or disciplinary measures at home or in the community. Some of these differences in the treatment of children are addressed in legislation within countries[442] and in an international convention on the Rights of the Child.[443] However, in spite of legislative measures, there is widespread concern in most countries about the abuse of children – whether it is sexual, physical or emotional.[444] [445]

Carrying out measures to protect children can become mired in the cultural values of the community; in the perceived rights of parents and other authority figures to discipline children; the use of children for their economic value for either labour or the sexual gratification of adults;[446] and the reluctance of members of the community to undergo the inconvenience of being involved with the legal process or to have disputes with their neighbours. This reluctance to be involved has led to calls for mandatory reporting of childhood abuse, by health care-givers and others working with children.[447' 448] However, mandatory reporting does not guarantee that the matter will be adequately investigated or that justice will prevail. It does however place the onus on responsible authorities to account for when tragedies occur such as the death of a child.

---

[442] Child Care Board Act, Laws of Barbados 1969 Section 46. rev 1981

[443] Convention on the Rights of the Child; UN General Assembly resolution 44/25; 1989

[444] Laws of Barbados LRO 1985; Prevention of Cruelty to Children Act; CAP 145

[445] World report on violence and health; Eds. E G. Krug, L L. Dahlberg, J A. Mercy, A B. Zwi and R Lozano Ch 3. Child Abuse And Neglect By Parents And Other Caregivers; http://whqlibdoc.who.int/publications/2002/9241545615_chap3_eng.pdfYou +1'd this publicly. Undo

[446] 'Setting 'Em Up': Personal, Familial and Institutional Grooming in the Sexual Abuse of Children; Anne-Marie Mcalinden, Social Legal Studies September 2006 vol. 15 no. 3 339-362

[447] Child Abuse: A Guide for Mandatory Reporters; 2011; http://www.dhs.state.ia.us/policyanalysis/policymanualpages/Manual_Documents/Master/comm164.pdf

[448] Child protection in Barbados: The need for a national reporting protocol; J Sealy-Burke, Consultant; The United Nations Children's Fund (UNICEF) 2007

The presence or absence of mandatory reporting, and the efficiency, or otherwise, of responsible authorities, should not absolve medical and social services professionals from investigating as widely as possible their suspicions of child abuse, particularly when a child's life is threatened. On the other hand, mandatory reporting by persons in the community or by family members, may either be used to harass others, or may not be done, to avoid involvement in the legal processes, and for fear of being harmed by those who have been reported on. The efficacy of mandatory reporting to the police also depends on the trained resources available to the police.[449]

The investigation of cases of suspected abuse has both a social and a medical component. A medical investigation starts with the recognition that the physical state or signs in the child do not match with the reported history of the injury/illness. The investigation must be thorough with visual recordings of both soft tissue and bony injuries, and microbiological or DNA evidence in the case of sexual abuse. In cases of bony injury, both old and new fractures must be noted. A psychological/psychiatric assessment of the child, its parents and other care-givers should be obtained, and the child removed from the suspected abusive environment for observation as required.

Persons making psychological assessments must be careful to not suggest or plant stories in children's minds, particularly when sexual abuse is suspected.[450] Psychological assessments are a very important part of an investigation but should not be used to override clear forensic evidence of abuse. Where there are contradictory findings, it is probably best to place the matter before the court, which ultimately has to accept responsibility for an abused child.

In the case reported the physical evidence of an abused child appeared clear on examination of the child. Medical and social worker referrals were made, as well as reporting to the Child Protection Agency. Without a thorough investigation the child is discharged home on the word of the social worker that the parents are to be believed. Unfortunately, the child is dead within two days of discharge from the consequences of an abdominal injury. There is nothing in the narrative given on the progress of the abdominal injury suspected on admission, and the post mortem report does not state whether the abdominal injury was a new one after discharge of the child.

---

[449] Child abuse - how the police investigate allegations, https://www.citizensadvice.org.uk/relationships/children-and-young-people/child-abuse/police-involvement/child-abuse-how-the-police-investigate-allegations/
[450] Recovered Memories of Sexual Abuse; J Hopper 2011

- *Lapses in management*

The management of an abused child involves the management of the entire family within their community. It is very important to try and prevent further abuse, of the child and other children, and hopefully to stop the child from becoming an abuser themself.[451]

The greatest lapse in management is that where the practitioner's responsibility ends when the physical ailments are ameliorated. A lapse in the physician's attitude may give others the impression that their responsibilities can also be discharged.

An investigation of abuse is seldom aided by an admission by the abuser or those in intimate relationships with them. Therefore, reliance should be placed on the medical forensic evidence, the previous record if any of the suspected abuser, and the witness statements of other members of the family, those in the neighbourhood or in the school environment, where appropriate. Where circumstances allow, covert surveillance with cameras should be done, and may even have to be deployed in hospital settings when the pattern of harm to the child continues whilst it is hospitalised.

Child protection agencies may have lapses in judgment, particularly when the facilities they control for the protection of children are overcrowded, or when the agency itself is a focus of accusations of abusive behaviour in the facilities under their control. In addition, the protection officers may turn a 'blind eye' to events to try and avoid time-consuming court processes, in which their integrity or expertise may be questioned or exposed to public scrutiny or lawsuits.[452]

In the circumstances described most of the parties involved can be judged to have performed inadequately. The medical personnel had made the diagnosis of non-accidental injuries, but then accepted an inadequate social worker report to discharge the child back into the abusive situation. The social worker made a definitive decision/recommendation on the basis of interviewing the parents and the child alone, and made no attempt to speak to or assess the other caretaker of the child, or the other children in the home.

As regards the Child Protection Agency to whom the matter was reported, there was no report of any action or investigation in the two weeks that the child remained in hospital.

---

[451] Long-term Effects of Child Sexual Abuse, P E Mullen, J Fleming; Issues in Child Abuse Prevention, 1998, no 9

[452] Are Public Social Workers Liable for Failing to Prevent Child Abuse? http://www.socialworkers.org/ldf/legal_issue/200411.asp?back=yes&print=1

PATIENTS AT RISK

Case report 1.

A 60-year-old man with a history of poorly controlled hypertension presented to Accident and Emergency with a history of feeling unwell and light-headedness of several hours duration. He was found to have an elevated blood pressure 150/125 mms Hg and a depressed level of consciousness - Glasgow Coma Scale 7/15. A CT of the brain showed a major left intra-ventricular bleed. The patient was intubated as the level of consciousness declined, and referred to the medical service. The medical service stated that according to their department protocols intra-ventricular and subarachnoid bleeds were to be seen by neurosurgery. The A&E department was unaware of this protocol and referred the case to the neurosurgery service. The neurosurgery service stated that they were unaware of such protocols and the case required management of the high blood pressure as the first priority and therefore should be managed by internal medicine.

The A&E consultant spoke to the consultants of both services without resolution as to which service would accept responsibility for the patient. The Director of Medical Services was asked to intervene with the contending departments. The patient remained under the care of the A&E department for another 36 hours before the medical service accepted responsibility for the patient's management. The patient died on the medical service with no further input from the neurosurgical service.

Case report 2.

A 90-year-old woman was brought to the A&E department with a three day history of rectal bleeding and vomiting on that day. She stated that she had had a previous bout of bleeding a few years ago, and was told that there was no need to come to hospital if it happened again. On examination, she was haemo-dynamically stable, the Hb was 4gms/dl, WBC raised at 20, and a CXR showed infiltrates in the right lung. The patient was referred to the surgical service.

She was seen by the surgical service who advised referral to the medical service, for blood transfusion and treatment of aspiration pneumonia. The medical service saw the patient and stated that lower GI bleeding was a surgical problem, and there was no respiratory distress necessitating admission. The surgery consultant was consulted and instructed that given the medical opinion, the patient should be transfused in the A&E department and discharged.

Several hours later the surgical intern brought three units of blood to the A&E department and asked the nursing staff to transfuse the patient and then she could be sent home. The nursing staff declared that there was no place to store blood in the department and told the intern that they were not going to administer the transfusion and he should take the blood away. The intern responded that he was not going to take the blood away and left the department. The nursing staff asked the orderly in the department to return the blood to the blood bank. The A&E staff rang the surgical consultant and said that they would not carry out the plan as stated, and the consultant responded that since there was no active bleeding the patient would not be admitted to the surgical wards and the medical department should be consulted. After two days and intervention by the Director of Medical Services, the medical department was persuaded to admit the patient.

Case report 3:
A 70-year-old man, with a history of diabetes presented having had a hypoglycaemic episode; his wife had found him sweating and unresponsive and measured a low blood sugar. He had been given his evening dose of insulin with a normal blood sugar and a sweetened drink before. His wife had attempted to get him to drink sugar water, but when he did not respond an ambulance was called and he was brought to the emergency department. He was known to be hypertensive, and had a history of asthma and prostatic cancer. He was reported to have had a wet unproductive cough over the last three weeks. There had been prior hypoglycaemic episodes, and a month previously he had been admitted, and his twice-daily insulin dosage had been reduced then. He was alert and oriented, in mild pulmonary distress and was noted to be wearing malodourous pampers.

The hypoglycaemia was assessed as complicated by possible pneumonia and urinary tract infection. Investigation showed him to be very anaemic, with a high blood sugar, but otherwise normal parameters. Chest X-ray showed bilateral pneumonia, worse on the right, and sclerotic and lytic bony lesions. He was referred for admission to the medical department and was seen by the junior doctor several hours later. After consulting his immediate senior over the phone, an antibiotic was prescribed and the insulin dosage was reduced, and it was advised that the patient be followed up in the polyclinic. He was discharged after midnight but returned the following day with shortness of breath and was again hypoglycaemic. He was referred back to medicine and admitted; he had an episode of vomiting blood the following day and died.

Issues raised

• ***Undesired patients.***
Patients may be unwelcome to a health professional for a number of
reasons and although most professionals may go through the motions
of dealing with such patients, there is an inevitable result of defects in
the care of the patient.[453] The defects in care may not rise to a legally
indefensible level, but are almost certainly felt by the patient, their
relatives and other health professionals involved. The factors that may
trigger these situations relate to the patient themselves, the attending
health professionals, and the institution in which they are treated.

Patient factors. - Age, ethnicity, nationality, social standing, behaviour,
appearance, possible contagion and having an 'incurable' condition may
all factor into making a patient undesirable. Elderly patients are often
discriminated against, and there is no standard definition of when a
patient becomes elderly, it being in the eye of the beholder. A person's
race and ethnicity may be subtle but major factors in some communities,
not-withstanding laws against discrimination. A patient's behaviour
and appearance often factor in with other social attributes and may act
as the precipitating factor in discriminatory actions. However, possible
contagion and an incurable condition are often the most important factor,
for that with other factors potentiates the attitudes and actions that the
undesired patient faces.

Institutional factors - time of day, work schedules of other health
professionals, bed occupancy, workload, and the availability of
equipment and supplies all factor into how a patient may be treated as
undesired. Patients, who present with emergencies late at night or in
the early morning hours, face a depleted staff some of whom may have
to be summoned into work. Full bed occupancy, including anticipated
elective admissions, and the availability of functioning equipment and
supplies are often the major factors determining when patients become
undesired.[454] Faced with such situations, patients are kept for long
periods in the emergency department awaiting admission, or awaiting
decisions by the admitting physicians[455]

---

[453] What Doctors Feel: How Emotions Affect the Practice of Medicine– 2014 by D Ofri
[454] The Effect of Hospital Occupancy on Emergency Department Length of Stay and Patient
Disposition; A J. Forster, I Stiell, G Wells, et al, Academic Emergency Medicine, 2003, Vol 10, Iss 2,
pgs. 127–133,
[455] Reducing Transfer Time from the Emergency Department to Inpatient Bed:
http://www.ihi.org/resources/Pages/ImprovementStories/
ReducingTransferTimefromtheEmergencyDepartmenttoInpatientBed
LeeMemorialHospital.aspx.

Professional factors. Both physical and mental issues factor into how health professionals treat patients, particularly those assessed as undesired for admission.[456] The commonest factor is tiredness after the stress of long hours of emergency duty imposed on a busy routine work schedule.[457] The health of the individual practitioner particularly related to substance abuse and/or their general physical fitness also play a role.[458] These physical factors commonly lead to, or are combined with, reliance on telephone reports and the assessments of less experienced staff. However, a not uncommon factor is the mental attitude associated with poor interpersonal relationships brought about by dissatisfaction with colleagues or the administration of an institution itself.[459]

In the first case report the patient is 'undesirable' because of the difficult to treat condition. The second patient is likely undesirable because of her advanced age and her condition, which could be difficult to resolve. In both cases, the patients required admission to hospital but there ensued a battle of who should be responsible. The dispute between the departments was conducted by senior staff through third parties.

In the third case report, there is no interdepartmental dispute but the decision to treat an elderly patient with pneumonia and an unstable blood sugar at home was untenable. The most junior doctor is on the frontline advising the patient, including the advice not to come back to the service for follow up.

* *Departmental differences.*
Whenever differences develop into tussles between individuals, departments or even institutions, there is often an expectation that there will be a winner and a loser. This expectation is usually related to differences in the perceived status of the parties in dispute. Differences in status become exaggerated when there is no practice of cooperation between individuals or departments. Lack of cooperation and poor governance leads to unilateral 'policy' declarations and inevitably to conflict in which patients are the likely losers. Professional differences are often expressed as policies; when unilaterally declared policies such as clinical protocols or guidelines affect other disciplines, conflict is inevitable.

In the first two case reports disputes arise between physicians from two departments about the responsibility for treating patients presenting as

---

[456] What Doctors Feel: How Emotions Affect the Practice of Medicine; D. Ofri; Beacon Press 2014
[457] Resident physicians level of fatigue and medical errors: the role of standardization. Z Stern, T Katz-Navon, O Levtzion-Korach, E Naveh; International Journal of Behavioural and Healthcare Research, 2009, 1, 223-233
[458] Impaired healthcare professional. Baldisseri MR; Crit Care Med. 2007; 35(2 Suppl): S106-16.
[459] Problems for clinical judgment: Introducing cognitive psychology as one more basic science. Redelmeier, D. A., L. E. Ferris, et al. 2001. Canadian Medical Association Journal 164 (3): 358-360.

emergencies. In one instance, the nursing staff also refused to administer needed treatment. In both instances, unwritten 'protocols' are used as justification for the refusal to treat.

In the third case, the treatment regimen is not well thought through, and no responsibility is shown in advising follow-up by an unrelated institution.

- *Clinical protocols and guidelines.*

A clinical protocol is a directive as to how a patient's condition should be treated. Clinical guidelines are intended to assist practitioners in coming to practicable judgments in patient care situations.[460] Both guidelines and protocols should be based on evidence and be subject to review as new evidence becomes available.

The care of difficult conditions involves more than one discipline, and establishment of protocols and guidelines should reflect that multidisciplinary involvement. It is therefore imperative that departmental guidelines or protocols be subjected to institutional scrutiny and made known to all the parties that may be involved. Failure of collaboration results in issues for referrals and the inefficient use of resources.

Effective collaboration must be based on genuine consultation, consensus building, and the distribution and monitoring of the guidelines/protocols. Monitoring is a quality control measure done by the collection of data, clinical audit, a review of peer-reviewed literature, and where appropriate and feasible approved research into the problem. Collaboration itself must be monitored at an institutional level by appropriate approval and oversight mechanisms.[461]

In the three case reports a referral has been made to a department for an emergency admission and is met by a statement that the referral should have been to another department, or in the third case can be handled without admission. In the first case the department invokes a new protocol that was unknown to the other departments.

---

[460] Clinical Practice Guidelines: Field MJ, Lohr KN (Eds). National Academy Press, 1990. http://www.openclinical.org/guidelines.html

[461] Clinical guidelines to improve patient care; Wollersheim H, Burgers J, Grol R. Neth J Med. 2005; 63(6): 188-92.

Refusing to Work

Case report:
A 30-year-old man, known to be HIV positive, attended the emergency department complaining of a dry cough for 3-4 days and fever for two days. At the time there was a Severe Acute Respiratory Syndrome [SARS] epidemic alert. The triage nurse saw the patient but did not ask any SARS-related questions. A temperature of 39°C was recorded and he was asked to sit in the waiting room. The patient was called into the department nine hours later but was not seen by a doctor until several hours later.

The doctor obtained a history that he had recently travelled from a SARS-affected city. Universal precautions were instituted; a chest X-ray was reported as an atypical pneumonia, and he was referred to the medical service as suspected SARS or PCP for isolation. The internist responded that he was unaware of a protocol for the management of SARS cases, and was informed by the A&E staff what the protocol was. When no arrangement was made two hours later, the A&E staff initiated the protocol arrangements to transfer the patient for isolation. Meanwhile, the A&E staff, including the clerks and the maid, refused to attend the patient or work in the areas where the patient had been. The staff had been briefed on the previous day about the need for special rooms with extractor fans but no such rooms had been prepared. The head of the emergency department addressed the staff, calm was restored and all staff completed their duty. The Hospital Director and the chairman of the medical staff committee were informed and they informed the hospital infection control officer, who responded that other than A&E the staff had not been briefed as yet. Briefings were done but several nurses 'went off sick,' and in the following days the hospital supplies officer expressed concerns that many departments were ordering large quantities of surgical masks, gloves, gowns and caps.

Issues raised

- *Background to fears*

SARS [severe acute respiratory syndrome] is caused by an avian flu virus; it spreads like influenza and has a high mortality rate.[462] The human immuno-deficiency virus [HIV] is the cause of AIDS which when it was

---

[462] Severe acute respiratory syndrome (SARS). Wong KF, To TS, Chan JK. Br J Haematol. 2003;122(2):171.

first described was highly fatal and was dubbed the gay plague; affected patients were heavily stigmatised.

Both of the conditions were reported in the case history, and caused panic amongst staff.

- ***Abandonment***

"Abandonment of a patient in danger without sufficient cause and without allowing the patient sufficient opportunity to retain the services of another practitioner;"[463]

Abandonment can be physical or emotional or by withholding advice and services. Patients with stigmatised diseases are frequently subjected to withdrawal of basic services involving direct or indirect contact. In emergency departments staff may claim to be attending to other emergencies, judged to be more urgent. It is not unusual for patients who are triaged as not urgent to wait several hours in an A&E department, apart from the fact that triaging decisions may be incorrect, the acceptance of several hours wait for care is an expression of poor functioning of an emergency department.

In the case described the triage staff, as well as other staff in A&E and on the ward, abandoned the care of the patient. In A&E the patient was left in a cold waiting room for nine hours, which is either an expression of poor professionalism or a conscious or unconscious act of 'abandonment'.

- ***Duty of care***

"The doing of or the failure to do any act or thing in connection with his professional practice, which is in the opinion of the council unprofessional or discreditable"[464]

It is a breach in their duty of care by a health professional who avoids contact with patients including feigning illness themself. Health professionals protect themselves from contracting illness by adhering to universal precautions, not on the basis of not caring for the patient. In the case of a respiratory illness the precautions are to wear masks and to wash one's hands after contact with the patient. As an additional precaution the patient should also be given a mask when the mouth and pharynx are not being examined. Isolation measures do not mean refusing care.

Nurses on the ward where the patient is admitted for isolation report sick; there is little doubt that such widespread illness of the staff from one ward is contrived in response to a suspected SARS case. If their illness is not genuine

---

[463] Laws of Barbados; Medical Registration Act Regulations CAP 171 Part V [2]
[464] Laws of Barbados; Medical Registration Act Regulations CAP 171 Part V [2]

the conduct of the staff is unprofessional, and if they have been certified as ill, the person or persons so certifying them may also be acting unprofessionally. Such action clearly breaches the duty of care to the suspected SARS patient and to other patients on the ward.

- **Has the threat and fear of the staff been properly addressed?**
In any condition identified as a deadly infectious disease, health professions leaders and ministry of health staff have a duty to define the threats and to determine and disseminate the means by which the threat can be met and controlled. Staff in the first contact areas such as A&E and the Medical Department must be targeted first, but not exclusively.[465] Management must also ensure that staff who do not work during 'normal' working hours receive the information and training required.

From the narrative given, procedures and management guidelines have been determined and some staff made aware of what should be done when a SARS case is suspected. However, the nursing staff working in the designated isolation ward were not briefed before the first case presented itself. Some of the A&E staff had been briefed but those who work at night as well as the non-professional staff had not received the briefing.

- **Have the measures decided upon increased the fear among the staff?**
When a deadly disease is announced in the public domain, fear is a natural consequence for members of the community. Health professions and community leaders have a responsibility to address the problem in a manner that would stop the spread of the disease. Unfortunately, rational actions do not always allay fears, and fears often lead to irrational actions.

In the narrative given no specific measures appeared to have been taken to address the fears that exist. In the A&E department staff were briefed on the need for special ventilation measures; however, these were unlikely to be in place in the short term. Instead of allaying fears this could have actually increased them, for the staff are now aware that they are working in 'inadequate' facilities.

- **Have health care staff circumvented directives from management?**
When dealing with a dispute at work, workers may resort to a strike or a sickout. Essential service workers such as in health and security may be prohibited by law from taking such actions, nevertheless effective action can be achieved by resistance or sabotage, and staff arranging to get certificates of leave of illness.

---

[465] Severe acute respiratory syndrome (SARS) in Hong Kong in 2003: stress and psychological impact among frontline healthcare workers; C W. C. Tam, E P. F. Pang, L C. W. Lam and H F. K. Chiu, Psychological Medicine 2004/ Vol 34 / Iss 07 / pp. 1197-1204

"Knowingly giving a certificate with respect to birth, death, state of health, vaccination, or disinfection or with respect to any matter relating to life, health or accidents, which the medical practitioner knows or ought to know is untrue, misleading or otherwise improper; "[466] It is unprofessional to knowingly give a false certificate of illness; but it is difficult for doctors to be sure of illness like severe headaches, backaches or tiredness.

In many countries health professionals have organised themselves into unions in order to negotiate with their employers, which may be government. As a union they may take industrial action to deal with disputes, although many professionals abhor such action. Industrial action by health professionals has occurred in many parts of the world and to avoid abandoning patients, provisions are usually made to deal with emergencies.[467] Unofficial work stoppage by a 'sickout' has become a weapon used by many unionised workers and when it occurs among health care professionals, the unprofessional act is compounded when such 'illness' is falsely certified.

In the case report given it appears that a number of nurses may have taken the route of sick leave to avoid caring for a patient with suspected SARS. Other non-professional staff have shown reluctance and resistance to dealing with the patient, but have not actually stopped working in the institution.

• ***Have the regulatory mechanisms for the professions been enforced?*** Enforcing regulations for the professions must be done through a process that is just, a process that relies on determination of the truth rather than on emotions, which in issues about serious illness are always near the surface. Little attempt has been made to enquire into 'sick-outs' or the 'false certification' that may accompany them. The situation will draw comment from employers, politicians and the press; but in spite of claims to know who is producing the false certificates there are usually no complaints to the regulatory bodies responsible for disciplining the doctors alleged to have issued such certificates.[468] The failure to enquire into such accusations must leave the impression that a sickout is a fool-proof way of protest and may encourage others to do the same. The fact that not all workers engage in sickouts is a testimony to their professionalism and the effectiveness of the training they would have received.

---

[466] Laws of Barbados; Medical Registration Act Regulations CAP 171 Part V [2]

[467] Nurses' sick out crippling hospitals; Only emergency cases being dealt with; D Hussey-Whyte; jamaicaobserver.com; Sept 03, 2010

[468] http//the-right-solutions.blogspot.com/2011/02/unprofessional-behavior-by.html

In the case described there appears to be a lot of informing at the administrative level being done, but little being accomplished at the level of the workers directly responsible for patient care.

- ***How can the fears of staff be addressed?***

The fears generated with SARS are similar to those with any deadly infectious disease, for even when the disease proves to be not spread by casual contacts, fear can persist and be disseminated if there are associated stigmatising factors, such as homosexuality and the HIV epidemic. As with the HIV/AIDS pandemic such fears can only be addressed with education and retraining of staff. One of the main things that has to be done is to stress that if patients are abandoned, that they cannot expect to be treated differently if they or their relatives became ill. Training should be aimed at addressing:

What is known about SARS and its modes of transmission? The measures that are to be taken to treat the patient and protect staff should be demonstrated by example within the limits of the existing circumstances. If staff are briefed to use facilities that do not exist, then more fear and anxiety are likely to be kindled and they are poor motivators to do what's correct.[469]

A reiteration of the ethical issues and how they can work to the benefit of staff. It should be made clear to staff that if they abandon patients then there is little reason why others should remain to look after them or their relatives if they became ill, whether it is with SARS or any other complaint.

In the situation described it appears that the bare bones of dealing with SARS patients had been addressed. No realistic plan had been put in place, either to address the facilities identified or to anticipate and address adverse staff reactions.

---

[469] Healthcare workers' attitudes towards working during pandemic influenza: Draper, H., Wilson, S., Ives, J., Gratus, C., Greenfield, S., Parry, J., Petts, J., Sorell, T. (2008). BMC Public Health, 8(1), 192

Restraining a Patient

Case report 1:
A 20-year-old man presented to the emergency department with multiple stab wounds to the chest. After waiting for some time to be seen, the patient left the department, but was brought back hours later by the police in handcuffs. Whilst waiting to be assessed he attempted to escape through a window and was restrained by all four limbs by uniformed police officers and an unknown assistant. The patient was sent for an X-ray and was found by another doctor coming in the X-ray department handcuffed to the bed by his upper limbs and by his lower limbs tied to the bed with crepe bandages. The doctor removed the restraints on the legs and on doing so the patient became extremely agitated and combative. He was then sedated by intra-muscular injection.

Case report 2:
A 25-year-old man presented to the emergency department agitated, unable to speak and shaking. The patient was seen and treated for a dystonic reaction to the medication he was taking. The patient was later seen to be wandering through the department and disturbing the nursing staff. The patient was then restrained to a bed by his arms, and was referred to psychiatry. The psychiatrist responded on the phone that they did not believe that the patient needed psychiatric evaluation at that time.

After a while the patient escaped from the restraints and was observed wandering through the department visibly shaking. He was reviewed by another doctor and was again referred to psychiatry, which in turn suggested referral to Internal Medicine. He spent three days in the emergency department restrained to a bed before he was admitted to a medical ward. He jumped from the balcony of the medical ward and sustained minor injuries. He was then transferred to the Psychiatric Hospital as an involuntary admission.

Issues raised

- *Use of restraints in agitated patients*

Patients become agitated for a variety of reasons[470]. In emergency departments the most important reasons are hypoxia and hypovolemic shock from injuries, acute psychiatric illness, and psychosis from drug

---

[470] The violent or agitated patient. Rossi J, Swan MC, Isaacs ED. Emerg Med Clin North Am. 2010; 28:235-256.

intoxication. The management of each of these causes is different and restraining such patients may result in harm from the restraints; or they may vomit and aspirate, as they are unable to turn and protect their airway. Restraint without a diagnosis in cases of hypoxia and hypovolemic shock could lead to a patient's death.

In patients with acute psychiatric illness, the use of appropriate sedative drugs in the correct dosage is essential. The use of restraints should be seen as temporary to facilitate administration of the appropriate medication.

In the patients described physical restraints are inappropriately used for long periods. The first case appears to have both injuries and an acute psychiatric illness and there is not enough information given about the injuries to decide how much they were contributing to the patient's agitation. Whatever were the circumstances in the emergency department, it appears that the patient is left in an agitated state for long periods without any health personnel in attendance. The diagnosis of a psychiatric illness and the use of appropriate sedation appears to have been unduly delayed.

In the second case the diagnosis of a psychiatric disorder is made, but there appears to be no department that wishes to take responsibility for the patient's care. The staff in the emergency department resorts to restraints as a method of stopping the patient disturbing the staff and presumably patients in the department. This goes on for three days and upon admission his psychiatric condition does not appear to have been treated until he jumps off a balcony on the ward.

- *Responsibilities in case referrals*

When referrals are made, and in particular in emergency situations, the patient and the referring doctors are entitled to a serious and in-depth consideration of the problem. It is unprofessional, as well as dangerous for the patient, to seek to evade responsibility by finding secondary issues that are then referred to other disciplines. In situations where there is a genuine reason for more than one discipline to be involved, each discipline should be clear about their management role and not shelve responsibility as if one problem should wait until the other is resolved. Usually medical problems in emergency situations are interconnected and should be treated together in a cooperative manner for the benefit of the patient.

In some systems referral patterns/protocols have developed for good reasons at some time in the past; such protocols are usually developed based on the availability of staff. All protocols should be kept under review so that when circumstances change outmoded systems do not continue to be used to the detriment of the patient.

In the first case described, it appears that some of the emergency department doctors are evading dealing with the patient and leaves the agitated patient to be restrained by the police. There is no mention of a referral being made and the assessment of the patient's wounds appears to be unusually delayed.

In the second case described, it is difficult to evade the conclusion that all three of the departments involved appear to have been evading responsibility in managing an acute psychiatric illness. The mismanagement goes to the point of restraining the patient for three days in an inappropriate place.

- ***Prior conditions and attitudes towards patients.***
There are several conditions and situations that may influence the attitude of staff to a patient. This may lead to misdiagnosis, delays in treatment and occasionally overzealous treatment when dealing with colleagues or celebrities.

The patients who are most likely to have delays in assessment, misdiagnosis and treatment are those who are dirty, unkempt and smelly; loud, abusive and disruptive, often associated with alcohol abuse; psychiatric patients, particularly those with disruptive or threatening behaviours; stigmatised and 'threatening' diseases such as HIV and lethal infectious diseases; known hypochondriacs; known or presumed criminals; and persons with stigmatised lifestyles, such as males with feminine behaviours, prostitutes, minority religious identification and modes of dress.

In the cases described enough information is given to diagnose psychiatric disorders, but there is not enough information given to positively recognise other stigmatising features. The first case, although he appears to be a victim, may also be involved in criminal behaviour and may have been known to the staff in the emergency department.

The second case appears to be known to the psychiatric staff, to the point that they decide over the phone that he does not need to be evaluated at the time; in fact, they only appear to take notice after the patient's attempted suicide.

Case report:

A 25-year-old woman referred to psychiatry after a failed suicide attempt was diagnosed as having a major depressive episode with psychotic features. She was 20 weeks gestation and was started on both antidepressant and antipsychotic medications. The patient's mother said she had 'problems and a difficult relationship with her boyfriend, the pregnancy and being HIV positive'. The patient confirmed that the father of the child in this pregnancy was also HIV positive. The psychiatrist called the HIV Reference Unit and spoke to a nurse who stated that the patient was known to them and due to commence HAART antiviral treatment shortly.

The patient was HIV negative during her second pregnancy nine years ago, and recorded as HIV positive during this pregnancy. The patient was followed as an outpatient and when the baby was born it was taken into care for adoption. In two years of follow-up she had four admissions for suicide attempts, and during one admission it was noted that she was not on HAART therapy; contact was made with the Reference Unit and the head of that unit stated that she was taken off medication because it was discovered that she was HIV negative. In explaining the circumstances, the head of the unit noted that when the patient tested positive she was started on therapy although her CD4 counts were normal and the viral load undetectable; she had taken part in a random rapid kit test survey and tested negative; confirmatory PCR testing was done and was found to be negative and HAART therapy was stopped. The staff at the unit and in psychiatry both acknowledged that they knew the patient was not using condoms and had ignored it since they were both HIV positive and felt it did not matter. When the psychiatry staff told the patient that she was HIV negative, she was shocked at the news.

Issues raised

- *Was HIV testing and counselling appropriately done?*

HIV testing is voluntary and any pregnant woman should have counselling and an HIV test. Counselling should educate the patient about HIV, dealing with its transmission particularly with the unprotected intercourse required to become pregnant again, as well as the problems related to an HIV positive infant. Effective counselling starts preparing the patient for the personal and societal reaction to a positive result.[471]

Post-test counselling reinforces and builds on the foundation of pre-test counselling for both the HIV positive patient and the persons who have been tested as contacts of HIV positive persons but have a negative result. One of the prerequisites for effective post-test counselling is to have confidence in the test result. The intensity of the counselling required should always be tailored to the scale of the patient's problem and their capacity to benefit. A patient's capacity is influenced by their ability to understand the issues; the nature of any mental problems they have; and the abilities and methods used by the counsellor. Judgmental attitudes of the counsellor may play a role and may depend on their religion and previous experience. Group counselling may also play a role, for members of the group may surrender their confidentiality in sensitive areas. In practical terms groups do surrender some confidentiality, and the question is whether an individual who agrees to join a group consciously gives up their rights to confidentiality, and what responsibility would the counsellor organising the group have for any breach that occurs.[472]

When services are busy, counselling may become perfunctory, particularly prior to testing and group activity. Follow-up counselling is often ignored when the test is negative, even for contact tracing, and repeat testing may not be done. Where 'routine' testing is done, it is most likely that the result may not be followed up when the patient has only briefly used the service. One manifestation of ineffectual counselling is the fact that in a service dedicated to prevention of mother to child transmission, 20% of pregnant HIV positive mothers had been pregnant before and in the prevention programme.[473]

In the report given the patient was 16 years old on her second pregnancy and was tested for HIV then. There appears to have been effective contraception advice given at that time for she had not been pregnant for several years but she subsequently became pregnant for an HIV positive man being followed in the HIV Reference Unit. What counselling was done did not prevent her from becoming suicidal on being told she was HIV positive.

When the patient was fortuitously found to be HIV negative after being treated as HIV positive for two years, this information is not passed on to the psychiatric service under whose care she has been for those two years. Although

---

[471] Pre-HIV test counselling; www.health24.com › ... › HIV/Aids › Counselling

[472] Is Confidentiality in Group Counselling Realistic? Davis, K L; Personnel and Guidance Journal, 1980,59,4,197

[473] KAP among HIV infected women with repeated childbirths in Barbados Kumar and St. John WIMJ 2001 Vol 50 supp 2; 16

the medication had been stopped, she remained confused and shocked when she is told that she was HIV negative by the psychiatric service. One must conclude that counselling was ineffective in the HIV Reference Unit for both the patient and her sexual partners.

- ***Confirmation of HIV positive status over the phone.***
It is hazardous for confidential information to be sought and given over the phone; fraudulent identification may be given by unauthorized persons to obtain such information, and phone lines to sensitive units may not be secure.[474]   The participants are difficult to identify with certainty, unauthorized persons may overhear conversations, and information heard may be mistaken for something else. Written communication although not perfect can be made more secure, but some nuances may be more difficult to convey than in a conversation.

HAART therapy is confidential information for it is given only for HIV/AIDS. The CD4 count and the viral loads are used to measure when the disease is advanced and monitor progress under treatment.[475] HAART is not the standard for antenatal therapy unless indicated for the treatment of the mother.[476] Sensitive information should be shared in a confidential manner between the persons responsible for treating the patient. Patients should know that confidential information is being shared and that there is the same level of confidentiality with other professionals.[477]

Staff other than the professionals that have confidential information available to them, should be trained and placed under a legal responsibility to keep such information confidential. A patient may feel that sensitive information coming from nursing or other staff has breached their confidentiality, and such information should never be delegated for transmission to non-health professionals, no matter what confidence the health professional has in that person.[478] When confidential information is passed between services it should be done at a senior level

---

[474] Florida investigates breach of confidentiality in HIV records. AIDS policy & law. 1996 (.18): 1, 10-1;
[475] Guidelines for the use of antiretroviral agents in HIV-1-infected adults and adolescents. Department of Health and Human Services. 2011; http://www.aidsinfo.nih.gov/
[476] Antiretroviral drugs and the prevention of mother-to-child transmission of HIV infection In resource-limited settings Report of a Technical Consultation, UNAIDS, Geneva, 2004 www.who.int/hiv/pub/mtct/en/arvddrugsmeetingreport.pdf
[477] AMA's Code of Medical Ethics; Patient Confidentiality; http://www.ama-assn.org/ama/pub/physician-resources/legal-topics/patient-physician-relationship-topics/patient-confidentiality.page
[478] GMC; Confidentiality guidance: Sharing information with a patient's partner, carers, relatives or friends; 2009; http://www.gmc-uk.org/guidance/ethical_guidance/confidentiality_64_66_sharing_information.asp

so that responsibility can be taken for any problems that arise.[479] When patients present with related problems to different departments it is important that each department has all the relevant information.

In the report given sensitive information is given over the phone; but no breach of confidentiality is apparent. The information was not passed at a senior level and vital information about process and sexual contacts is left out. Whether this lapse is due to lax work, or that the staff in the unit felt some responsibility knowing that an HIV negative person became positive as a sexual partner of the HIV positive patients under their care. The failure to communicate to the psychiatric department when the patient is found to be HIV negative after two years of HAART treatment and with repeated suicide threats cannot be justified.

The dichotomy in attitudes probably contributed to the poor outcome described; for instead of the patient's mental status improving on hearing that she is not HIV positive, she continues to be disturbed including a further suicide attempt.

- **Was the testing ordered in the ward warranted or done as a 'routine'?**

An HIV positive test and antiviral treatment should be known on admission to hospital and further testing is not warranted unless there is some doubt expressed, or the result is not known. 'Routine' testing is advocated on the grounds that one can test more persons, by doing the test on everyone who attends health facilities, and pick up more asymptomatic HIV positive persons. This should enable such persons to be followed, counselled and treated earlier than if they came for testing on their own volition. This is a change in policy from what voluntary counselling and testing that had been advocated before, and raises ethical and legal questions re consent for testing and the counselling required.[480]

There is a legal liability for an incorrect result, if there was sufficient information to warrant a review of the result, or a confirmatory test is the standard and neither is done. The kind of information that may warrant review is an unexpected result given the clinical information, or other results that do not correlate with the test result. Confirmatory tests for HIV are usually more time consuming or difficult, but are more reliable than the standard test as regards false positive or false negative results.

HIV testing falls into the category that a positive should be confirmed, and if clinical information warrants it, a negative test should be repeated

---

[479] Sharing patient information between professionals: confidentiality and ethics; A J Braunack-Mayer and E C Mulligan; Med J Aust 2003; 178 (6): 277-279

[480] Desperately seeking targets: the ethics of routine HIV testing in low-income countries S. Rennie, F Behets Bull World Health Organ 2006 vol.84 no.1

after several weeks to make sure that the window period has been covered or viral load testing done.

The case report suggests that the testing done on admission was routine and illustrates that the professionals may go through the 'routine' but do not necessarily follow through on the result. The routine test result is not recorded and therefore did not pick up a problem of conflicting test results. Furthermore, repeated 'routine' normal CD4 counts and absent viral loads did not influence the decision to start HAART therapy or prompt a review of the HIV test result. The subsequent negative test came about inadvertently when she was being used to test a new rapid testing method; it is only when this unexpected result occurs that the full rigour of confirmatory testing is done.

- *What role has the HIV status played in the patient's psychiatric condition?*

Stigmatized AIDS and HIV positive persons are well known to go through severe mental distress including anger, severe depression and suicidal ideation. In addition, patients with HIV disease may become demented before there is any other evidence of progression to AIDS.[481] These severe psychiatric reactions were the primary reason why pre- and post-test counselling assumed such importance in managing HIV.

Although there has been some hard-fought-for change in attitudes, stigmatization of HIV positive persons and homosexuals remains a factor in handling HIV affected patients. Persons with intractable attitudes, particularly against homosexuals, have justified them on religious grounds. Some countries have invoked their constitutions and enacted broad antidiscrimination statutes to try and influence community attitudes and actions.[482] Others have chosen to keep discriminatory laws against homosexuality, on the basis that male homosexuals are the primary reason for the spread of HIV. Some countries have gone further and sought to criminalise the transmission of HIV whether intentionally or not.[483]

In the report given the patient on being told that she is HIV positive makes a suicide attempt. This occurred on a background of having been tested negative at least twice before in the HIV Reference Unit. This raises questions about the skills of the staff in the reference unit re the efficacy of the preventive counselling provided.

---

[481] Natural history of neuropsychiatric manifestations of HIV disease. Atkinson, J. H; Grant, I; Psychiatric Clinics of North America, 1994,Vol 17(1), 17-33.
[482] South Africa; Employment Equity Act; 1998
[483] R. V. Cuerrier, [1998] 2 SCR 371 (Supreme Court of Canada);

- *Should the effectiveness of counselling at the Reference Unit be assessed?*

All services should be assessed for their effectiveness by looking at their overall results, as well as critical incidents occurring in a service. Such audits should be initiated internally, but may also need to be examined independently when incidents threaten the integrity of the service or the institution of which it is a part. It is equally vital that the broad results of an audit should be available outside of the service if support for any necessary change is to be obtained.

Where a service has engaged the public to change behaviours and to take medications as preventive measures, it is imperative that the public should be informed of the results and effectiveness of such measures.

In the case described there are several issues that are in need of a critical review:
- *The false positive test, did the error occur in the laboratory, or in the identification of patients?*
- *The institution of HAART therapy outside of departmental guidelines.*
- *The transmittal of confidential information between services; and*
- *The effectiveness of counselling for behaviour modification.*

- *Should possible childhood sexual abuse/statutory rape be ignored?*

There is little doubt that childhood abuse whether physical, mental or sexual has a profound effect on the behaviour of the abused child well into their adult life. Such persons often become abusers themselves, or become sexually irresponsible. It is therefore necessary in tackling such behaviours in adults to recall their entire history, not necessarily for any legal action but for an understanding of the patient and for the counsellor to know of the origins of the behaviour and why it should be changed.[484]

In the case described there appears to have been no enquiry into the early history of the patient in spite of having two pregnancies around the age of 16 years. Her continued promiscuous behaviour with more than one known HIV positive man suggests a possible pattern of childhood sexual abuse that should have been explored.

- *Are there legal means to curb the deliberate/reckless spread of HIV?*

Since the advent of AIDS and the widespread stigmatization of HIV positive persons, concern has been expressed that HIV infected persons may deliberately or recklessly spread HIV, particularly through

---

[484] Impact of child sexual abuse: A review of the research. Browne, A; Finkelhor, D; Psychological Bulletin, 1986 Vol 99(1), 66-77

unprotected sexual intercourse.[485], [486] Counselling of HIV positive persons and others about the use of condoms is often counterbalanced by religious objections to condoms, on the basis that protection from the spread of HIV encourages sexual activity outside of marriage, or other sinful activity such as prostitution and sodomy. When such prohibitions fail, calls are made to break the confidentiality of HIV positive persons or to prosecute them for criminal activity.

Warning third parties of a mortal risk is well established in judicial precedent.[487] The risk to the third party must be a mortal one; HIV/AIDS once fell into this category, but with the advent of HAART therapy it could be argued that HIV/AIDS is no longer a fatal disease. The patient whose confidentiality is to be broken must know of their condition and how they place the third party at risk. When the risk behaviour is unprotected sexual intercourse, one can only know of the behaviour from the patients themselves.[488] The deliberate or reckless spread of HIV/AIDS can be viewed as a criminal act, and some countries have enacted specific criminal statutes in relation to the transmission of HIV; others have used existing statutes such as attempted murder.[489] As in any other criminal trial evidence would have to be presented that transmission occurred and that it was done deliberately or recklessly.

In the narrative described there was no need to warn the patient, for she appears to know that she was having sex with HIV positive persons; what was necessary was to impress upon her the danger of unprotected sex. There does appear to have been reckless endangerment by the HIV positive men in having unprotected sex with the patient, no matter what they considered her HIV status to be.

---

[485] Global Network of People Living with HIV/AIDS Europe, Terrence Higgins Trust (2005). "Criminalisation of HIV transmission in Europe: A rapid scan of the laws and rates of prosecution for HIV transmission within signatory States of the European Convention of Human Rights".
[486] Center for Disease Control & Prevention, HIV Transmission: Can HIV be transmitted through a human bite? (2010) http://www.cdc.gov/hiv/resources/qa/transmission.htm
[487] Tarasoff v. Regents of the University of California, 17 Cal. 3d 425, 551 P.2d 334, 131 Cal. Rptr. 14 (Cal. 1976)
[488] A Legal and Ethical Analysis of Third Party Notification of HIV; N S. McKinney The AABSS Journal, 2012, Volume 16; http://aabss.org/Journal2012/05aabssLegalAndEthicalAnalysis.pdf
[489] Knowingly Exposing Another to HIV, J. Grishkin; Yale Law Journal, Vol. 106, 1997

Responsibility for Defects

Case report:

A 56-year-old man is admitted vomiting blood profusely for four hours.
He was alone at home and had tried to no avail to get his doctor. His
wife returned an hour later and found him slumped over the toilet. With
the aid of a neighbour she moved him to the bed, tried ringing for an
ambulance but none was available. His wife tried to reach their doctor
and was told to get him to the emergency department. The neighbour
rang a private ambulance and they said that they needed to have the fee
when they came.

The patient was taken to the hospital where he was unresponsive,
pale and clammy with no perceptible pulse. An intravenous line was
started and four units of O negative blood ordered urgently. A junior
doctor is dispatched to the blood bank to bring back the blood right
away and is told that there are only two units of O negative blood in
the bank, it has not been tested and he would have to wait until other
tested blood is cross-matched. Whilst waiting in the laboratory for the
blood to be ready the doctor receives a call from his senior asking 'if he
has got lost'. He explains that the technician insists that the blood be
cross- matched and had just told him that the patient is O positive and he
is cross matching the blood that is there. The senior doctor demands to
speak to the technician and stresses that he should obey his order for the
uncross-matched blood, and is told by the technician that he is wasting
his time on the phone. The blood is delivered an hour later, is started
but the patient dies shortly thereafter. A letter of protest is written to the
head of pathology department responsible for the blood bank. One month
later a circular is sent out stating that no blood will be issued from the
department without being cross-matched and that no untested blood will
be issued without a written consent form from the patient or their next
of kin.

Issues raised

- *Complaining about services.*

Complaints about services come from any quarter; the complaints by staff
in relation to the treatment of patients are most likely related to:

Blood Transfusion Services - particularly related to emergency requests
for un-cross-matched or untested blood in desperate life-threatening
situations. The use of universal donor O negative blood is accepted as a

substitute for cross-matching in desperate situations.[490] The use of blood untested for pathogens is more controversial; however, it is recognized that in desperate situations such blood could be used with the written authorization of the treating physician.[491] With transmissible disorders such as HIV where the testing procedure may have a false negative rate, donors may undergo further screening. There are other difficulties where donors are few relative to the demand, and service may be denied to those who are unable to recruit donors. These difficulties create tensions between staff and may result in complaints about the service provided.

Equipment availability or failures are a common cause for complaint. The frequency of complaints relates to the type of equipment, its maintenance, and the availability of capital for replacement of out-dated equipment. Poorly maintained equipment may fail or malfunction during a procedure and place a patient at risk; sometimes staff feel pressure to proceed in an emergency or perceived urgency and risk using equipment that they are doubtful about. This is difficult to defend if something goes wrong and the patient is harmed.

Environmental conditions, particularly air-conditioning is of importance to both patients and staff for temperature control and comfort. However, it can be hazardous to health if through poor maintenance it disseminates bacteria or fungi.

In the case described the patient is in severe shock and blood transfusion is required immediately. The physician has judged that the patient's condition cannot await an emergency cross-match and requests universal donor blood; what is available is untested for pathogens. The technician decides to cross-match blood for the patient and a confrontation and complaint ensues.

The subsequent departmental memorandum seeks to absolve the department from any responsibility for having untested blood and tries to put the responsibility for its use on the patient or their next of kin.

- ***Untested blood in life-threatening situations.***

A physician should accept responsibility for using untested blood in life-threatening situations; such orders should be made in writing preferably on a previously agreed institutional form. Blood stored in a bank or blood products should have been tested for pathogens, and the responsibility is that of the blood bank if any problem is subsequently discovered.[492]

---

[490] Guidelines on the management of massive blood loss. Stainsby D, MacLennan S, Thomas D, Isaac J, Hamilton PJ. Br J Haematol 2006; 135(5): 634-41.

[491] NSPBCP Guideline for Massive Transfusion in Nova Scotia November 18, 2010

[492] Strict Liability, Negligence And The Standard Of Care For Transfusion-Transmitted Disease; 1994; 36 Ariz. L. Rev. 473 M J. Miller

In urgent but not immediately life-threatening situations where untested blood is the only blood available, the patient, guardian or surrogate should be asked to consent after the circumstances and risks are fully explained. However, should something go wrong it could be argued that consent was forced on the patient.

In the situation described the physician has asked for universal donor blood to avoid the need for cross-matching, and would not have been aware that the blood available was untested. When made aware of this the physician and the technician engage in a confrontation over their authority rather than the needs of the patient.

- ***Defective equipment / supplies / drugs***

The use of defective medical resources/supplies presents problems which include-

Knowledge of the defect. Equipment may have been observed to have malfunctioned or to be poorly calibrated; supplies may have been observed to be poorly stored, inadequately sterilized or have surpassed an expiry date; drugs may have gone past their expiry date or have been recalled or warnings issued. These and similar circumstances carry the responsibility to report the defect and to accept responsibility for using the defective equipment etc. if something goes wrong.

Life-threatening situations call for any measure available to save a patient's life. If there is defective equipment, supplies or drugs and no alternative can be found, the physician may decide to accept the risks in an attempt to save the patient's life. Whatever the outcome it is important to record the known defects and the circumstances that led to its use, in case an accusation of negligent conduct was subsequently made.

Health professionals other than physicians do not carry the legal responsibilities of a physician to patients, and although they have important responsibilities, it is imprudent of them to ignore the requests of a competent physician in life-threatening situations.[493]

Urgent situations which are not imminently life-threatening should not be used as an excuse for the use of defective materials. If the situation cannot be remedied before the urgency must be dealt with, and no alternatives can be found, the patient or guardian should be made fully aware of the situation and asked whether they are prepared to accept the risks involved in proceeding.

---

[493] Physician-nurse conflict: can nurses refuse to carry out doctors' orders? Frederich ME, Strong R, von Gunten CF. J Palliat Med. 2002; 5(1): 155-8

Non-urgent/elective situations. The use of defective materials is unwise
even with the 'knowledge and consent' of the patient. In situations where
it appears that the situation cannot be remedied, then the responsible
institution or authority should be asked to acknowledge responsibility for
the use of the defective materials in addition to the informed consent of
the patient.

Environmental hazards may abound in health care institutions. Hazards
arise from air-conditioning, piped and bottled gases, smoking on the
premises, and the use of asbestos for a variety of purposes. Similar
considerations apply as to the use of defective equipment; however,
cause and effect may be more difficult to establish when a problem arises.
Knowledge of the environmental problem before it is obvious is not
always clear to everyone, and risks may be taken depending on whether
the situation is life-threatening, urgent or elective.

*In the case described the blood bank technician is aware that the available
blood requested is untested for pathogens and therefore presents a risk for
transfusion. However, the technician completely ignores the desperate nature of
the request, proceeds in spite of protests along routine lines and the opportunity
to save the patient's life is lost.*

An Impaired Physician

Case report:
A 60-year-old physician was brought to the emergency department because of 'strange behaviour.' His family reported symptoms indicative of paranoid delusions and auditory hallucinations. He was belligerent, agitated and lacked insight into his symptoms. There was a previous diagnosis of schizophrenia and he was not consistently compliant with medication. A few months previously the physician had a death in his office and the emergency technicians called to the scene, publicly questioned his ability to carry out resuscitation.

The patient was initially reluctant to be admitted to the psychiatric hospital but eventually agreed to voluntary admission. His son, a physician, was reluctant to have him involuntarily admitted out of concern that when he recovered he would see it as a betrayal by his family. In hospital he agreed to take medication after much discussion and persuasion. A few days after admission he declared that there was nothing wrong with him, he would no longer take any medication and left the ward against advice. At the time he was assessed as still having psychotic symptoms without insight into his illness.

The psychiatrist had two immediate concerns: one to find the patient to effect an involuntary admission for his self-protection, and a fear that he might attempt to resume practice. In addition to observing the usual protocols established for patients who lack capacity, the psychiatrist also wrote to and called the Medical Council expressing concern that should the physician attempt to practise, the public would be endangered.

He was subsequently located by the police and was admitted involuntarily. After a few weeks he was released from hospital and was said to be compliant with the medication prescribed.

Issues raised

- *What constitutes an impaired physician?*

An impaired physician is one who has a condition that interferes with their proper conduct of patient care.[494] The impairment may be related to a physical or mental condition, or the adherence to cultural or religious viewpoints and/or practices that result in unethical or illegal conduct in relation to patients. Physical impairment may be related to substance abuse or to medication, and mental states may be spontaneous or

---

[494] Impaired healthcare professional Baldisseri MR1. Crit Care Med. 2007; 35(2 Suppl): S106-16.

induced, and include the various forms of dementia, uncontrolled mental illnesses, and sociopathic and psychopathic personality disorders as well as the disorders of substance abuse.[495]

The behaviours associated with the impaired physician that may not be labelled as a mental disorder, include substance abuse; abusive or offensive behaviour most often in racial, ethnic and religious matters; wilful professional misconduct; and habitual unprofessional or criminal conduct within or outside the practice of medicine.

In the case report given, the physician has an acute mental disorder that would preclude him from the conduct of any ethical or safe professional practice.

- *Diagnosis of the impaired physician*

The diagnosis of an impaired physician usually starts with observations of behaviour or conduct by colleagues, other workers, patients or relatives of patients, and the wider community.[496] Some of the observations include: late for appointments, increased absences or unknown whereabouts; unusual and unannounced rounding times; increase in patient complaints about missed appointments, quality of care and careless medical decisions; increased secrecy, overt alcohol intoxication and concealing of needle marks; decrease in productivity or efficiency, including incorrect charting or writing of prescriptions; increased conflicts with colleagues, with increased irritability and aggression; an erratic job history in applications for posts.

The formal process of labelling a physician as impaired has implications for their livelihood as a practitioner and although a diagnosis of a particular illness is made, the diagnosis of an impaired physician should be made in the larger context of the practitioner's ability to practise medicine. Institutions should have a confidential and independent panel with powers to grant or withdraw privileges and to monitor progress where privileges have been retained.[497] When the impairment is not a physical one, it can be hazardous to choose one type of practice over another for an impaired practitioner. Any choice of continued practice should be accompanied by a broad monitoring regimen.

Regulatory bodies should have a confidential mechanism to enquire into and regulate the practice of an impaired physician; unlike

[495] The Sick Physician Impairment by Psychiatric Disorders, Including Alcoholism and Drug Dependence; JAMA. 1973; 223(6): 684-687
[496] Identification of Physician Impairment; Pham JC1, Pronovost PJ, Skipper GE. JAMA. 2013; 22; 309(20): 2101-2.
[497] Four years experience of a hospital's impaired physician committee. Schwartz RP, White RK, McDuff DR, Johnson JL. J Addict Dis. 1995; 14(2): 13-21.

institutions who have the power to modify the practice of a physician, a regulatory body has the rather blunt powers of stopping the physician from practising, issuing warnings and in some instances setting up mechanisms for monitoring a practitioner's practice.[498]

The legal mechanisms for determining who is impaired can only be invoked when there has been an infraction of the law, such as a death thought to be the result of gross negligence or the deliberate action of the practitioner.[499] Legal proceedings unlike those in institutions cannot be kept confidential and outcomes are punitive rather than redemptive.

There was no issue in making a diagnosis in the reported case; the physician had been treated before for the mental disorder, and now has obvious incapacitating symptoms.

- ### *Reporting the impaired physician.*

Observation by colleagues is usually the starting point in diagnosing the impaired practitioner and initiating some action that would benefit the practitioner and protect the patients they are treating. What to do with the observations made is sensitive and it is tempting to do little else than gossip about it with other colleagues. Many do not want to be involved in case they are themselves attacked or accused, and also fear the loss of friendships and deterioration in working relationships.

The concerning behaviour should be noted in an objective manner in personal or patient's notes, and is almost certain to be challenged for its accuracy. If a personal approach is decided upon, it is best done through a senior, respected and independent person, whether that person is a colleague, a religious or other community leader. Reporting is best done through a confidential mechanism, which would be defined in an institutional code of conduct for staff, or in the regulations of the professions regulatory body.[500] Institutional and regulatory bodies should also have a confidential system for enquiry into these complaints, and a flexible system of dealing with the severity of the problem. Only flexibility and confidence in the fairness of the system will give fellow practitioners the confidence to report issues with a colleague.[501] The public also has greater confidence in regulatory systems that include persons from outside the profession.

---

[498] Regulation of the medical profession: fantasy, reality and legality; A Samanta, and J Samanta; J R Soc Med. 2004; 97(5): 211–218

[499] The Shipman enquiry http://webarchive.nationalarchives.gov.uk/20090808154959/http:/www.the-shipman-inquiry.org.uk/reports.asp

[500] Reporting Impaired, Incompetent, or Unethical Colleagues; AMA Code of Medical Ethics; http://www.ama-assn.org/ama/pub/physician-resources/medical-ethics/code-medical-ethics/opinion9031

[501] Identifying and Assisting the Impaired Physician; Boisaubin, E V.; Levine, R E. American Journal of the Medical Sciences: 2001; Vol 322; 1; pp. 31-36

Reporting of the physician in the case report to the regulatory body only occurred when the patient absconded from care and it was feared that he might attempt to practise.

- **Treatment of the impaired professional**

Because of the implications for the public, treatment of the impaired professional should be acceptable to a broad body of professionals, with monitoring of progress by a diverse group along with credible and appropriate laboratory testing. Monitoring is crucial where the practitioner is allowed to continue practising, and with regulatory oversight may involve testing in instances of substance abuse, or checking compliance with medication.

The treatment of this practitioner patient was within the standard of care for the ailment diagnosed. However, there had been no effective monitoring of compliance with the medication, leading to a psychotic breakdown.

- **Confidentiality of the practising professional**

The confidentiality of an ill practitioner is as important as that of any ill person. However, given their responsibility for patients if the practitioner's health places patients' lives at risk, confidentiality should be broken to the appropriate body that can prevent them from practising; in doing so one must determine that the risk to others is a mortal one. [502] Breaking the confidentiality of an impaired professional should be done to the appropriate regulatory body rather than to individual patients or in a public forum. It would be for the regulatory body to take appropriate action to protect the public.

In the instance described the treating physician became concerned about breaking confidentiality, when there was a fear that the absconding practitioner/ patient might attempt to practise, and sought the advice of the professional regulatory body.

- **When should an impaired practitioner be allowed to practise?**

Many practitioners make the decision for themselves as to when they are fit to work. In an institutional setting it may be sanctioned by a departmental head on the recommendation of the practitioner's personal physician. These mechanisms are not appropriate when dealing with the impaired physician who should have their work regulated by an institutional or professional regulatory body, with powers of formal

---

[502] Tarasoff et al. V. The regents of the University of California et al. Supreme Court of California. 17 Cal. 3d 425; 551 P .2d 334

monitoring and of withdrawal of practising privileges.

In the case reported the practitioner had been diagnosed previously and was non-compliant with medication. There was nothing said as to whether the regulatory body had been involved in the decision to allow him to continue practising, and if so what informed that decision.

Case report:
A 60-year-old woman attended a general practitioner complaining of malaise, anorexia and weight loss. She was diagnosed as being anaemic (Hb 10.2 g/dl). Six months later she attended the clinic with an additional complaint of abdominal pain. An ultrasound was ordered and it showed a heterogeneous abdominal lesion; further evaluation with contrast-enhanced CT was advised as soon as possible and was requested. The patient was advised that she would be called to be given a date for the scan to be done.

Three months after the patient had complained of her abdominal pain and had been investigated, a referral letter was addressed to the 'On-call general surgery consultant'. The letter contained the results of blood tests showing elevated cancer screening levels and a note that a CT scan had been ordered. The records department gave an appointment for four months later.

Three months later and one month before the scheduled outpatient appointment, the patient presented at the emergency department with worsening abdominal pain, shortness of breath and palpitations. The patient said she had lost 15Kgm in weight and had not received a date for the CT scan that was ordered six months previously. The patient had a palpable abdominal mass, which was shown on a CT scan ordered in the emergency department to be invading the adjacent abdominal wall. She was admitted and underwent an urgent exploratory laparotomy. However, her postoperative course was complicated by a pulmonary embolus and she died one week after her operation. When the hospital notes were reviewed for the surgery department audit, there was an outpatient clinic entry stating 'Absent from clinic'.

Issues raised

- *The early diagnosis of cancer*

The early diagnosis of a cancer is either done by screening or by the physician recognizing the early symptoms and carrying out the appropriate diagnostic measures.[503] [504] It is appropriate to ask what role

---

[503] Alarm symptoms in early diagnosis of cancer in primary care: cohort study using General Practice Research Database; R Jones, R Latinovic, J Charlton, and M C Gulliford; BMJ. 2007; 334(7602): 1040.
[504] Screening Tests for Cancer - National Cancer Institute; https://www.cancer.gov/about-cancer/screening/screening-tests

the primary care physician should play in the diagnosis of cancers?[505]
Where the health care system restricts direct access to specialist care,
both primary care physicians and specialists should be involved in the
early diagnosis of cancers, and that there must be suitably responsive
mechanisms for the referral of patients for specialist care.

*In the report given the patient presented to the primary care physician with
symptoms that should lead to a suspicion of a cancer diagnosis. The symptoms
were incorrectly attributed to a mild anaemia, until more troublesome symptoms
arose six months later.*

- ***The role of the primary care physician in investigating patients***
A patient on attending any doctor expects a diagnosis to be made, and
when required, to be referred as early as possible. The primary care
physician is expected to have sufficient knowledge to initiate the correct
diagnostic procedures, but not necessarily for initiating additional
investigations that may be required by the specialist physician.[506]

The specialist investigations initiated by a primary care physician are
often repeated when there has been a waiting period for the specialist
appointment. Repeat investigations may be at a cost to the patient in
terms of any risks of the procedure, the expenditure to the patient or
to the system of care. It is appropriate that a primary care physician
orders diagnostic/screening investigations such as mammograms or
colonoscopy, but should refrain from ordering staging investigations
such as MRIs or CT scans unless done in consultation with the treating
specialist. Such strictures do not negate the wider role the primary care
physician should play in the management of patients with cancer.[507]

*In the report given the primary care physician missed the opportunity
of screening for common cancers at the initial consultation. On the second
consultation, the investigation ordered showed obvious disease and should
have precipitated an urgent referral. What followed instead was a request for
a staging investigation and a routine letter of referral that resulted in a four-
months appointment.*

- ***The urgent referral***
Patients with urgencies dealt with in emergency departments are

---

[505] The Role of the general practitioner in the diagnosis of early cancer; JG Walsh - 1958 onlinelibrary.
wiley.com/doi/10.3322/canjclin.8.3.83/pdf
[506] Impact of investigations in general practice on timeliness of referral for patients subsequently
diagnosed with cancer: analysis of national primary care audit data; G P Rubin, C L Saunders, G A
Abel, S McPhail, G Lyratzopoulos, and R D Neal; Br J Cancer. 2015; 112(4): 676–687.
[507] The Role of Primary Care Physicians in Cancer Care; C N. Klabunde, A Ambs, N L. Keating, et al; J
Gen Intern Med. 2009; 24(9): 1029–1036.

prioritized in a triaging system,[508] and the less catastrophic urgencies may be subject to delays that may vary from hours up to a day.[509] This type of delay in emergency departments is exhausting for the patient and their relatives, but is not as long as obtaining a specialist appointment. Getting a specialist appointment is usually quicker in private than in public systems, where appointments may vary from weeks to many months.[510] Therefore, there should be systems to enable urgent appointments to be made to specialist clinics.[511] Most systems of appointment depend on non-professional staff that are asked to deal with letters or phone calls from physicians or their assistants. Such staff usually have no special training as to when an urgent appointment should be given and inevitably depend on some direct guidance from the specialist concerned. It is therefore appropriate that urgent requests be handled by some direct communication between the referring physician and the specialist, the most direct means of achieving this is via telephone contact and to a much lesser extent be email. Both of these have their own difficulties, with telephone contact depending on the efficiency of the telephone as well as the availability of both the referring physician and the specialist involved. When telephone contact is frustrated, a letter delivered by the patient is often used; such letters should have some prominent display of the URGENT nature of the request. The letter should be couched in such terms that the lay staff might either agree with the judgment of urgency, or seek guidance from the specialist service.

Referral systems and including those dealing with urgencies should be subject to periodic review and be modified as necessary.[512] This should avoid patients falling through the cracks, and avoid an indefensible legal claim.[513]

In the report given the only evidence of urgency given is addressing the letter to 'the on-call general surgeon'. There is no indication that the lay staff seeks the advice of the 'on-call general surgeon' or discerns that the information requires an urgent appointment. It is ironic that the appointments staff do not recognize that the patient has been admitted and died, and records the patient as being 'Absent from clinic' when the appointment was due.

---

[508] Emergency department triage: an ethical analysis | RP Aacharya BMC Emergency Medicine 2011... bmcemergmed.biomedcentral.com/articles/10.1186/1471-227X-11-16

[509] Triage and patient safety in emergency departments; S Oredsson, BMJ 2011; 343:d6652

[510] Wait Times for Specialist Appointment - The Commonwealth Fund Www.commonwealthfund.org/interactives.../wait-times-for-specialist-appointment

[511] NHS waiting times in England - NHS Choices; www.nhs.uk/NHSEngland/appointment-booking/Pages/nhs-waiting-times.aspx

[512] Medicare physician referral patterns. D Shea, B Stuart, J Vasey, and S Nag; Health Serv Res. 1999; 34(1 Pt 2): 331–348.

[513] GPs advised on avoiding missed cancer diagnoses - The MDU 2015 - https://www.themdu.com/.../latest.../gps-advised-on-avoiding-missed-cancer-diagnose...

- *Ethical and legal responsibilities in delayed care*

Professionals carry both ethical and legal responsibility for a breach in the standard of care of the patient that results in avoidable harm.[514] The administration of a clinic or an institution may also carry legal responsibility for breaches in care.[515] Delays in care may be brought about by staff failing to follow guidelines for appointments and procedures; [516] and by a failure to maintain equipment making it unavailable in a timely manner. Delays are also brought about by a failure to diagnose a patient's condition, but only carry legal responsibility when such failure can be demonstrated to have been due to an inadequate history and examination, or the lack of investigation or follow-up when warranted.[517]

In the report given, the primary care physician carries some responsibility for the lack of diagnostic measures undertaken at the first consultation, by not seeking an urgent appointment when there was no doubt about the diagnosis. There is also the culpability of the radiology department that fails to give an appointment for six months; this administrative indolence is mirrored in the appointments department. The surgery department should examine their system for dealing with urgent referrals for it could have contributed to the failure to get an urgent outpatient's appointment.

- *The responsibility of patients in referral systems*

It is in a patient's interest to be involved in the care they receive, and when referrals are being made should make sure they understand what is expected. Physicians must bear in mind that what is being said to patients is likely to be unfamiliar to them and may be confusing. It is therefore appropriate to reinforce instructions and ask the patient to report back if they have any difficulty. Some patients faced with serious illness go into denial and may not follow instructions or faced with a delay in service assume that the condition is not so serious.[518] Patients may be intimidated by the systems they face and accept appointments for much later than they were told was necessary.

---

[514] The Ethics of Delay: A Good or a Bad? M Berstein Bioethics.net
www.bioethics.net/2014/06/the-ethics-of-delay-a-good-or-a-bad/
[515] Medical Malpractice: When Can Patients Sue a Hospital for Negligence? C Boeschen; nolo.com
[516] Guideline for referral of patients with suspected colorectal cancer by family physicians and other primary care providers; M. E Del Giudice, Can Fam Physician. 2014; 60(8): 717–723.
[517] Rapid diagnostic pathways for suspected colorectal cancer: views of primary and secondary care clinicians on challenges and their potential solutions; M T Redaniel, M Ridd, R M Martin, F Coxon, M Jeffreys, J Wade; BMJ Open. 2015; 5(10): e008577.
[518] Denial: When it helps, when it hurts - Mayo Clinic; www.mayoclinic.org/healthy-lifestyle/adult-health/in-depth/denial/art-20047926

The patient also has a right to seek a second opinion when they are in doubt; physicians should make patients aware of that right and to facilitate them in doing so.[519]

In the report given, a referral was made for a CT scan and the patient told they would be called for an appointment. The call did not come for a further six months, and the patient or the physician made no enquiry two months later when an urgent referral was made. It is not clear how urgent the investigation or referral was instilled in the patient.

---

[519] Code of Conduct; Caribbean College of Surgeons; Other opinions sect 2.6; http://www. caribbeancollegeofsurgeons.com/documents/Caribbean-College-Of-Surgeons-Code-of-Conduct.pdf

CRIMINAL CASES

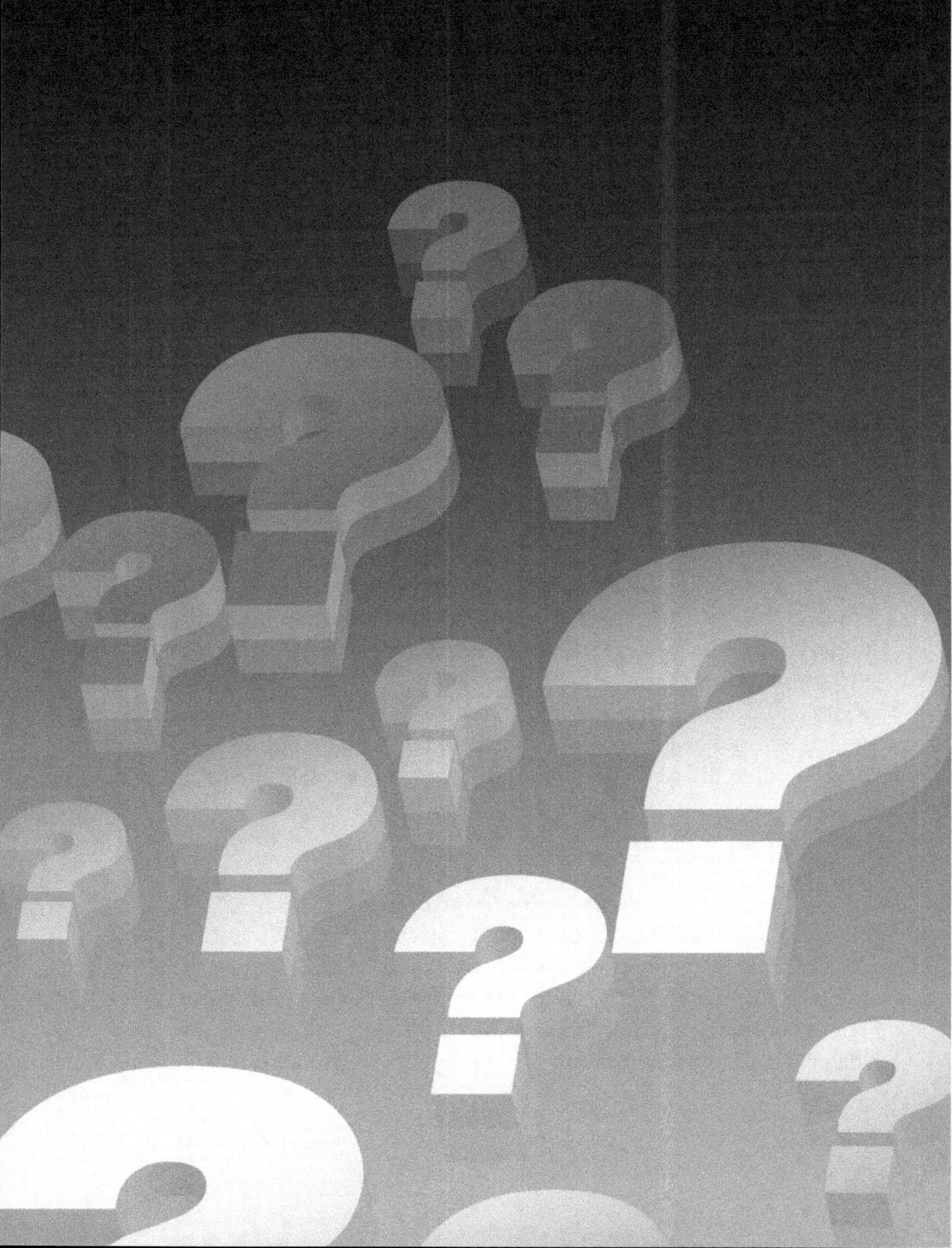

Case report:

A 20-year-old man was admitted with multiple gunshot wounds and treated for chest and limb injuries. He threatened to discharge himself after he saw one of his assailants visiting the ward. The chest drain was removed after two days and he discharged himself the following day. He returned to the ward that day with severe chest pain and a chest drain was reinserted. Two nights later shots were fired outside of the hospital and he told the staff that he had a visitor earlier that day who he felt had come to assess where in the ward he was located. The following morning he was transferred to a private room to reduce the security risk to staff, patients and visitors.

Four days after the transfer he became abusive and threatened the nursing staff; this 'pugnacious' behaviour continued for another two days when he was discharged, but continued when he returned to the ward for dressing reviews. His dressing reviews were changed to another ward and his behaviour improved. Two weeks later while waiting on the corridor outside the ward, he was shot at; in the ensuing pandemonium he seized a passing nurse, used her as a shield and ran away from the hospital. His assailant also escaped on foot.

He was brought back a few hours later with a gunshot wound to the abdomen and was scheduled for emergency laparotomy. The operation was delayed as staff requested armed escorts to accompany the patient at all points and that he be moved to the Defence Force medical facility for his post-operative course. After operation he was readmitted to a private room and access to the ward blocked. He was discharged in the care of the police who said that he had a conviction for drugs two years earlier, had been sent for drug rehabilitation, but absconded from the programme.

Issues raised

- ***A patient who seeks to discharge themself***

Discharging oneself from care is the legal right of any mentally competent patient unless they are being lawfully detained.[520] Factors that influence self-discharge usually relate to dissatisfaction with treatment and fear. There is usually a poor relationship with the health staff, but in some instances alternative treatment is being sought. Every effort should be

---

[520] The patient who threatens to self-discharge, J S Zaman; British Journal of Hospital Medicine 2006; 67(5): 230 - 1

made to persuade the patient to stay, but if they insist on leaving they
should be asked to sign a self-discharge form. A self-discharge form
should include specific statements that the reasons for advising staying
were explained to the patient and that they understood what had been
said to them.[521] If the patient is thought to be not mentally competent a
psychiatric opinion should be sought.

A patient who discharges themself from care and returns is entitled to
the same care and attention, no matter how annoying the circumstances
may have been to staff. Any thought of punishing the patient must
be avoided.

*In the report given the patient has been injured by gunfire and felt that
another attempt was going to be made on his life whilst in hospital. After
discharging himself he returns shortly after with worsening chest pain from his
injury and treatment is resumed. The patient expresses a fear that he is being
stalked and is moved to a less public ward. His relationship with the nursing staff
in the ward is poor, and he is discharged for dressing reviews in another ward.
His worse fears are realized whilst waiting outside the ward for review, when he
is shot at and uses a nurse as a shield to escape his assailant.*

- *The role of the police in injuries occasioned by interpersonal
violence*

Article 3 of the Universal Declaration of Human Rights states " Everyone
has the right to life, liberty and security of the person."[522] When a patient
expresses fear for their life and is credible, the police should be consulted
right away through the head of the institution. In addition, when
practitioners are aware from a patient's injuries that a felony has been
committed the staff have a duty to inform the police of the matter. If the
patient is in a position to understand they should be told that their injury
is being reported to the police. If the patient objects to the disclosure
it could be considered a breach of confidentiality and the practitioner
should seek legal advice before disclosure, or be prepared to justify
their decision if challenged.[523] Laws vary in jurisdictions on the duty
and what to report, and in some instances the failure to report is treated
as a misdemeanour.[524] Practitioners should provide the police with any
material/evidence they obtain in the course of treatment while ensuring

---

[521] Patient self-discharge from the emergency department: who is at risk? V L Henson, D S Vickery,
Emerg Med J 2005;22:499-501
[522] The Universal Declaration of Human Rights www.un.org/en/documents/udhr
[523] Confidentiality and the Duty to Report: A Case Study; R E. Watts; http://www.sagepub.com/
lippmanstudy/articles/Watts.pdf
[524] Misprision of felony, Sykes v. Director of Public Prosecutions [1962] A.C. 582 //OHIO REVISED
CODE

that the police or person to whom the material is handed is identified and that the item or its container is identifiable subsequently. Practitioners are often reluctant to get involved in cases that may go to the courts; however, not reporting a felony will not avoid this responsibility.

In the report given there is no account of the felony being reported to the police. Involvement of the police may or may not have averted the subsequent attempts on the patient's life whilst attending the hospital.

- *Secure facilities in a health care institution*

Secure facilities in an institution depend on the nature of the threat. Patients who may need to be secured from outside threats include public figures or those who have had attempts made on their lives. Prisoners need to be secured from being able to escape; and violent mentally ill patients may need to be secured to prevent them harming themselves or others. If a patient is to be moved to a secure facility there should be a plan known to the staff and be such that both the staff and the patient feel confident in the security of the facilities provided. Security in a health care institution must be effective without compromising the care of the patients. It is easier to secure a private room rather than an open ward; however, staff must have confidence in the security personnel as well.

In the report given shooting from outside of the hospital was meant to intimidate and needed demonstrable and credible security. The second attack did not materialise until he was in an unsecured part of the hospital.

- *The patient allegedly threatens a nurse*

Patients seldom threaten professional staff for they fear victimisation by other staff and possibly incorrect treatment; on occasion threats are issued to obtain treatment or priority in treatment.[525] A patient may be disturbed from mental illness including senility, fear, drugs [including those prescribed], toxicity from their illness, pain, alcohol intoxication or withdrawal, and their reaction to perceived wrongs. Well-trained professionals should be able to recognise when medical causes are operating and can usually discern what the perceived wrong is. Reactions associated with medical factors are not always clearly irrational and may be acting in combination with a perceived wrong.

Most patients in control of their emotions, even while in pain, are reluctant to challenge doctors or nurses face to face, for they have a perception that they are vulnerable to neglect or some wrongful action on

---

[525] Educating staff to manage threatening paranoid patients. Di Bella GA. Am J Psychiatry. 1979; 136(3): 333-5

the part of the individual or the group of professionals complained about. Patients, rather than confront doctors or nurses, complain to someone they trust and will often ask for the complaint not to be brought to the attention of the offending parties for fear of victimisation.

Staff related factors. Staff may be unsympathetic to a patient because of race, colour, class, religion, perceived or known criminality, how the illness or injury occurred, antisocial behaviour, such as urinating or defecating in the bed and excessive or trivial complaints. The staff member may be impaired by mental illness, drug or alcohol dependency, intoxication, tiredness, dissatisfaction with their conditions of service and this is being reflected in their treatment of the patient. Most of the professional factors operate at a subconscious level, however, for those who do not the patient has usually been made aware of the professional's attitude by both word and deed.[526]

Previous incidents. An untoward incident with a professional and a patient may have occurred, and may or may not have been recorded, but is usually known. The untoward incident may have occurred with a relative or a friend and the current incident appears to parallel what the patient may have heard before. Sometimes previous incidents are associated with a ward rather than with an individual professional and when that occurs the leadership on the ward has usually been involved in the incident itself or has failed to deal with the issue to the satisfaction of the patient or their relative, or has blamed the patient. Sometimes the incident may not be related to the individual patient but may have been widely publicised or discussed in the community. It is not known how previous incidents may determine patient or professional's behaviour and therefore untoward incidents need to be looked into in depth before coming to a conclusion, and to try and deal with any issues that may linger.

Societal factors. A society may become acculturated to making threats as a matter of course.[527] Examples can be found in the spheres of political, religious, media and other community leadership styles and actions. Threats often lead to counter threats particularly when the threats are seen to be ineffectual, misplaced or have been misunderstood as real threats. This opens for discussion a wide number of issues in the society including the criminalisation of substances widely used in the community and not considered as seriously harmful.

---

[526] Impact of the threatening patient on ward communications; Am J Psychiatry 1980; 137:616-619

[527] Aggressive behaviour in children and youth: When is it something to be concerned about? Centre for Addiction and Mental Health http://www.camh.net/About_Addiction_Mental_Health/Mental_Health_Information/agg_behav_childyouth.html

The situation described in the report case suggests that the patient had no trust that he would be kept safe by the staff in the hospital. His mental state and previous history had not been looked into and may have given insight into his behaviour. Perceived criminality would almost certainly have had a bearing on the attitude of staff to the patient, and this would have been made worse when he used a nurse as a shield in the attack in the hospital. The institution appears to go into a reactive mode, and no attention appears to have been given to the patient's mental state.

- *How should a patient's threat be handled?*

When a patient issues a threat an empathetic approach by the person or persons seen by the patient to be in charge of their care will usually resolve the problem. This approach gives a better opportunity to find out the basis for the behaviour, and seek to resolve it. Unfortunately, most professionals prejudge the situation when they disagree with the way in which the patient or relative has chosen to express themself and tend towards disciplinary solutions. Resolution of problems should not always have to involve a disciplinary action even though some professionals believe that to be told that their behaviour could have been different is in itself a disciplinary action.[528]

Hierarchical structures exist and should deal with situations such as threats, although such mechanisms should only be invoked after an empathetic personal approach has sought to resolve the problem. Within the institution there should be a complaints mechanism available to both patients and staff, which should deal with issues in a confidential manner. In some settings such a mechanism relies on one individual such as an ombudsman. The nature of the threat would determine whether it is necessary to bring into play the police.

The police are the societal agency responsible for dealing with persons who threaten each other. The head of the institution should only bring in the police after consultation with the persons responsible for the care of the patient. In most instances the institution would be unwise to seek to get rid of the patient, for anything that goes wrong with their care after that could be the subject of legal action.

In the report given the fact that the patient's alleged previous threat was used to seek to justify not caring for the patient suggests that the approaches of conflict resolution were not used to deal with the alleged threat when it occurred.

---

[528] A Measure of Styles of Handling Interpersonal Conflict; M. Afzalur Rahim The Academy of Management Journal 1983, Vol. 26, No. 2 pp. 368-376

- *A patient is threatened*

A staff member, another patient or another person may threaten a patient.[529] Staff must be cognisant of the vulnerability of the patient and must take into account that what the patient is experiencing may be the most disturbing and possibly frightening experience in their life and therefore they may not behave in a normal manner. Furthermore, a threat from a patient may be related to alcohol, drugs or mental illness. Any threat from a staff member to a patient must be taken seriously and dealt with promptly through an institutional complaints mechanism.

A threat from another patient should be dealt with initially by those persons in charge of the patient issuing the threats. A threat from another person unrelated to the institution should be dealt with by the security mechanisms of the institution and the community depending on the nature of the threat.

The nature of the threat. Threats may be verbal or physical including those that are life-threatening. When threats are obviously dangerous, the police should deal them with whether they are issued by a staff member, another patient or any other person.

Security in public institutions must be appropriate to the role of the institution whilst allowing the public to use the institution for its unique purpose.[530] The regulation of staff, patients, visitors and visiting to patients must all be thought out so that staff and patients are secure and feel secure but there is no interference with patient care and the ability of the staff to function effectively. To do so security staff should be trained related to the unique nature of the institution, to know the pivotal roles and the persons who play them and to know when to use their discretion.

Should staff provide their own security is a debated point in some places, where threats and personal firearms are common.[531] Staff must press an institution to provide them with adequate security. Carrying personal firearms to work is unlikely to be effective protection in the kinds of roles / tasks that professionals perform and may even set the professional up as a target by a determined criminal.[532]

Transferring a patient because of a threat to them should never be done to the detriment of the patient. Patient transferral may be construed as a victory for the person issuing the threat, particularly if a staff member or another patient did the threat.

---

[529] Conflict in the health care workplace; M A. E. Ramsay, Proc (Bayl Univ Med Cent). 2001; 14(2): 138–139.
[530] Designing Hospital Security 2001, S Slahor, http://securitysolutions.com/mag/security_designing_hospital_security/
[531] Should Doctors Have Guns? http://brainblogger.com/2008/05/09/should-doctors-have-guns/
[532] Murder in the Hospital: A Lesson from an Actual Security Event P. Carter http://www.saione.com/articles/Murder_in_the_Hospital.pdf

In the report given the patient appears to under a continuing threat from persons outside of the institution and an earlier involvement of the police appears to have been warranted.

- ***The role of army and prison hospitals as 'secure' institutions.***
The role of an army hospital in peacetime is probably to give army personnel continuing practice in the care of the ill so as to be able to provide battlefield care and security for army personnel. A prison hospital is there to provide security for inmates during the treatment of an illness. Although both institutions are supposed to supply security it is for a specific class of persons and would set a poor precedent to admit persons except they had a unique treatment capability.

In the instance described a bad precedent would be set in transferring the patient to an army facility as was suggested by staff. This is particularly so since the facilities available at the institution were thought to be inadequate to treat the injury at hand.

- ***Does fear justify a normally inappropriate action?***
More often than not fear as a motivator of action leads to panicky and wrong decisions. [533] In patient care fear and panic is likely to lead to unprofessional decisions frequently with the abandonment of the patient. Staff have an obligation to protect themselves as well as the patient in life-threatening situations. When it is thought necessary to evacuate the institution both the patients and staff must be evacuated along with any life support measures for those in need of them. The Geneva Code states, "I will maintain the utmost respect for human life even under threat."[534]

There is no doubt that the staff had good reason to be afraid for the shooting occurred in the corridors of the hospital. In dramatic situations like the one reported an immediate police or security presence is necessary and reassuring, but actions that interfere with the patient's care were unwarranted, including an early discharge of the patient 'in the care of the police.'

---

[533] Decision-making under stress: Scanning of alternatives under physical threat; G Keinan, N Friedland, Y Ben-Porath, Acta Psychologica, 1987, Volume 64, Issue 3, Pages 219–228
[534] WMA International Code of Medical Ethics 57th WMA General Assembly, 2006 http://www.wma.net/en/30publications/10policies/c8/

Treating a Prisoner

Case report:
Mr B was remanded to prison by the magistrate to face a charge of
stealing items from a supermarket. The next day prison officers bring
him to the emergency department with multiple abrasions on his face
and trunk. When he is asked what caused the injuries, the patient looks
nervously at the prison officers and says he fell down the stairs at the
prison. The officers intervene and says that they were told by the last
shift that the other prisoners in the cell had attacked him. When being
examined in the examination room, with the prison officers outside, the
prisoner says that he was beaten by the police before he was taken to
court, and when he was remanded they put him in a cell with three other
men and said 'He is all yours'.

Dr Goodbar, who is seeing a prisoner for the first time, had been upset
when she heard her colleagues talking about cases of beatings and rape
among the prisoners they had seen. During her examination she tells the
patient that she wants to do a rectal examination and he refuses to have
it done, saying that he does not want anything more than his bruises
treated. Dr Goodbar wishes to be thorough, as she knows she will be
called upon to write a report, and she is not certain that the prisoner or
the guards have told her the truth. When she insists that she needs to do
a thorough examination, the prisoner says 'Only if you admit me to the
hospital'. Dr Goodbar rings the surgical service on call and asks them to
see the patient for an intra-abdominal injury.

Issues raised

- ***The duty of a health professional in suspected abuse***
A practitioner must seek the information necessary to make an accurate
diagnosis and enable the treatment of the patient, both physically and
mentally. When the information leads the practitioner to the conclusion
that the patient has been abused, whether they are police, teachers,
priests, parents or colleagues, they have a duty to collect the evidence to
support their conclusions and to present their findings to an appropriate
authority in a confidential manner.[535]

---

[535] Principles of Medical Ethics relevant to the Role of Health Personnel, particularly Physicians, in
the Protection of Prisoners and Detainees against Torture and Other Cruel, Inhuman or Degrading
Treatment or Punishment; The Office of the United Nations High Commissioner for Human Rights;
Adopted by General Assembly resolution 37/194, 1982; http://www2.ohchr.org/english/law/
medicalethics.htm

A confidential report on abuse should take into account the need to protect the victim from further harm. The practitioner should be aware that both abusers and their victims may not speak the truth as self-protective mechanisms and that the careful collection, documentation and interpretation of physical evidence are the best way to present and defend their findings. Practitioners should be wary of allowing their relationship with persons in authority, or with colleagues, to interfere with or influence their professional conduct and standards.

In the case described the practitioner recognises that the narratives of the parties involved are irreconcilable, and determines to do a thorough physical examination. The patient resists a sensitive examination and bargains to get out of prison, if not out of custody; the practitioner responds by shifting responsibility for the patient to another plausible service.

• **Should a practitioner accede to a patient's view on treatment?**
A patient's wishes should always be taken into account when they are being examined or treated. However, a practitioner should not accede to wishes which they consider unreasonable; that would compromise their professional integrity; or would put the patient or others at risk. Patients are entitled to consent to any examination or treatment and it is the practitioner's duty to give enough information and explanation to allow the patient to consent to what is being suggested. Intimate examinations are particularly sensitive because of embarrassment, discomfort, and the sense of being sexually violated.

In the case described the practitioner may have a number of reasons for doing a rectal examination but has not explained why she wants to do so. The patient may have his reasons for not wanting this examination done and bargains with the doctor who responds by shifting responsibility and refers before completing the assessment.

• **What does one do if abuse is detected in police custody?**
Since the Nuremberg Trials at the end of the 2nd World War in 1945 and the Declaration of Tokyo 1975 [revised in 2006], it is a tenet of medical ethics that medical practitioners should not take part in the abuse or torture of prisoners.[536], [537] This principle applies to all acts of abuse by the police, the military, in education and religious institutions, and within

---

[536] "The Nazi Doctors and Nuremberg: Some Moral Lessons Revisited". Pellegrino, E. 1997. American College of Physicians 127 (4): 307–308.

[537] Declaration of Tokyo; Guidelines for Medical Doctors concerning Torture and Other Cruel, Inhuman or Degrading Treatment or Punishment in relation to Detention and Imprisonment; http://www.wma.net/en/60about/70history/02declarationTokyo/

health care. If accusations or suspicions of abuse or torture prove to be well founded, the perpetrators and their colleagues or institutions will not easily accept the stain on their character. Both the persons responsible and their institutions may seek to suppress the accusations by doing further damage to the victims as well as to the person who brings the problem to light. It is therefore prudent before any accusation or action is taken to gather all the evidence available, such as obtaining photographs of injuries, and keep copies of notes and investigations made at the time. It is also best to know what is the best route to follow in a particular case, and if not, to enquire of one's seniors, representative organisation or any institutional mechanisms that exists.

There will be occasions when an incident of abuse is being pursued by the press, and the confidentiality of patients should not be broken without their consent. Further specific information on patients should be given to the press by an institution's public relations office. The law requires that the identity of children should not be publicised in abuse situations.

In the case reported, the instinct of the practitioner to get the patient admitted rather than be returned to an abusive or dangerous situation is an admirable one, but may fail if sufficient evidence has not been garnered to warrant admission.

- ***Should a hospital be used as a sanctuary?***

Hospitals are used as a place of safety for children who are abused during the acute phase of any physical or emotional injury. As soon as they are well a determination should be made through the child protection services for their further safety.[538]

Hospitals are also used as a place of safety for the mentally ill to protect them and others. Mental health or similar acts prescribe how patients are to be admitted involuntarily, and how they can be treated.[539] Courts may also remand people to be incarcerated and treated in mental health institutions. Prisoners should only be in hospitals for their illness and during such illness should be guarded but not physically restrained without the consent of the medical staff.

Apart from mental health institutions there are specialty hospitals which have acted as sanctuaries. Usually these patients have illnesses or disabilities that carry a severe stigma, and have included leprosy and tuberculosis establishments, and more recently HIV specialist facilities. The use of acute care hospitals as sanctuaries for the elderly is often

---

[538] L.R.O. 1991 Protection of Children CAP. 146A; Laws of Barbados
[539] A comparison of mental health legislation from diverse Commonwealth jurisdictions; E.C. Fistein, A.J. Holland, I.C.H. Clare, and M.J. Gunn; Int J Law Psychiatry. 2009; 32(3): 147–155

resented by the staff of those institutions and may lead to the neglect of those patients.

In the report given the patient clearly feels that the hospital could be a place of sanctuary and the practitioner appears sympathetic to this and shifts responsibility to others.

- ### *How should the sensitive situations be resolved?*

When conflicting stories become apparent in health care settings the attending practitioner should ensure privacy for the patient, assure them of confidentiality and get their story in detail. In abusive situations, the patient should be assured that their records will remain private until either the patient or the court asks for them.

A detailed history is essential if a forensic examination and recording for evidence purposes is to occur. Photographs should be taken of injuries, copies or photographs of X-rays be taken and forensic tests done for rape, alcohol or drug ingestion. It is prudent for a practitioner to make copies of the original notes and investigations for their own use. Sensitive notes have an uncanny way of disappearing, and this can leave the practitioner looking as if they are trying to hide something. If after all diagnostic and treatment measures are initiated or carried out, and it is clear that abuse or torture has occurred, attention should then be given as to how and when the abuse or torture should be reported to the appropriate authority.

Referrals to another service should be done with all of the information obtained and should avoid the appearance of passing the buck. Competitive buck passing leaves all those involved looking incompetent, in addition to harming the patient. In cases involving children the diagnostic process should involve social services personnel, and reporting done to the Child Care authorities. In other cases within an institution it is important to deal with the matter through institutional mechanisms and confidential correspondence. Practitioners who are not working within an institutional mechanism should seek legal advice, particularly that available through representative organisations.

Some practitioners may feel that institutional mechanisms are too slow or tend to hide issues and wish to express their conscience on the issue in public. When and how this is done should be carefully considered.

In the instance reported, difficulties related to possible abuse are emerging with an inexperienced practitioner demonstrating a lack of clarity about how to proceed.

Case report:
A 17-year-old presented stating that a piece of crack cocaine was stuck in his left ear. He had attempted to remove the object multiple times over a four-month period before seeking medical attention. When seen, he appeared agitated and was speaking in a child-like manner, and a decision was made to remove the object under general anaesthesia. The surgeon consulted the hospital lawyers who informed the narcotics division of the police. A police officer appeared and was allowed to be present in the operating theatre, where he purported to inspect the instruments to be used in the procedure. The removal of the foreign body was accomplished without difficulty and was handed to the policeman present without any further identification of the object. When the patient recovered the police took him away. He eventually appeared in court where he was fined a substantial sum.

Issues raised

- ***Duty of confidentiality and reporting a suspected crime***
The duty of confidentiality is an ethical, professional and legal obligation between the doctor and a patient.[540] This obligation should only be broken with the clear consent of the patient, to other professionals involved in the patient's treatment or to lawful authorities. Breaking the confidentiality of a patient to any other third party can only be justified if the patient by their action, or intended action, constitutes a clear mortal danger to that third party.[541]
In breaking a patient's confidentiality to other health professionals, the primary physician must ensure that in sensitive matters, the other professionals understand their own duty to preserve the confidentiality of the patient. In breaking confidentiality to lawful authorities, such as reportable contagious disease or criminal matters, the physician should make it clear to the patient what the physician's lawful duty is. In such situations the physician should, as far as they can, describe what the medical consequences of such decisions will be.[542] For example, in cases of contagious disease the patient may have to be isolated in a facility whilst

---

[540] WMA International Code of Medical Ethics; http://www.wma.net/en/30publications/10policies/c8/
[541] Tarasoff v. Regents of the University of California, 17 Cal. 3d 425, 551 P.2d 334, 131 Cal. Rptr. 14 (Cal. 1976)
[542] GMC Confidentiality; http://www.gmc-uk.org/guidance/ethical_guidance/confidentiality.asp

being treated, or be quarantined for a defined period. All such decisions should be based on scientific evidence.[543]

In situations of suspected crimes such as gunshot wounds and knife injuries, the patient should be made aware that it is the intention of the attending physician to make such a report, and why. Should the patient not consent to such disclosure, then a report should only be made when there is a clear and present danger to the patient themself or to others. In other situations where evidence or medical reports are being sought by the police or the court, the patient should be made aware that their confidentiality is being broken under force of law. They should also be told that only relevant facts to the police enquiry or the court order will be revealed, and that all other confidential matters related to them will remain confidential.

In the case reported the patient's confidentiality has been broken on the grounds that there is a statute in the country, compelling a report to the police of the possession of illegal drugs. However, at the time of the report being made the only evidence of such crime was the patient's description of the foreign body, without any confirmation that he was in possession of an illegal substance or of the requisite illegal quantity. The report led to the virtual arrest of the patient whilst undergoing treatment.

- ***Reporting to authorities without consent***

Reporting of births, deaths and contagious diseases is statutory requirements. The reporting must be accurate and uninfluenced by any patient's or their relatives' wishes for confidentiality. When a patient does not consent to reporting of their condition to authorities, the physician has a duty to explain the steps that the doctor is lawfully obliged to follow, and the consequences to the patient.[544]

In reporting of suspected felonies there are jurisdictions that have statutes that require reporting without the patient's consent. In many countries. physicians are required to report child abuse and neglect, and in others, the reporting requirements may be more extensive for matters such as domestic violence or illegal drug possession. In every case physicians should know the local laws and consult their medical professional advisors where appropriate.[545] Whatever the law, a physician should not put a patient's life at risk by arranging for the arrest/detention

---

[543] The Ethical Quagmire of Quarantine; https://www.scu.edu/ethics/focus-areas/bioethics/resources/the-ethical-quagmire-of-quarantine/

[544] When Patient-Physician Confidentiality Conflicts with the Law; K E. Schleiter, AMA Virtual Mentor. 2009, Vol 11, No 2: 146-148.

[545] Mandatory and Permissive Reporting; http://www.cpso.on.ca/policies-publications/policy/mandatory-and-permissive-reporting

of a patient before life-saving treatment is carried out, and the physician is satisfied that the arrest/detention of the patient will not endanger their life or worsen their condition. These conditions are equally applicable to patients who have already been detained by the authorities.

In the report given, the patient or his guardian has not been told what is being reported, and found that having sought medical attention he is arrested at the instigation of the practitioner, and before the alleged crime can be confirmed.

- ***Treatment of suspects of criminal actions***

Physicians are not ordinary citizens in the communities they serve, for they have special legal and ethical obligations to their patients; obligations that the ordinary citizen does not have to another. In particular they are obliged to respect the autonomy of the patient, particularly in respect of their confidentiality and to consent to the treatment that the physician will perform on them.[546] The ethical principle of Do No Harm, applies to all aspects of patient care whether it be physical or emotional; this applies equally to the principle of Beneficence. As regards the principle of justice, this means the equal treatment for all regardless of the social standing, criminal status, race, ethnicity, sexual orientation, religion or political affiliation.[547]

The physician who suspects that a patient's condition or an incidental finding may be the result of criminal action on the patient's part or that of another person, must consider the ethical principles of their profession, rather than those of the ordinary citizen. Findings that suggest a criminal action has occurred may either be that the patient is the victim of such action, or that it has occurred during the patient's commission of a criminal act; the physician's duty to the patient remains the same whatever has been the circumstance. Physicians might expect to come across criminal actions by patients in relation to injuries, poisoning, adverse affects of illegal drugs or controlled substances. In some countries there are some sexual acts or practices that are in criminal statutes, and physicians in the course of going into the history of some illness may ask about the practice of acts such as sodomy. In every situation the patient's interests must come first, with a careful recording of the facts, the gathering of suspicious evidence during the course of treatment and the preservation of such evidence should it be required by the police or the court.

---

[546] Some limits of informed consent; O O'Neill - Journal of Medical Ethics; 2003; jme.bmj.com Vol 29, No 1

[547] Justice - The four common bioethical principles - Definitions and ... www.alzheimer-europe.org/Ethics/Definitions...bioethical.../Justice 2010

The patient must be treated confidentially whether they are brought for attention by authorities as a convicted criminal, a person under investigation, or is a person who the physician suspects has been involved in criminal activity. The police, or other security personnel have no right to be present at the confidential communication and examination of any patient. Any presence of the police or security personnel must only be at the invitation of the physician where the patient is threatening the health personnel and cannot be controlled otherwise.

As regards the violent patient, the physician should always keep in mind that violent or threatening behaviour may be the result of the patient's medical condition, and that securing the patient is only a means towards dealing effectively with the patient's condition and not to 'imprison' them. Police or security personnel have no place in the treatment room, although they may be permitted to be on the outside of such rooms in case there is an attempt by the patient/criminal to escape lawful custody.

Except under specific statutes, a physician has no duty to report a suspected crime, except with the consent of the patient. However, there are circumstances where the community may feel that the physician should act otherwise. Indeed, many physicians feel that they are obliged to remove bullets for the purpose of ballistic evidence for the police. A bullet should only be removed when it is in the best interest of the patient to do so, and when the procedure will not cause further harm to the patient. Once the bullet is removed it should be placed in a container, labelled, signed and dated by the operating surgeon and sealed. It can then be handed to the police if the patient is already in their custody. If the patient agrees that they should report the matter to the police, the police can then be informed that the evidence is available to be collected. It is imprudent to give possible evidence to the patient or to other persons to hand to the police.

In cases of poisoning or intoxication, the physician has the responsibility for identifying the offending substance with or without the help of a forensics laboratory. Possession of illegal drugs usually comes to the attention of the physician, when the effects of an overdose become apparent.

Child abuse and domestic violence pose special problems in reporting. The physician and an appropriate team should collect all evidence, particularly photographic and x-ray evidence and preserve them. In domestic violence situations the patient/victim may be reluctant to admit that such violence has occurred. Most child abuse is done at home and the responsible adult, who may be the parent or guardian, will not consent to self-incrimination. Fortunately, in most countries there are specific statutes in place to protect children and they can be placed in care and protection, without the parents or guardians being able to block the reporting of the suspected abuse. Some jurisdictions have passed specific statutes to try and compel reporting of child abuse, [548] domestic violence and the possession of illegal drugs, irrespective of the wishes of the patient. These statutes do not work well without specific provisions for the protection of the patient and the physician, from irate accused persons.

If the physician is unclear about the course of action they should take, they should seek ethical and legal advice, preferably from their medical indemnity source, their regulatory body or from a formal ethics resource. In an institutional setting there should be a protocol set out for these circumstances. Such protocols should be formally drawn up with legal, ethical and professional input and be formally agreed, adopted and distributed. If no such protocol exists in an institution, the physician should be wary of off-the-cuff legal advice, particularly where such persons are not the responsible persons for the defence of the physician in matters of professional misconduct.

In the case reported, the patient's confidentiality has been broken on the basis of mandatory reporting of the crime of possessing an illegal substance. The patient has been arrested before treatment is carried out and the 'illegal' substance identified.

---

[548] Mandatory Reporters of Child Abuse and Neglect; https://www.childwelfare.gov/topics/systemwide/laws-policies/statutes/manda/

CULTURE AND RELIGION

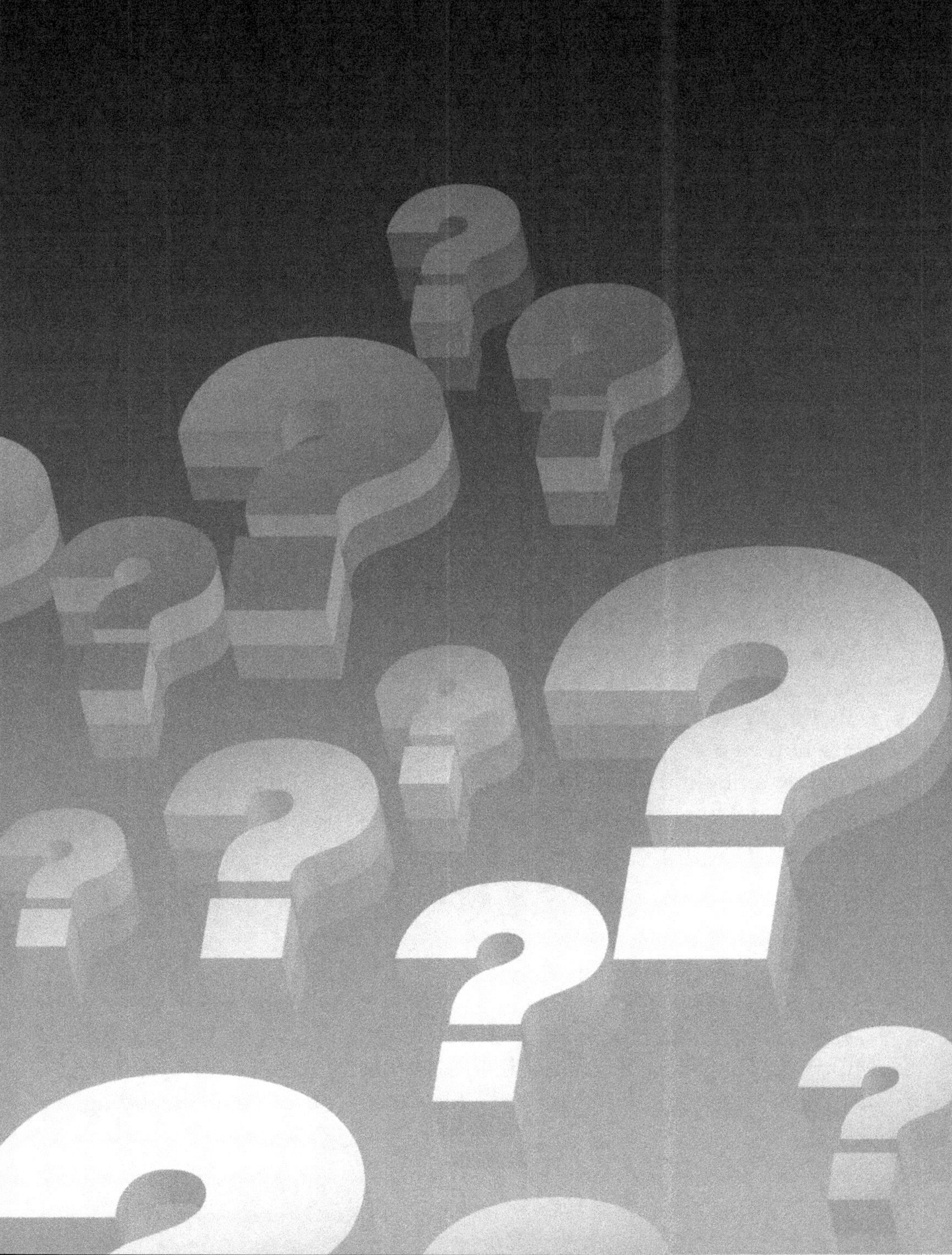

Case report:

A three-month-old infant with Down syndrome and a complete atrio-ventricular canal defect, presented with a three-day history of laboured breathing and darkening around the lips. The child's parents were Jehovah's Witnesses and were aware of the need for an open cardiac operation. They decided to seek to have the operation without blood transfusion and were advised that it was not the current practice anywhere.

On admission, the child was treated for cardiac failure in the Intensive Care Unit and improved but relapsed after three days and was readmitted to the ICU and placed on a ventilator and pressor support. When the haemoglobin fell to 7.7g/dl the decision was made that a red blood cell transfusion should be given and the parents made their objection to transfusion clear. The child remained unstable and the paediatrician decided to seek a court order to override the parent's refusal. A report was written for the hospital attorney's use before the court, and after three days the doctors were informed that the court order had been made. There ensued a contention between the paediatrician and the attorney as to who was to inform the parents of the court's decision. The attorney spoke to the parents about the court's decision.

The transfusion was given three days after the court decision to do so, but the infant remained critically ill and died two days later. On the day of the infant's death, a meeting was held with the parents, who expressed their anger over the transfusion and stated that they did not appreciate how they were made to feel by the attorney, as though by refusing their consent they did not care about their child's well-being. They also stated that they thought their child had become more ill, and were under the impression that once she had received the blood transfusion, she would be able to be removed from the ventilator.

Issues raised

- *Religious freedom, its limits*

In most countries religious freedom is guaranteed in the country's constitution and is contained in Article 18 of the Universal Declaration of Human Rights. However, an individual's freedom can be constrained by law, particularly when its exercise affects the rights of others including those of children.[549] The common religious practices that impinge on medical practice are, the rejection of blood transfusion by Jehovah's Witnesses; prohibition of contraceptive use by Catholics; a variety of denominations objecting to termination of pregnancies; ritual male circumcision in Jewish and Muslim communities;[550] female circumcision, otherwise called genital mutilation, in some cultural/religious groups;[551] and the performance of post-mortems.[552]

When these issues arise in medical practice. the individual doctor has a duty to present to the patient/surrogate normal medical practice and customary conduct. They also have a duty to listen to the patient's wishes and where possible to accommodate those wishes within the standards of safety of the procedure, but not at a high risk of loss of life or an incapacitating complication. Where there is a high risk of loss of life, and the procedure advised could substantially reduce that risk, then recourse to the courts should be contemplated particularly when these decisions are being made for a minor or an incapacitated patient.

Courts when faced with life and death issues, will most likely listen to sound professional opinion that speaks to a meaningful life or cure from disease.[553] Except in emergency determinations, courts should give a hearing to the contending parties, and a number of landmark decisions have been made in favour of patients and their surrogates at such hearings.[554]

In the report given, the religious belief of parents impacted on the treatment of a gravely ill infant, and recourse to the law to remove the parents' right of consent was invoked. However, the treatment proved futile and resulted in further alienation of the parents.

- *Treatment without consent, why, where and when*

Treatment without consent must be undertaken in life-threatening emergencies; as a result of an order of the court in urgent but life-threatening situations; and for 'mature' minors, in their best interests. In all of these situations, treatment is undertaken when a practitioner determines that it is in the best interest of the patient to do so.[555] Life-

---

[549] Religious Objections to Medical Care; American Academy of Pediatrics; Pediatrics, 1997.Vol 99, 2: Pgs 279-281

[550] History of Circumcision; www.d.umn.edu/~mcco0322/history.htm; University of Minnesota, 2004

[551] Religion or Culture? Stop FGM Middle East; www.stopfgmmideast.org/background/islam-or-culture

[552] Religious and Cultural Considerations for Autopsy; www.ohsu.edu/.../Religious-and-Cul... Oregon Health & Science University; Burton EC, Gurevitz, Stacy A. Religions and Autopsy. 2010.

[553] Law and Medicine: Pediatric Faith Healing; K Abbott; Virtual Mentor. 2009, Vol 11, 10: 778-782.

[554] Twenty-five years after Quinlan: Cantor NL. J Law Med Ethics. 2001; 29(2): 182-96.

[555] Exceptions to Informed Consent in Emergency Medicine; K M. Hartman, Bn A. Liang, Hospital Physician March 1999; http: //www.turner-white.com/pdf/hp_mar99_emergmed.pdf

threatening emergencies, such as a cardiac arrest or severe external bleeding, can be diagnosed by a variety of health professionals and acted upon, particularly by those with training to do so acting within their competencies.

Life-threatening situations that are urgent, rather than immediate, should have the consent of the competent patient, parent, or guardian. In situations where the patient is not competent, consent should be asked of the next of kin, although this right has been removed in one jurisdiction.[556]

In situations where consent is not given, there may be a variety of reasons including religious doctrine, or strongly held beliefs that are not in accordance with prevailing standards of medical treatment. Where all reasoning fails and the practitioner can make a strong case that it is in the best interest of the patient to be treated, the matter can be presented to the court. Courts normally favour professional opinion over lay opinion, and providing the court can be convinced that the proposed treatment is in the patient's best interest. Quality of life determinations is less applicable in urgent situations, but can be an important factor in court determinations of ordering treatment without consent. When minors are involved, the courts may order the removal of parental authority for the duration of treatment only. The best interest standard is the determining issue when treatment without consent is applied to mature minors, and is applied under judicial precedent referred to as the Gillick principle.[557]

In the case described, the court was asked to override the parental refusal to give a blood transfusion on the basis of their religious belief. In spite of the transfusion being administered death occurred shortly thereafter, this left the parents further aggrieved.

- ***Best interests standard***

The best interest of a patient is not easy to determine in a patient who requires difficult or hazardous treatment. The interests of the patient must be the prime consideration and be divorced from the interests of others whether they be parents, doctors or priests. Best interest is often equated with the expected quality of life and should not be confused with the prolongation of life. An objective determination of the expected quality of life is not easily made in urgent situations, particularly when cure of disease is not possible. These determinations are more difficult in children, for the quality of life will depend on family and community

---

[556] Mental Capacity Act 2005 (c. 9) - Legislation.gov.ukwww.legislation.gov.uk/ukpga/2005/9/contents
[557] Gillick v West Norfolk & Wisbech Area Health Authority [1986] AC 112

support factors that may change. As has been said, "The family of a severely limited young infant may evaluate their QL very differently to the population who have never been in that situation".[558]

In making such decisions views may be clouded by previous experience, religious and cultural views, as well as hearing about treatments from sources that are out of context to the situation. When there are unresolved viewpoints it is best to have an independent advisory panel that can hear the points of view and try to seek a resolution between the parties.[559] When such mechanisms fail and the practitioners still feel that it is in the best interest of the patient to be treated, the patient, parent or surrogate may be taken to court for a determination.

In the situation described, both the short-term and corrective long-term treatment would require blood transfusion to be administered. There was no independent mechanism in place, or deployed, to convince the parents to agree to a blood transfusion, and in spite of the short-term measure of the blood transfusion, and the lack of a long-term plan the practitioners decided to put the matter before the court.

- *Taking parents/patients to court*

Taking patients to court over their refusal of treatment is most likely done in psychiatric illness, and most jurisdictions have mental health laws to allow for the involuntary treatment of the mentally ill who may be a danger to themselves or others.[560] Getting a court to overturn refusal of medical treatment on religious grounds is uncommon in a mentally competent patient.[561] Not so rare is when parents refuse treatment for their children on the basis of the parents' religious beliefs.[562]

When a patient or a parent is taken to court over refusal of treatment, it is best done by an institution. Emergency access to the courts is best done when it is a choice between life and death. Choosing between death and cure of disease, or the suffering of a child, is best done in proceedings where argument can be heard from all sides.[563]

---

[558] The quality of life of young children and infants with chronic medical problems: review of the literature. Payot A1, Barrington KJ. Curr Probl Pediatr Adolesc Health Care. 2011; 41(4): 91-101
[559] Ethics Committees and Ethics Consultation: https://depts.washington.edu/bioethx/.../ethics.h..2013
[560] A comparison of mental health legislation from diverse Commonwealth jurisdictions; E.C. Fistein, A.J. Holland, I.C.H. Clare, and M.J. Gunnb; Int J Law Psychiatry. 2009; 32(3): 147–155.
[561] Adult: Refusal of Medical Treatment; [2002] 2 All E R 449; Comm by M Stauch; J Med Ethics 2002; 28:232-233
[562] Faith-Based Decisions: Parents Who Refuse Appropriate Care for Their Children; Commentary by R Orr, W E. Novotny, and R M. Perkin, Virtual Mentor. AMA J. Ethics 2003, Vol 5, 8 http://virtualmentor ama-assn.org/2003/08/ccas1-0308.html
[563] Overriding Parental Decision to Withhold Treatment, Michael Woods http://virtualmentor.ama-assn.org/2003/08/hlaw1-0308.html

In the report given, the court proceeding was done as an emergency proceeding. and the parents were not given an opportunity to put their case. Nevertheless, the transfusion was not administered for a number of days after the court decision because of a dispute as to who was responsible for informing the parents of the court's decision.

- ### *Legal hazards of parental disapproval*

The legal hazards of parental disapproval of a doctor's decision vary from a charge of battery for treating without consent, to that of criminal negligence where the child dies as a result of the treatment. A suit of negligence may be brought, particularly if the risks of a disputed treatment are not all explained, and even a remote risk is realized with damaging consequences.[564] Parents may also file suit alleging abuse of the child or defamation by any remarks made about their care of the child.

In the report the parents felt that the attorney defamed them before the court.

---

[564] The duty to warn patients about risk. Chester v Afshar [2004] UKHL 41; [2005] 1 A.C. 134; [2004] 3 W.L.R. 927; [2004] 4 All E.R. 587

Case report:

A 50-year-old woman was referred to the surgical service with a lump in the right breast. A needle biopsy was done and she was counselled about the likely diagnosis of cancer. The biopsy confirmed the diagnosis, and she was counselled about her therapeutic options; she chose to have the breast removed. She kept her appointment for surgery, but in the operating theatre informed the surgical team that the lump was not there any more. She was re-examined and asked to feel the lump herself and agreed that it was present. However, she said that there were no more cancer cells in the lump, for the prayers said for her had healed her and she requested a re-biopsy. The surgical team counselled her that the diagnosis was not in doubt, but she remained adamant and was given an appointment to return to clinic for further discussion. The appointment was not kept, but she returned about a month later and said that her previous doubts had been resolved and she wanted to have the surgery done.

Issues raised

- *Alternative/ complementary medicine*

There are many forms of traditional, alternative or complementary medical practices that exist alongside the worldwide practice of 'western' medicine. Many of the practices predate 'modern' western medicine, and claim the capability of holistic healing which are superior to that of western medicine. The hallmark of the success of western medicine has been the application of reproducible medications and technologies, with the results of treatment subjected to statistical analysis. Nevertheless, objective outcomes in medicine are only part of the patient experience, and subjective symptoms such as pain or feeling well are much more difficult to measure objectively. It is in this important area of the subjective that alternative and complementary medical practices claim their place, alongside, or even as being superior to western scientific medicine.

However, there are some forms of alternative medicine; e.g. meditation which can be shown to alter physiological parameters such as blood pressure and heart rate, which can be measured and therefore compared to western medicine. Unfortunately, there are no known studies that show a positive statistical effect of alternative practices on proven tumours.[565]

---

[565] Prayer and healing: A medical and scientific perspective on randomized controlled trials; C Andrade Indian J Psychiatry. 2009 Oct-Dec; 51(4): 247–253.

In the case reported there is no information elicited about the healing practice other than prayers were said. The surgeons were not prepared to humour the patient by doing another biopsy to show the tumour was no longer present, and made no enquiry as to what changed her mind when she returned for surgery.

• *Prayer – alternative or complementary medicine?*

Prayer is common to all religions and cultures and takes a variety of forms. When applied to medical problems, the claims for the efficacy of prayer are seldom made in isolation from other forms of therapy. Nevertheless, whenever an improvement occurs and prayers have been offered there are those who will claim that prayer has been the indispensable part of the improvement. The effect of prayer as an independent variable with other treatments, has not been verified or debunked in clinical trials.

When claims are made for the efficacy of prayers alone, they may be made for prayers in absentia or by a presence with or without some form of contact, including sexual contact.[566] There are some highly dramatized shows of healing by prayer that are widely publicised, however, objective study of such instances is not available.[567] In many cases prayers are offered for both the patient and the treating practitioners.

• *Ethical and legal issues*

In most countries the healing professions are regulated by law, and are required to go through a recognized training programme, obtain qualification and be registered to practise. Many practitioners of alternative medicine are not so recognised, but are enabled to pursue their practices legally on the basis that the law allows the practice of home remedies. Religious practice, except specifically banned in law, frequently involves itself in complementary or alternative medicine practices through prayer and other practices, without any training or registration to do so.[568]

There are many in the healing professions who are deeply religious and may profess to be only in their healing profession in fulfilment of their religious beliefs. While this is generally laudable, it would be unethical, and may in some circumstances be unlawful, for such practitioners to impose their religious beliefs on their patients.[569] Such an

---

[566] The Healing Powers of Sex | Psychology Todayhttps://www.psychologytoday.com/blog/.../the-healing-powers-sex
[567] Faith Healing. American Cancer Society. 2013-01-17.
[568] Obeah scholar.library.miami.edu/slaves/.../religion.html; University of Miami
[569] Religion and medical ethics. Green RM. Handb Clin Neurol. 2013; 118:79-89.

imposition can be considered a breach of the autonomy of a patient, and imperils the legal principle of informed consent.

As regards the right of the patient to their religious beliefs, this may be constrained in law when the practice is illegal, unhygienic, imperils the health or safety of others, particularly children or other dependants, and when it is in the public interest.

The patient expressed her beliefs but had sufficient doubt about them or respect for the surgeons to attend the surgery on the appointed day. The surgeons did not seek any details about the patient's beliefs and reiterated what treatment was necessary.

- ### *In the Public Interest*

A patient's autonomy may have to be constrained in the public interest for reasons such as the prevention of suicide, the spread of contagious disease or the endangerment of the life or well-being of another. Stopping the use of alternative medicine in the public interest would have to be done through court action that seeks to deny the competence of the patient to make a reasoned decision in the face of the particular illness.

The decision for public health departments in the case of contagious disease is a simple one, for the remedies are encoded in the law. Such laws may be written in specific terms but with general clauses that gives authorities the leeway to act in new diseases or situations.[570] This occurred when ebola emerged as a threat in Africa and contacts in countries outside of Africa were quarantined sometimes under controversial circumstances.[571] The problem becomes difficult when there is a serious disease transmissible by interpersonal contact, and the patient refuses to accept conventional medical advice and relies instead on alternative medicines or modalities such as prayer. Public health authorities may then resort to contesting the matter in courts using existing laws or even enacting new ones. Such a situation emerged with the HIV/AIDS pandemic and was made all the worse in the early years when there was no effective conventional medication available, and some countries criminalised the transmission of HIV.[572] A plethora of alternative medicine claims emerged, but with the consistent high mortality, religious groups made few claims for cure or alleviation. Instead many religious persons turned on those affected, blaming

---

[570] Specific Laws and Regulations Governing the Control of Communicable Diseases; CDC Quarantine and Isolation Laws and Regulations

[571] Ebola and Quarantine; JM. Drazen, R Kanapathipillai, EW. Campion, et al; N Engl J Med 2014; 371: 2029-2030

[572] The Case Against Criminalisation of HIV Transmission; S Burris; E Cameron, JAMA. 2008; 300 (5): 578-581.

them for their irreligious behaviour in both contracting the disease and spreading it to others, and instead of supplications for healing, condemnation was offered as the wrath of God.[573]

In the case presented there is no public interest that requires official intervention.

• *The effectiveness of alternative medicine*

The effectiveness of alternative medicine can be measured by its popularity and its consistent use as complementary to western medicine. In addition, some alternative practitioners are allowed to advertise in markets where medical practitioners are forbidden from doing so. On the other hand, the constant emergence of new forms or the revitalisation of old forms may also be due to be the ineffectiveness of any one form.

The persistence of western medicine as the standard of care is the result of continuing improvements, based on statistical analysis of new treatments in clinical trials. Statistical analysis is applied both in the short term and to the long-term survivals going over 5-10 years and more. There have been no comparable statistical studies when new forms of alternative therapies are introduced, and none with long-term results.[574]

The report given suggests that the alternative therapy of prayer was ineffective and was readily demonstrable by the persistent presence of the mass in the breast.

---

[573] AIDS and the Wrath of God (1994). Baggett, DJ Faculty Publications and Presentations. Paper 157. http://digitalcommons.liberty.edu/sor_fac_pubs/157

[574] Assessing the Effectiveness of Complementary & Alternative Medicine P Curtis, https://www.med.unc.edu/phyrehab/pim/files/Effectiveness.pdf

LEGAL JEOPARDY

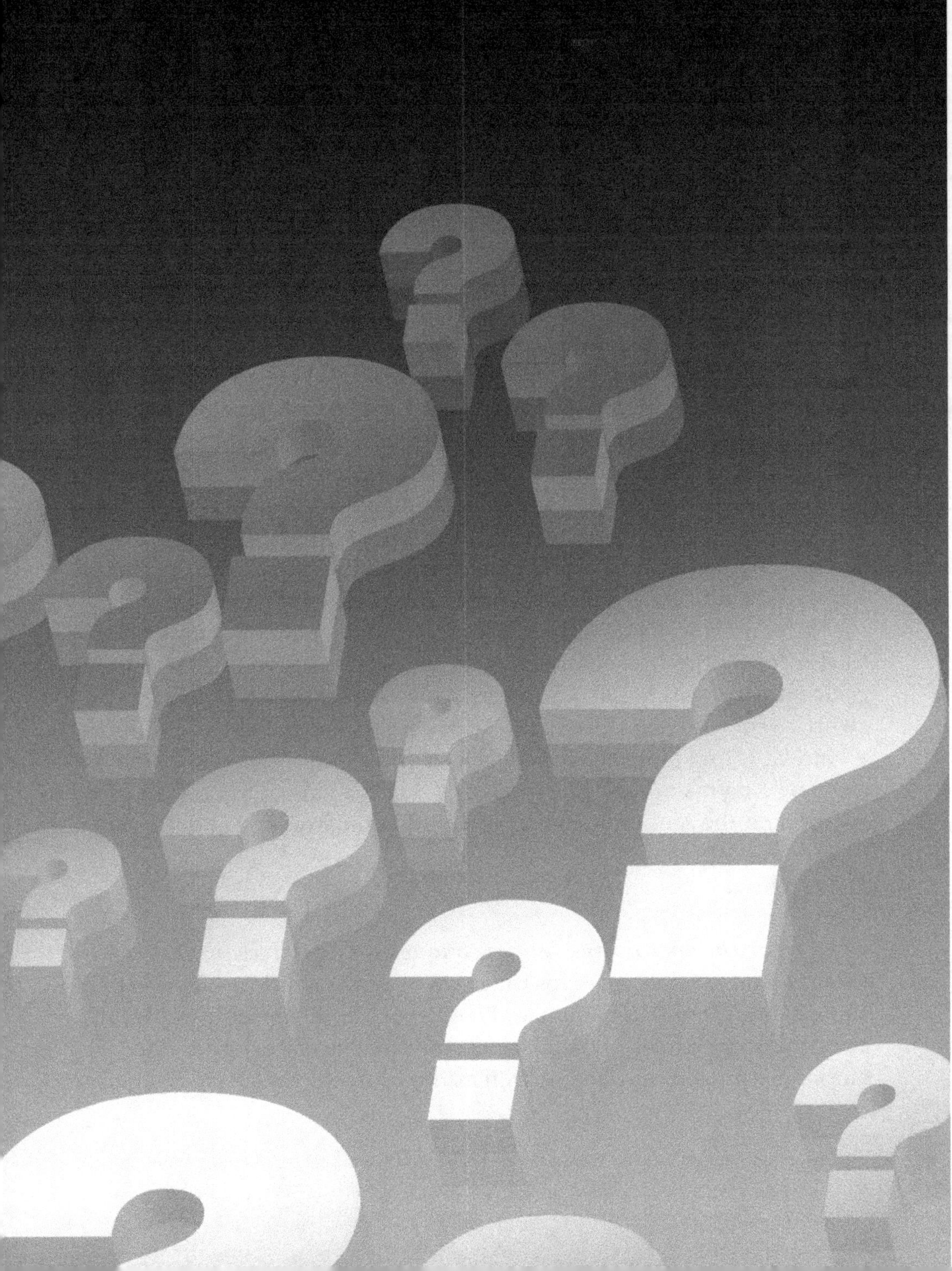

Retained Surgical Swab

Case report:

A 20-year-old man admitted with acute appendicitis was scheduled for operation. The intern is told by his senior to do the operation, has difficultly finding the appendix and asks to get his senior. After some time, the senior cannot be found and no other surgeon is available and the intern finishes the operation. The patient is told that 'nothing wrong' was found and he can go home the next day. On the consultant's ward round the patient asked 'Doc, if it wasn't my appendix what was it?' The intern responds that there was no sign of inflammation so he closed the abdomen.

When the patient returns for suture removal, he tells the nurse he had a fever and chills. The sutures are removed and the temperature taken, which is normal. The patient returns two days later, complaining of night fevers, pain, diarrhoea and pus from the wound. The intern orders an abdominal X-ray and tells the patient he may have to go back to theatre to drain the abscess. He speaks to his senior who looks at the wound and asks for forceps, which he plunges into the wound and pus gushes out. The intern orders an injection for the pain and the patient is sent for the X-ray. Later that day the intern gets a call to say that the X-ray shows a swab in the abdomen. The intern calls his senior and is told 'You better schedule him to get it out right away. You realize if he finds out you could be in big trouble!' The intern speaks to the patient, arranges the theatre, and rings his senior about the arrangements and he is told: 'You clear up your own mess'. The intern calls another registrar friend, and the swab is removed and discarded. After surgery the patient asked the nurse what was found and she replied: 'The theatre nurse said something about a swab being taken out'. The following day the patient asks: 'Can I see the swab?' and the senior blurts out 'Who told you anything about a swab?'

Issues raised

• *Have the doctors and nurses conducted themselves professionally?* Professional conduct involves the many ways in which professionals should interact with a patient and colleagues both ethically and legally.[575] The ethical principles of beneficence, non-malfeasance, justice and autonomy must be applied as well as the professional's legal obligations.

---

[575] WMA International Code of Medical Ethics; http://www.wma.net/en/30publications/10policies/c8/

Professionals have a legal duty of care that should be carried out at the standard of the ordinary trained professional; this includes the obligation to provide the facts necessary for the patient to give informed consent to the treatment prescribed.

In the report given the intern as the most junior doctor on the surgical team, had conducted himself well in relation to seeing the patient and arranging for her care; but decides to carry out a procedure which he was not experienced enough to be doing on his own. When difficulty arises he seeks help from his immediate senior, who cannot be found. When another problem arises, he is again told by his senior that he is on his own. While he seeks help, he also accepts advice to hide the problem from the patient.

The senior on the service has displayed unprofessional and unethical conduct throughout the treatment of the patient. He abrogates his supervisory role in not checking the diagnosis of his junior, and delegating his junior to do an operation without supervision. This behaviour is compounded by not being available when his junior needs help. In a further demonstration of unprofessional conduct, he decides to show his junior how to deal with an abscess, and demonstrates a total disregard for the patient's feelings. He distances himself when another problem arises, and refuses to supervise his junior when the problem needs surgical correction; and in addition he gives highly unethical advice to deceive the patient. When he thinks his advice about deceiving the patient has not been followed, he directs a rather aggressive question to the patient.

The consultant as the ultimate supervisor on his team does not appear to exercise this role except on ward rounds for there appears to be no expectation of supervision from the consultant since when difficulties arise, no one thinks to call him.

The registrar who agrees to assist the intern with removing the retained swab, whilst acting with the best of motives in assisting a junior colleague, appears to go along with the unethical advice to hide the fact of a retained swab by discarding it.

The nurse who checked the patient's wound and temperature acted within the level of skill expected of her level of training. It could be argued that when the patient complained of pain and a fever, she should have asked a doctor to assess the patient. Nevertheless, the instructions about returning if problems continued were appropriate.

The nurses who responded to the patient's questions about what was happening should have referred such questions to the doctor and not act on speculation or hearsay.

- ***Has there been negligence on the part of any of the persons involved?***
The legal standard for negligence in medical treatment rests on three

pillars. The professional involved must have a duty of care to the patient; has carried out the care of the patient outside the normally accepted standard of care within the profession; and the patient must have suffered compensable harm[576]. The normally accepted standard of care can be related to the local circumstances and the local body of professional opinion. However, such standards may be argued by expert opinions of persons in the field[577]. Compensable harm can be physical or mental and it may be immediate or delayed. A suit of negligence must usually be brought within a specified time limit, which varies in jurisdictions. However, the statute of limitation may take effect after the patient becomes aware that harm has occurred, and evidence of harm may become manifest many years after the care event.

In the case reported, all of the doctors and nurses involved have a duty of care to the patient. The patient has suffered pain and suffering as well as any losses from further surgery related to a retained swab. Although the direct burden of the retained swab falls on the intern who undertook the procedure, a share of that burden falls on the operating theatre nurses, who would have shared responsibility for counting the swabs, but also on the intern's supervisors, for failing to supervise the conduct of the operation.

- *What is a breach in professional standards?*

The legal standard for a breach of the normal professional standard is whether the conduct of the practitioner or nurse falls outside the standard expected of their level of training and responsibility. All practitioners are expected to be able to take a history and do an examination of a patient and diagnose common conditions; this can also be expected of a nurse but not to the same level of discrimination as the doctor. All doctors are expected to be able to do simple operative tasks such as the suturing of wounds, but are not expected to undertake more complex surgical procedures without further training.

In the case reported the intern did not meet the standards expected at his level of training when he agreed to undertake an operation unsupervised; and did not attempt to elicit the help of other senior persons having failed to contact his immediate supervisor. Although a swab and instrument count is usually delegated to the staff assisting at the operation, the responsibility is ultimately that of the operating surgeon. It was unethical to deceive the patient about the retained swab, and a definite breach of professional standards if the record is falsified.

---

[576] Bolam v Friern Hospital Management Committee [1957] 1 WLR 582; UK
[577] The Standard of Care in Medical Negligence — Moving on from Bolam? H Teff; Oxford J Legal Studies (1998) 18 (3): 473-484.

The operating theatre staff bear some responsibility if they failed to do an accurate swab and instrument count, and any other measures that are usually employed by staff to ensure that swabs and instruments are not left behind.

The registrar/senior resident's professional conduct must be judged not only by what he does but also by what he does not do. He breached the standards of the profession by failing to supervise the treatment of the patient by a junior. Not making himself available to his junior when called upon and giving bad advice to deceive the patient further aggravates the abrogation of the supervisory responsibility.

The consultant as the most senior person responsible for the care of the patient can be held responsible for failure to adequately supervise the junior staff. This failure is illustrated where the staff makes no attempt to contact him when assistance is needed, and suggests an established pattern of unavailability.

The nurse responsible for removing the sutures may be implicated in any claim related to a delay in the diagnosis of the complication, if it could be shown that the nurse acted outside of the responsibility delegated to her.

Claims of Negligence

Case report 1:
A 25-year-old man with a complaint of lower abdominal pain treated
himself with home remedies and prayers. After three days of worsening
pain he experienced intermittent fever, diarrhoea and three episodes
of vomiting. After two weeks he collapsed at home and was taken to a
health centre where he was recorded as being conscious and coherent
but was dehydrated with a pulse rate of 120/min, temperature 35° C
and BP 100/50 mms Hg and mild abdominal tenderness. A diagnosis of
dehydration due to gastroenteritis was recorded and IV fluids started.
After three hours and two litres of IV fluids, his pulse was 100, BP 110/70
and T37.6°C. The patient felt better and he was discharged home. Eight
hours later, he collapsed again and was taken to hospital where he
was diagnosed as septic shock due to an acute abdomen. After further
resuscitation, a laparotomy was done which revealed a generalised
purulent peritonitis due to a gangrenous perforated appendicitis.

Post-operatively, he required ventilation for three weeks, during which
time he had pulmonary and kidney complications. He was discharged
from hospital after four weeks.

The family sued the doctor and the health centre for misdiagnosing
their relative resulting in his life being endangered. Damages were
being claimed for undue suffering and the cost of hospitalisation. Expert
opinion was sought as to whether the diagnosis of gastroenteritis was
negligent, resulting in the prolonged hospital stay.

Case report 2:
A 65-year-old professional man was gifted an executive medical profile
examination at his retirement function. When examined he was found to
be in "perfect health" except for a prostatic specific antigen of 6 [normal
<4]. Rectal examination was normal but an ultrasound examination
showed a hypo-echoic focus in the right lobe of the prostate, which
was biopsied. The biopsy result showed a carcinoma of the prostate.
After further investigation he was offered brachytherapy or surgery.
He opted for brachytherapy, which was performed by the urologist he
had consulted. Three months later he developed frequent and painful
urination, and he became impotent. In spite of numerous visits to the
urologist, with lab investigations, cysto-urethroscopy and medication,
the symptoms persisted for a year, when he noticed he was passing
air in his urine. He consulted another surgeon, who noted no urine on
catheterisation of the bladder and that the catheter was in the rectum on

rectal examination. A 4 cms communication was palpated between the rectum and bladder. A suprapubic cystostomy was done.

By this time, his wife had left him and he required paid help at home. Many of the symptoms persisted and a year later a rectal exam showed the fistula to be larger at 6 cms. Intermittent diarrhoea became more frequent and blood stained. After further consultation and discussion, a sigmoid colostomy was done. By this time, he had lost his house, in paying for his medical expenses, and was admitted to a geriatric home for care where he died 18 months later at the age of 68 years.

His 40-year-old son sued the urologist for failing to advise the patient on the pros and cons of conservative vs. surgical vs. radiation treatment, and for delayed recognition and poor management of his father's injury that led to excessive suffering and death, as well as losses for medical expenses.

Case report 3:
A 35-year-old woman had consulted an ENT surgeon for the previous five years about a swelling in the neck. The swelling, diagnosed as a non-toxic multi-nodular goitre, had grown larger in the last year. It was agreed that she should have surgery and was admitted to hospital under the care of the ENT surgeon and was subsequently seen by a general surgeon. A subtotal thyroidectomy was performed and the operation note listed the general surgeon as the surgeon and the ENT surgeon as the assistant. Immediately after surgery the patient developed difficulty in breathing and was re-intubated. The comment made on the anaesthetic chart was *"Stridor on extubation, cords visualised partial closure not complete movement."* On the following day after a further attempt at extubation, the ENT surgeon performed a tracheostomy. After four days the tube is removed for cleaning and it is stated in the nursing notes *"breathing is still somewhat laboured."* On day 5, she is recorded as having a good voice with the tracheostomy tube in situ. On day 6, the tracheostomy is removed and the nursing notes state *"Good breathing"* and she is discharged home that day.

The patient is followed as an outpatient by the ENT surgeon who notes one month after discharge from hospital that there is *"sluggish movement of both cords R > L but not to full abduction."* One year later, she is seen by another doctor for wheezing and is noted to be having stridor. An opinion is sought from another ENT surgeon who notes, *"the vocal cords are fixed in the midline due to bilateral recurrent laryngeal nerve damage"*, and advises that an urgent operation is necessary and remarks that the patient ought to sue the surgeon who did the operation. The first ENT surgeon received a writ suing for negligence, and responded in defence that the general surgeon performed the surgery.

Issues raised

- ***The basis for claims of negligence***

The practice of medicine carries inherent risks for the patient and in some instances for the practitioner. When complications arise resulting in harm to patients, some patients will seek to be compensated for that harm. Since the complication that occurred was unintended, there exists a framework that determines when fault can be that of the practitioner. There are three pillars established in law on which a claim of negligence may be determined to be on the practitioner's part. – there must be a duty of care; a breach in the current standard of care; and a causal link between the breach in the standard of care and the harm to the patient.

The duty of care is a concept of expectation where the practitioner is trained for the service they purport to deliver, and the patient understands what service that practitioner can deliver. A breach of this duty in carrying out a medical service can be considered a battery in criminal law.

The standard of care is that where the practitioner must meet the expectations given to the patient, and also the standard expected for that service by a responsible body of the practitioner's peers, also known as the Bolam test.[578] This standard applies to the ability to diagnose and investigate a patient, as well as to the medical treatment or procedure recommended and carried out. A breach in the standard of care where no harm results, may be considered a -'there but for the grace of God' moment.[579] However, when something goes amiss and it can be directly attributed to a breach in the standard of care, a claim of negligence may succeed. If something goes wrong and it cannot be attributed to a breach in the standard of care, then a claim of negligence should not stand.

The harm that occurred must be compensable, and includes pain and suffering, bereavement, loss of consortium, as well as medical expenses and loss of income both current and future. Claimants will spread the net as widely as possible. Only spouses or the parents of a minor child of the deceased, or previously dependent parents of the deceased may be allowed to claim for bereavement. Funeral expenses may be claimed if

---

[578] Bolam v Friern Hospital Management Committee [1957] 1 WLR 582
[579] John Bradford (1853). The writings of John Bradford Volume 1. Cambridge: Cambridge University Press.

they were paid for by dependents of the deceased.[580]

In the three case reports, there is a duty of care by the doctors being sued, a misdiagnosis is questioned, and there is a question about a breach in the standard of management.

In the first two cases the claimants for compensation are not the patients and their entitlement to make the claims for damages would have to be established.

• *Responsibility for a patient's care*

Responsibility for a patient's care in an institution is usually reflected in the assignment of admitting and procedural privileges to the professionals working there.

Admitting privileges. Not all practitioners who work in the institution have admitting privileges. Consultants or senior staff in accident and emergency, in anaesthesia and in pathology may not have admitting privileges, as they are not expected to take care of the patient's entire illness.

Procedure privileges. It is difficult to have clearly defined procedural privileges for professional staff in the evolving fields of medicine. Hospitals or insurance agencies may define procedural privileges by either giving named privileges to a professional or by only disbursing payment for specific procedures to particular professionals. Specialist titles, training, qualifications and professional registers provide a guide but do not fully satisfy the demand for determining specialist expertise. Other tests of competence include showing how many of the procedures have been done by an individual, and what the results of those procedures have been.

Public vs. private services. Public services are organised by and paid for by a government run entity and care is the responsibility of teams headed by a senior practitioner. The junior members of the team carry out care under supervision, either direct or indirect. Private patients expect their care to be carried out by the person they pay for such service, and when private patients are treated in government run entities, the responsibilities and demarcations for care must be made clear to avoid confusion about where responsibilities lay. When a patient contracts a specific practitioner to provide a service and another professional is going to do the service, the patient should give explicit consent for this to be done. The public patient has a contract with the institution to provide competent professionals to do the service but not necessarily a specific professional.

---

[580] Fatalities – the effect death has on a claim for compensation; http://www.thompsons.law.co.uk/clinical-negligence/effect-death-compensation.htm,

Charging fees. The professional who charges and receives a fee is considered responsible for the patient's care. Splitting a fee among professionals for referral of a patient is unprofessional and illegal in some jurisdictions e.g. *'The division with any person who is not a partner or assistant of any fees or profits resulting from consultations or other medical or surgical procedures without the patient's knowledge or consent'.* [581] If care is undertaken jointly the patient should know the different roles of the professionals.

In the first case reported, the primary care practitioner has no admitting privileges to hospital, and determined that three hours of clinic observation was sufficient to determine if the patient should be referred for admission. The safety of the decision would be judged by the observations made and recorded in the clinic notes.

In the second case reported, there is nothing said to determine whether the urologist was qualified to calculate the dose and administer the treatment given.

In the third case, the patient is under the impression that she was operated on by the ENT surgeon she has been attending; however, when a claim is made against that practitioner he states that another doctor did the operation. Although the patient was visited by another surgeon prior to surgery the patient clearly understood the ENT surgeon to be doing her surgery and the care undertaken after surgery supports the patient's understanding.

- ### *Defending against claims of negligence*

The best defence against claims of negligence is to ensure that they do not occur, that the claim has no basis in fact, that there was no compensable harm, or that the claim was not related to a breach in the standard of care. This involves delivering the best clinical practice, keeping patients and their relatives truthfully informed at all stages of care, and if something does go wrong to apologise to the patient and determine a plan for dealing with the matter. The patient record is the best legal defence and if good records are kept of the interaction between the doctor and the patient, most suits are defensible.

In some jurisdictions there is a time limit in which a claim can be brought, and this may be adjusted to start when the patient discovers that the injury was due to the treatment given. If a suit does come, copies of the patient record should be secured and the practitioner's insurer informed at the earliest opportunity. Consent forms, although not an unbending legally binding contract, are indicative of what the patient understood was to be done and by whom.

---

[581] Laws of Barbados; CAP 171 The Medical Registration Act Regulations 1972 Part V; 21 (2) (f)

Malpractice insurance will cover the expenses of defending a suit.[582] Sometimes insurance companies settle a defensible claim to avoid the expense of claims that attract differing opinions. Claims should be responded to without rancour and with reference to the original records. Any alteration or correction of records should be dated and timed for memory cannot be relied upon as a truthful witness.[583] A claimant will subject the answers given to expert opinion and the practitioner is entitled to have their own expert opinion.

In the first case report expert opinion may be sought as to whether the primary care practitioner examined the patient thoroughly and interpreted the history and findings properly. Expert opinion may also be sought as to whether the eight hours delay in getting appropriate treatment significantly contributed to the claims being made.

In the second case expert opinion will be sought on whether the radiation treatment was properly administered, and whether the patient was properly investigated when adverse symptoms developed, and whether the delay in diagnosis made a difference to the subsequent course.

In the third case the ENT surgeon has tried to deflect the claim by stating another doctor did the operation. This should lead to an expansion of the suit rather than avoiding responsibility, for at all stages the ENT surgeon appeared to be in charge of the treatment. The consent form should be indicative of whom the patient understood would do the surgery and the operation note should be explicit about the roles undertaken by the surgeons, as well as the details about the procedure.

- ***Was the patient warned about the possible complications of surgery?***

When consenting to a procedure, patients should be warned about the likely risks and outcomes of the procedure and informed about the available alternatives. Professionals must make a judgment between warning a patient about all possible risks, which may so alarm the patient that they decide against doing a necessary procedure. In all cases a specific and dangerous risk of the procedure should be mentioned to the patient so they can understand and balance those risks against the benefits of the procedure. Practitioners should also be prepared to answer questions about their own experience with the proposed procedure. In the words of a judge, to get informed consent the patient must be told about 'material facts, risks, complications and alternatives

---

[582] Malpractice Insurance; B Sage; personalinsure.about.com
[583] Medical records MPS Fact sheets May 2011

to the procedure that a reasonable person in the patient's situation could consider significant in deciding whether to consent, but a physician need not disclose all information'.[584]

Warning of specific risks should be recorded in the notes and in some cases the patient should be asked to sign a declaration as to what they have been warned about. For example, in the procedure of thyroidectomy patients should be warned of the risks of recurrent laryngeal nerve damage and the possible alteration of their voice; and where applicable the risk of damage to both nerves and not being able to breathe normally. In such instances it would also be prudent to document the functioning of the vocal cords before surgery, and if the operation is being done on a professional singer, the possibility of voice alteration must be mentioned and discussed.[585]

In the reports given, there is no mention that the specific risks of the procedures undertaken were discussed with the patients.

- ***What do the notes state about the treatment and procedures carried out?***

Medical records, including operation notes, should be as full as possible noting any positive or negative findings, and are a guide to sorting out postoperative problems in the short or long term and can be used in defence in a court of law in regard to the standard of care given.[586] When problems arise, a differential diagnosis should be made and the actions taken will determine the standard of care given to the patient. Negligent conduct is determined by a complication that caused harm to the patient as a result of the action of the practitioner that fell outside the normal standard of care.[587] Appropriate diagnostic and procedural actions will be judged on the testimony of expert witnesses who have special knowledge and experience of the condition.[588] However, the standard of care is that of any professional in the field in the prevailing circumstances, and would be different for the professional who has had special training in the condition being treated.[589] These issues are determined by an examination of the notes made at the time, by the effects of the condition

---

584 Gouse v. Cassell (615 A.2d 331) 1992
585 'Medico-legal aspects of Informed Consent' L.M. Nova, R.J. Rembert; Neurological clinics 1998; 16; No1
586 The use of an aide-memoire to improve the quality of operation notes in an orthopaedic unit; R Din, D Jenna, BN Muddu; Ann R Coll Surg Eng. 2001; 83: 319-320
587 The Four Elements of Medical Malpractice. Yale New Haven Medical Center: Issues in Risk Management. 1997. http://info.med.yale.edu/caim/risk/malpractice/malpractice
588 General Medical Council - Acting as an expert witness - guidance for doctors; http://www.gmc-uk.org/guidance/ethical_guidance/expert_witness_guidance.asp
589 Bolitho v. City and Hackney Health Authority [1997] 4 All ER 771

on the patient, and on any other independent observations. If the observations or opinions of two professionals differ, any independent evidence such as photographs could be used as evidence.[590]

In each of the reports given, the notes of the practitioners would be the most important evidence of the standard of care given. In the third report there is no mention of the recurrent laryngeal nerves being identified at operation; however, the immediate postoperative problems and observations made were suggestive of bilateral recurrent nerve injury.

- **What are the legal responsibilities of those taking part in a patient's care?**

Anyone who takes part in care, whether they be anaesthetists, nurses or assistants of various types, has a responsibility to act professionally, with due diligence and can be sued related to their specific roles. However, the professional in charge of a procedure carries the primary responsibility, including the delegation of specific responsibilities.

The ethical problem for a professional, such as a surgeon, is if they were unable to show that they saw and explained to the patient what was going to be done at the surgery. A surgeon can be sued for battery if a patient can credibly claim that they were not aware that that surgeon was going to do their operation, and therefore had done so without their consent. If a surgeon states that he was asked to do the operation by another, then the defence must rely on the terms of the written consent, and the notes made as to his own actions before, during and after the operation. It is legally hazardous to walk away from procedures undertaken and take no further responsibility in the patient's care.[591]

In the reports given, the doctors are being sued for negligence in the treatment given. In the third report the surgeon being sued claims in defence that he was the assistant. However, the surgeon on record took no part in the postoperative care and follow-up.

- *Expert opinions*

The standard of care is usually represented in legal proceedings as that given by expert witnesses who are usually chosen from the area of practice that is under examination, or from an area related to the claims being made. Experts may differ and are usually drawn from experienced practitioners, often with an academic background. Expert opinion can be challenged, and a court has held that a doctor could be liable

---

[590] Legal aspects of documenting patient care; Ronald W. Scott 2nd Ed 2000
[591] American College of Surgeons: Code of Professional Conduct; http://www.facs.org/fellows_info/statements/stonprin.html#top

for negligence in respect of diagnosis and treatment despite a body of professional opinion sanctioning his conduct, if the Court is satisfied that the body of opinion relied on was not reasonable or responsible.[592]

Some jurisdictions have established specific criteria on which to be qualified as an expert witness, and courts prefer balanced opinions rather than the biased report of a 'hired gun'. Some jurisdictions after hearing the expert opinions from the parties, will require them to agree on a single expert on whom the court can rely. Expert opinion should be supported by the scientific literature, and because of the long time it may take for cases to progress to adjudication, the literature quoted should have been available at the time of the incident. Similarly, opinions should take into account local conditions, given the assurance that the consent to treatment has been informed as to the relevant local conditions and expertise.

In the first case expert opinion from a primary care practitioner should be sought as to whether it was within the standard of care for the practitioner at the clinic to miss an unusual presentation of acute appendicitis. The opinion will turn on whether a thorough examination of the abdomen was done, particularly whether bowel sounds were recorded and whether a digital rectal examination was done.

In the second case reported, the question of delay in diagnosing the complication is unlikely to be contested by experts. However, whether an earlier diagnosis would have made a difference to the subsequent course of the patient may well be argued.

In the third case expert opinion will rest on whether the operation note recorded that the surgery was carried out with the requisite skill, and whether the postoperative diagnosis for the breathing difficulty was properly made and appropriately handled.

- *Claims after death*

Death cannot always be staved off by medical treatment; however, when death occurs during treatment questions about the efficacy of the treatment may be raised. Legal claims in relation to death can be criminal or civil. Criminal claims relate to intentional deaths; i.e. murder;[593] or criminal negligence where the practitioner's care was so outside the normal standard of care that it caused the death of the patient.

There are questions as to who can bring a civil claim after death, and what sanctions can be imposed in such suits.[594] A claim of professional misconduct may be brought before the regulatory body, but if there

---

[592] Bolitho v City & Hackney Health Authority (1997) 4 ALL ER 71
[593] 62 R. v. Harold Frederick Shipman, 2000
[594] Proving Wrongful Death in a Civil Case; nolo.com

is also a criminal case being pursued, regulatory bodies will try to defer action until the criminal case has been determined. Nevertheless, because there may be long delays in the criminal courts, the regulatory body will come under pressure to complete their own enquiry with a view to the protection of patients who may come under the care of the accused practitioner.

After death, spouses, the parent of a 'legitimate' minor child of the deceased, and the dependent parents of the deceased may bring a claim. Claims for damages vary substantially after death and may include bereavement, medical expenses, loss of earnings including pensions, and funeral expenses.[595] Economic damages may include the value of the financial contributions the deceased would have made to the survivors, such as loss of the expected earnings, pension or other benefits. In some jurisdictions, damages may be given for the survivors' mental anguish; loss of the care, protection, guidance, advice, training, and nurturing from the deceased; and loss of love, companionship and consortium from the deceased. Punitive damages may be awarded for especially bad conduct, but does not usually apply in medical malpractice suits. However, there are instances where treble damages have been recovered against nursing homes for elder abuse and death.[596]

In the second case reported, a claim of wrongful death would have to be proven whether it was considered negligent in the management or the delayed diagnosis of the complication of treatment. The deceased would probably have had a compelling case during his lifetime, particularly claims for pain, suffering and loss of consortium with his spouse. After death only the estranged wife or the beneficiaries of his estate would be entitled to claim for expenses incurred during treatment. The son is not a dependent, and unless he is a beneficiary of the deceased's estate may not be entitled to make a claim.

---

[595] 10 Things You Want To Know About Medical Malpractice; D Cheeks; www.forbes.com
[596] Forensic Psychiatry: Clinical, Legal and Ethical Issues, J Gunn, P Taylor, 2014- Pg. 54

Illegal Restraint?

Case report:

A 40-yr-old woman was brought by her live-in companion to the emergency department; there had been a domestic dispute and she had drunk Pinesol and alcohol. Her companion had induced vomiting and brought her to the emergency department. She was tearful and did not answer questions about the event, but in her previous history she had been admitted before with a parasuicidal episode and diagnosed as psychotic, but had defaulted from attending the psychiatric clinic. Her physical examination and basic investigations were normal, and she was cooperative including drinking activated charcoal.

She was referred for admission to the medical service and whilst waiting she became more tearful and wanted to go home. She was counselled about the need for admission but still attempted to leave. Two orderlies were asked to hold her whilst an intravenous sedative was administered. Her companion became very upset and was asked to leave while the doctor attempted to administer the sedative with the patient standing and resisting the orderlies. Her companion protested that the patient was being assaulted, and left saying she was going to call her sister who was a lawyer.

The patient was lifted onto the bed and sedated. A call came from a lawyer who said that she was being restrained unlawfully and should be allowed to sign her own self-discharge. The doctor responded that the lawyer had no say in the decisions made by the doctor and that the patient was in no fit state to sign her own self-discharge.

The emergency consultant advised that the psychiatrist should see the patient. The doctor on call for psychiatry [an intern] came, and advised that the patient should be allowed to sign her own self-discharge and attend the psychiatric outpatients.

Issues raised

- *Definition and legal status*

Parasuicide is where a person does themselves harm, not to the point of causing death but mimicking a suicide attempt.[597] It is distinct from attempted suicide where the intention was to die. When there is any doubt, the initial diagnosis should be an attempted suicide. Suicide

---

[597] Parasuicidal Behavior; M. M. Cornette; http://www.springerreference.com/docs/html/chapterdbid/61531.html

is illegal in the sense that it may invalidate some legal claims that the person's estate may make to life insurance. To attempt suicide is not illegal in most jurisdictions but there are some where it is an offence; e.g. in India where self-immolation related to dowry payments has been a cultural practice.[598]

In the case reported, doing the act in the presence of someone else, coupled with the previous episode made it almost certain that this was a parasuicide episode.

- ### *Appropriate referral*

Suicides and parasuicide attempts should be referred to a psychiatrist; if there is a judgment that concurrent medical or surgical treatment is required, the appropriate simultaneous referrals should be made. The decision to make a medical referral should be made on the condition of the patient, knowledge of the substance taken and the anticipated treatment required.

In this case, there is a referral to the medical service for treatment of the toxic condition before referral to the psychiatrist. The psychiatrist was only consulted after the patient had refused admission and was forcibly restrained and sedated. However, the patient had cooperated with all of the emergency treatment offered and when she wanted to go home, the diagnosis of being of unsound mind to the point of needing to be restrained could be challenged.

- ### *Restraint of a patient or an assault?*

A patient can refuse treatment at any time and can only be lawfully restrained if they are a danger to themself or others. Forcing treatment on a patient who is clearly conscious and is declaring that they do not want to be treated can only be done if the patient is diagnosed to be psychotic or mentally ill and requires urgent treatment for that mental disorder. Urgency to treat is determined by whether the patient is an imminent danger to themself or others. There are specific provisions in mental health acts that state what patients may be restrained, under what circumstances, and how this should be done.[599] In such acts patients may be medically recommended by two doctors, one of whom must be a psychiatrist; or an order by the court where the police are notified to apprehend the patient and take them to a place of safety.

In the case described, the emergency physician appears to have made a diagnosis of an attempted suicide rather than parasuicide, and determined

---

[598] Indian Penal Code 1860 section 390; http://en.wikipedia.org/wiki/Indian_Penal_Code
[599] Mental Health Act of Barbados 1989 Cap 45

that the patient should be restrained from going home to complete the act. Any challenge to that diagnosis should be made by a psychiatrist.

- **Method of restraint.**

Persons who are required to restrain patients should be trained and should at all times be under the supervision of a senior person. In the case of the police, that seniority is placed at the sergeant level. There is nothing that defines the level of seniority of doctors who can notify the police that restraint of a patient is needed. If a patient is injured while being restrained, questions may have to be answered as to the training of the persons doing the restraining, and their supervision at the time of the incident.[600]

In the case described, orderlies were used to restrain the patient and the question could be raised as to what training they had. The scene described of a patient being restrained in front of relatives, whilst an attempt is made to give a sedative intravenously whilst standing, should draw very critical comment.

- **Dealing with relatives and other relations**

Unless relatives can assist with the patient, or are required as a chaperone, it is prudent to ask them to leave when treatment is being administered. If a mentally competent patient asks for a relative or friend to stay, the health professional must consider such a request, but has to make a judgment as to whether it is in the best interest of the patient or the relative/friend to remain, and give an opinion accordingly.

In the case described the 'relative' is present when the patient is being restrained by orderlies in order to administer a sedative intravenously. The 'relative' perceives that an unlawful restraint is being perpetrated and goes to get legal advice. The legal intervention precipitated other advice about how the situation should be dealt with.

- **A legal challenge**

A legal or other opinion cannot direct how a patient should be treated but should be considered as a flag to remind one to review the course of action being taken, and that there may be legal action taken subsequently. Any action must be justifiable in a court of law as the normal standard of care of the general body of physicians acting in a similar situation.

In the case reported, the question of unlawful restraint hinges on the diagnosis of the patient being of unsound mind and likely to be a danger to herself. The fact

---

[600] 'Use of force by mental health workers violated due process' Davis vs Rennie. JLME 2001; Vol 30; 1 114-6

that a psychiatrist was not called initially may be used to question the diagnosis of being of unsound mind and the need for forceful restraint.

- **The role of the police**

The Police are entitled to take into custody anyone who has, or is suspected of having committed a crime; or who appears to be a danger to themself or others. There are usually specific provisions in mental health acts for the police to be informed by a mental health officer and take into custody a mentally ill patient and take them to a mental hospital or a place of safety for treatment.

In the case reported the doctor in Emergency made a decision that the patient was suicidal and required to be forcibly restrained from leaving hospital. This course was challenged by a call from a lawyer, and psychiatric advice was then sought. The psychiatric opinion was that it was safe for the patient to be dealt with as an outpatient. If the psychiatric advice had been that the patient would be a danger to themself by not being treated, the police could have been asked to assist in securing the hospitalization of the patient.

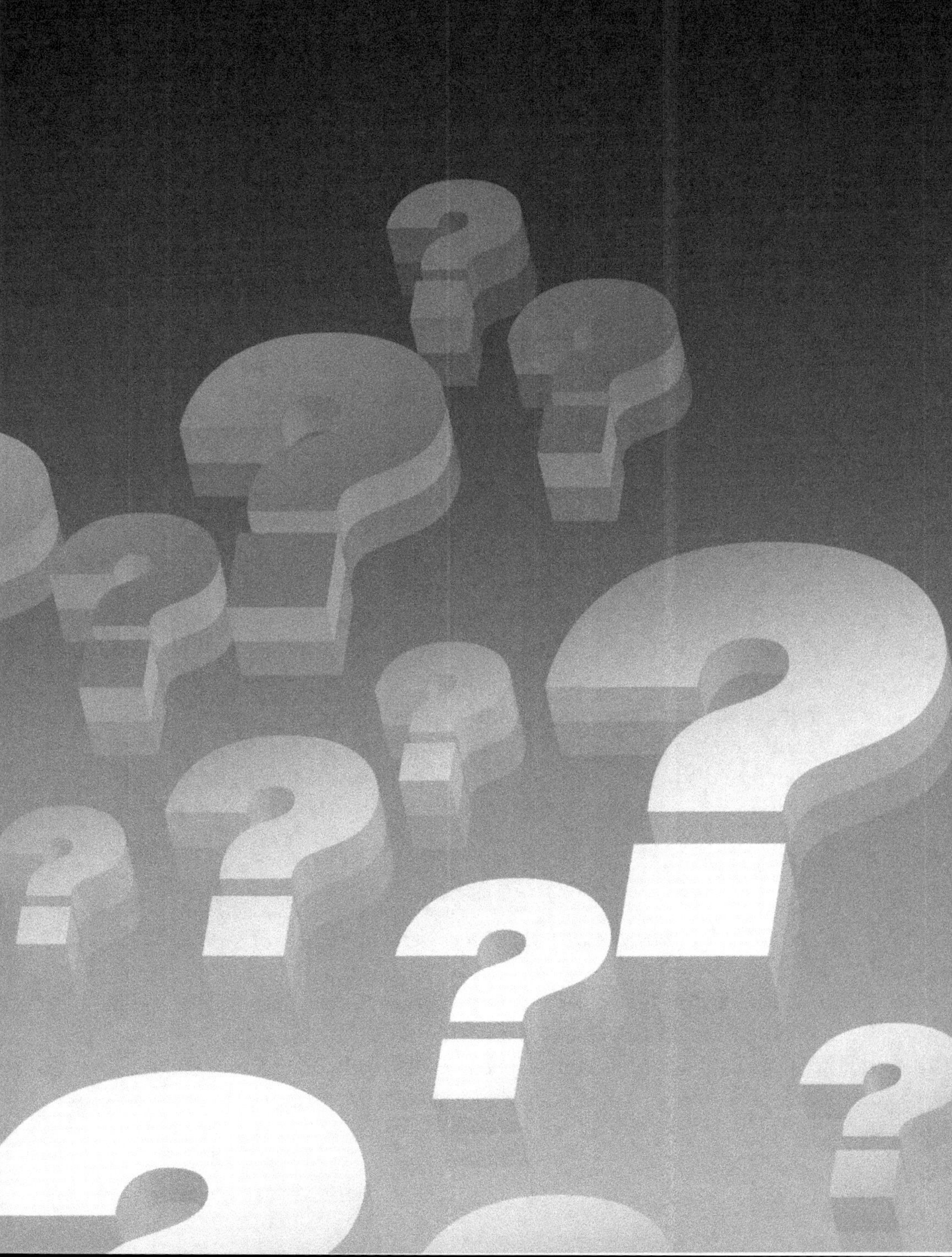

PUBLIC HEALTH

Case report:

A resident of a public long-stay facility was hospitalized with an extensive skin rash. She had a severe anoxic brain injury as an adolescent, and had been in the facility for ten years. She was diagnosed with a severe scabies infestation, and was isolated and treated. The facility from which she came was notified of the scabies diagnosis.

A public health officer identified several other cases of scabies at the facility and those affected were quarantined, and visiting family of the residents were informed that there was a contagious disease affecting several residents. Concern was expressed on the radio call-in programmes, and the public health officer released a statement stating that there was an outbreak of a severe skin rash at the facility and that the one person who required admission was 'doing well'. The information that the patient was doing well was not obtained from the treatment team, and at the time of the release the patient's condition had deteriorated having developed a staphylococcal bacteremia.

The public release precipitated many calls to the patient's mother wishing her daughter well, and the family becomes frustrated by the story in the press and the deteriorating condition that they are seeing. The family asks to speak to the physician in charge and is told that they must ring the physician to make an appointment. The patient's mother feels that there is some deception going on and consults an attorney who writes a letter demanding that the physician in charge of the patient provide the family with information regarding the patient's condition. Meanwhile the treatment team and the nursing staff are receiving calls from the long-stay facility demanding 'updates' on the patient's condition. The senior physician speaks to the family only to report that the patient's condition has continued to deteriorate, and she died a few days thereafter.

Issues raised

- *What is the purpose of public health notification of a patient's illness?*

Notification of illness to public health authorities must be distinguished from notification of illness to the public. Notification of illness to public health authorities is to inform those professionals of the presence or trends in certain diseases and enable them to take appropriate collective actions to safeguard the health of the public.[601] There is no role for a practitioner to go to the public to inform or warn them about a patient's illness.

The purpose of publication of individual illness would be to warn or sensitise the public about the unwitting spread of dangerous diseases such as HIV/AIDS, Ebola, food contamination, or vector-borne diseases such as dengue and zika.[602] General statistical information of diseases may also be released to influence public behaviour. Such statistics may vary from transmissible disease such as HIV and dengue to the 'lifestyle' conditions of non-communicable chronic diseases, and the behavioural ones such as motor vehicle accidents.[603]

There may be occasions when release of a patient's illness to the public is of high public interest, such as the illness of national leaders. However, such release of information is only warranted with the clear consent of the patient or family and must be done by a responsible designated spokesperson. Such spokespersons should either be part of the treatment team or be a conduit from the team.

In the instance described it was appropriate that the public health authorities be notified of an outbreak of scabies in a residential institution, but there was no rationale for general public notification of such an outbreak. Patients are often easily identified in small communities and the public notification led to multiple calls to the family. The family was distressed since the information in the public notice did not comply with the patient's condition, and created a wall of distrust between the family and the treating physicians.

- *Limiting public information*

When isolation of a patient is needed for the protection of the patient or others, that information should be transmitted to the family and visitors whether the isolation is done in an institution or at home. Such information can be given by word of mouth, and supplemented by a written notice if an institution has had to be closed. Notices may be time limited; e.g. for a chicken pox patient,[604] be treatment limited; e.g. the protection of the immuno-deficient, or the protection of others in antibiotic resistant skin infections.[605]

---

[601] 2016 Nationally Notifiable Conditions - Centers for Disease Control https://wwwn.cdc.gov/nndss/conditions/notifiable/2016/

[602] Outbreak Communication - World Health Organization www.who.int/csr/resources/publications/WHO_CDS_2005_32web.pdf

[603] Journalists can play a key role in raising awareness of non-communicable diseases thecommonwealth.org/.../journalists-can-play-key-role-raising-awareness-non-commu...

[604] CDC Emergency Preparedness and You | Understand Quarantine and ... emergency.cdc.gov/preparedness/quarantine/qa.asp

[605] Isolation Precautions | Guidelines Library | Infection Control | CDC https://www.cdc.gov/infectioncontrol/guidelines/isolation/index.html

The circumstances described justified limited information being given to the families and visitors to those persons who were 'quarantined' within the institution. There was no justification for information to be given to the public about the patient who was admitted; such information turned out to be misleading and led to considerable distress in the patient's family who were easily identifiable in a small community.

• *Can authorities break the confidentiality of a patient without their consent?*

A patient's confidentiality should not be broken unless the patient poses a mortal threat to another person, and the threat cannot be managed without the cooperation of the patient.[606] Any other breach of confidentiality should only be done with an order of the court.[607] In the disclosure of anonymous information, account must be taken of other identifying factors that may breach the confidentiality of a patient, particularly in small communities. Whether intended or not, breaches in confidentiality that bring distress or harm to the patient and their family may be subject to civil legal action.[608]

In the report given, the patient has not been named in the public notification made, however, the identification of the institution in a small community was enough to identify the patient, and precipitated multiple calls to the family. Unfortunately, the information released proved to be misleading and caused a great deal of distress for the family. The distress was such that the family sought legal advice to find out the true nature of the patient's progress.

• *What role do attorneys have in doctor-patient communication?*

Attorneys play an indispensable role in defending as well as prosecuting practitioners when a patient or their guardian feels that something has gone seriously wrong. The things that can go wrong vary from the patient feeling that they have not been treated with sufficient courtesy, to harmful treatment and up to the criminal death of a patient.[609]

Most legal interventions can be avoided by a good doctor-patient relationship in which the patient and their relatives are kept fully informed about the illness being treated and the progress or lack thereof

---

[606] Tarasoff v. Regents of the University of California, 17 Cal. 3d 425, 551 P.2d 334, 131 Cal. Rptr. 14 (Cal. 1976)

[607] Patient confidentiality: when can a breach be justified? K Blightman, SE Griffiths, C Danbury, Contin Educ Anaesth Crit Care Pain (2014) 14 (2): 52-56.

[608] Medical confidentiality: an intransigent and absolute obligation; M.H. Kottow; J Med Ethics, 1986,12,117-122

[609] Handling requests from attorneys; R G. Thornton, Proc Bayl Univ Med Cent). 2003 Apr; 16(2): 249–252.

being made. When complications occur the patient/guardian should be made aware of it as soon as possible, and when necessary an apology should be tendered even when there has been no harm done by a mistake made. In procedural disciplines, checklists should be followed in order to minimize mistakes.[610] Checklists are also appropriate in other branches of medicine, e.g. ascertaining the allergic status of patients before prescribing drugs, and thinking through the possible harm to patients/ guardians and relatives of revealing/discussing individual illness in public.[611]

In the report given, the guardians/family of the patient become frustrated by a public report that the patient is doing well whilst they are observing deterioration in the patient's condition. A request to speak with the treating physicians is met with a response to 'make an appointment'; their frustrations bubble over and they seek legal advice as to what to do. The resulting letter from the attorney precipitated the desired contact with the treating physician who explains the deteriorating state of the patient, but also has to explain that they had no role in the misleading publicity given to their relative's illness.

---

[610] Do Safety Checklists Improve Teamwork and Communication in the Operating Room? S Russ, S Rout, N Sevdalis, K Moorthy, A Darzi, and C Vincent, Ann Surg 2013; www.annalsofsurgery.com
[611] What Is Public Health Ethics? - Centers for Disease Control
https://www.cdc.gov/od/science/integrity/.../student-manual-final-073012-508.docx